# Rhinoplasty

*State of the Art*

# Rhinoplasty

## *State of the Art*

## EDITORS

*RONALD P. GRUBER, M.D.*
*Clinical Instructor of Plastic Surgery*
*Stanford University Medical Center*
*Stanford, California*

*GEORGE C. PECK, M.D.*
*Chief, Department of Plastic and Reconstructive Surgery*
*Beth Israel Hospital*
*Passaic, New Jersey*

Illustrations by
Wendy Beth Jackelow

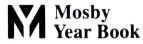 **Mosby**
**Year Book**

St. Louis   Baltimore   Boston   Chicago   London   Philadelphia   Sydney   Toronto

# Mosby
# Year Book

Dedicated to Publishing Excellence

Sponsoring Editor: James D. Ryan
Assistant Editor: Karyn Fell
Associate Managing Editor, Manuscript Services: Deborah Thorp
Production Manager: Nancy C. Baker
Proofroom Supervisor: Barbara Kelly

1  2  3  4  5  6  7  8  9  0   CL/CL/WA   97  96  95  94  93

**Library of Congress Cataloging-in-Publication Data**

Rhinoplasty: state of the art / [edited by] Ronald P. Gruber,
   George C. Peck,
      p.   .cm,
   Includes bibliographical references and index.
   ISBN 0-8016-6277-X
   1.  Rhinoplasty.  I.  Gruber, Ronald P.   II.  Peck, George
      C., 1927-   .
   [DNLM: 1.  Rhinoplasty—methods.   WV 312 R4738]
RD119.5.N67R484  1992                         92-18736
617.5'230592—dc20                             CIP
DNLM/DLC
for Library of Congress

*This book is dedicated with love and affection to our wives, Gloria and Cathy.*

# Contributors

**Paul W. Black, M.D.**
*Atlanta Plastic Surgery*
*Scottish Rite Children's Medical Center*
*St. Joseph's Hospital*
*Atlanta, Georgia*

**Mark B. Constantian, M.D.**
*Adjunct Assistant Professor of Surgery*
*Plastic and Reconstructive Surgery*
*Dartmouth Medical School*
*Hanover, New Hampshire*
*Active Staff*
*Department of Surgery (Plastic Surgery)*
*Nashua Memorial Hospital*
*Nashua, New Hampshire*

**Eugene H. Courtiss, M.D.**
*Associate Clinical Professor of Surgery*
*Harvard Medical School*
*Chief, Division of Plastic Surgery*
*Newton-Wellesley Hospital*
*Boston, Massachusetts*

**Rollin K. Daniel, M.D.**
*Clinical Professor of Plastic Surgery*
*University of California at Irvine*
*Irvine Medical Center*
*Irvine, California*

**Gary D. Friedman, M.D.**
*Clinical Instructor*
*St. Francis Hospital*
*San Francisco, California*

**Robert M. Goldwyn, M.D.**
*Clinical Professor of Surgery*
*Harvard Medical School*
*Head, Division of Plastic Surgery*
*Beth Israel Hospital*
*Boston, Massachusetts*

**Mark Gorney, M.D.**
*Associate Clinical Professor of Surgery*
*Stanford University*
*Chief of Plastic Surgery*
*St. Francis Memorial Hospital*
*San Francisco, California*

**Ronald P. Gruber, M.D.**
*Clinical Instructor of Plastic Surgery*
*Stanford University Medical Center*
*Stanford, California*

**Bahman Guyuron, M.D.**
*Chief of Plastic Surgery*
*Clinical Professor*
*Case Western Reserve University*
*Chief of Plastic Surgery*
*Mt. Sinai Hospital*
*Cleveland, Ohio*

**Steven M. Hoefflin, M.D.**
*Assistant Clinical Professor*
*Division of Plastic Surgery*
*UCLA School of Medicine*
*Senior Attending*
*UCLA Medical Center*
*Los Angeles, California*

**Jose Juri, M.D.**
*Plastic Surgery*
*Professor, Post-Graduate Course of Plastic Surgery*
*The Medicine University-Argentina*
*Buenos Aires, Argentina*

**Henry K. Kawamoto, M.D., D.D.S.**
*Clinical Professor*
*Division of Plastic Surgery*
*UCLA School of Medicine*
*Los Angeles, California*

**BERNARD L. KAYE, M.D.**
*Clinical Professor of Surgery (Plastic)*
*University of Florida College of Medicine at*
  *Jacksonville*
*Active Staff*
*Baptist Medical Center*
*Jacksonville, Florida*

**CARSON M. LEWIS, M.D.**
*Assistant Clinical Professor of Plastic Surgery*
*Department of Plastic Surgery*
*University of California at San Diego*
*Senior Staff Member*
*Scripps Memorial Hospital*
*San Diego, California*

**WILLIAM A. MATHEWS, M.D.**
*Senior Attending Anesthesiologist*
*Hoag Memorial Hospital, Presbyterian*
*Newport Beach, California*

**RODOLPHE MEYER, M.D.**
*Former Professor*
*University Hospital of Lausanne*
*Centre Hospitalier Universitaire Vaudois*
*Centre de Chirurgie Plastique*
*Lausanne, Switzerland*

**LORELLE N. MICHELSON, M.D.**
*Clinical Assistant Professor*
*Department of Surgery*
*Division of Plastic Surgery*
*University of Medicine and Dentistry of New Jersey*
*New Jersey Medical School*
*Newark, New Jersey*

**FERNANDO ORTIZ-MONASTERIO, M.D.**
*Professor of Plastic Surgery*
*Graduate Division*
*Universidad Nacional Autonoma de Mexico*
*Mexico City, Mexico*

**DOUGLAS K. OUSTERHOUT, M.D., D.D.S.**
*Clinical Professor of Plastic Surgery*
*University of California at San Francisco*
*Attending Plastic Surgeon*
*Davies Medical Center*
*San Francisco, California*

**GEORGE C. PECK, M.D.**
*Chief, Department of Plastic and Reconstructive*
  *Surgery*
*Beth Israel Hospital*
*Passaic, New Jersey*

**GEORGE C. PECK JR., M.D.**
*Attending Plastic Surgeon*
*Beth Israel Hospital*
*Passaic, New Jersey*

**JOHN W. SIEBERT, M.D.**
*Assistant Professor of Surgery*
*Director of Microsurgery*
*New York University Medical School*
*Chief of Plastic Surgery*
*Bellevue Hospital Center*
*New York, New York*

**JAMES M. STUZIN, M.D.**
*Clinical Instructor of Plastic Surgery*
*University of Miami School of Medicine*
*Attending Physician*
*Mercy Hospital*
*Miami, Florida*

**EDWARD O. TERINO, M.D., L.L.D.**
*Director, Plastic Surgery Clinic of Southern California*
*Westlake Community Hospital*
*Thousand Oaks, California*

**BARRY M. ZIDE, D.M.D., M.D.**
*Associate Professor of Surgery (Plastic)*
*New York University Medical School*
*Bellevue Hospital Center*
*New York, New York*

# Foreword

Aesthetic rhinoplasty is clearly one of the most difficult operations in plastic and reconstructive surgery. Any text that disseminates information to make that operation more successful is a welcome edition to a plastic surgeon's library. Drs. Gruber and Peck's book is one such text that brings the very latest techniques to both the beginning surgeon and the seasoned rhinoplastic surgeon who wishes to fine tune his or her skills.

It is always a monumental task to bring together the ideas of many experts in a given field into a cohesive, smoothly flowing text. This book, which combines the ideas of no less than 23 authors, manages to do just that. Each author discusses his or her particular area of expertise, and yet one chapter is allowed to visually flow into another. The schematics of all chapters are done by one artist to maintain this visual continuity.

The purpose of the book is evident in the book's subtitle: "State of the Art." Despite the unavoidable delay from conceptualization of the book to actual printing, the latest ideas in rhinoplasty and ancillary procedures are available to the reader. These ideas are presented in a fashion that does not "talk down" to the novice or neglect the detail required by an expert rhinoplastic surgeon. The individual authors place a special emphasis on their own preferred method of analysis and treatment, rather than provide a generic literature review. The reader, therefore, gets the benefit of their experiences. Some of the ideas and techniques are first being presented in this book.

An extremely wide variety of rhinoplasty topics are covered, beginning with anatomy, anesthesiology, and operation planning—topics that are often neglected. Primary and secondary rhinoplasty is, of course, one of the major focuses of attention, but special attention is paid to both the open and closed approaches without creating an unnecessary debate as to which approach is better. The non-Caucasian nose gets special attention, as well it should. Airway obstruction is also given special attention, and deservedly so, since this is one of the complications that surgeons tend to minimize. The short nose chapter presents an unusually clear and precise method of treatment for one of the most difficult types of rhinoplasty problems. Although a separate chapter on rhinoplasty complications is not allotted for, rhinoplasty complications are dealt with by various authors in the latter part of their chapters. The cleft lip nose chapter provides the reader with one author's personal experience, including some very long-term follow-up results, which are always appreciated. Of special interest are the ancillary procedure chapters. Procedures for the chin, cheek, and forehead are covered in a very thorough manner, giving the reader a full appreciation of how important they can be for the overall effect of the nose.

After 28 chapters, more than 500 pages, and over 900 illustrations, it becomes obvious that this book is an in-depth analysis of rhinoplasty by a number of the world's experts. This book, therefore, becomes a wonderful source of practical information that the surgeon can rely on prior to surgery or when trying to analyze preoperative and postoperative problems. It has certainly found a special place in my library.

NORMAN COLE, M.D.

# *Preface*

Rhinoplasty is one of the most difficult technical procedures in plastic surgery. A quantum improvement in the achieved results occurred in the mid-1970s when the concept of augmentation by cartilage grafting was emphasized. A second quantum leap occurred in the mid-1980s with the advent of the open technique. The open approach made it possible for the surgeon to execute many of the maneuvers that had previously been described but were simply too difficult to carry out. Since that time the rhinoplasty operation, like so many other procedures in plastic surgery, has gone on to exhibit continuous improvement, from the standpoint of diagnosis, planning, newer techniques, and execution. The purpose of this book is to bring the reader up to date with all of the factors that go into producing an exceptionally fine rhinoplasty result.

Part I considers basic techniques, and allows the reader an opportunity to see the anatomy of the nose from a clear and more precise perspective than ever before. Nasal proportions are also discussed. Without this in-depth analysis of the relationship of one part of the nose to the other, and the nose to other parts of the face, it is impossible to get a good grasp of what should be done at surgery. Patient selection is also an extremely important issue. As everyone knows, a satisfactory result on an unhappy patient is worse than an unsatisfactory result on a happy patient. Nasal analysis and operative planning is gone into in great detail and depth. This is often an overlooked area of plastic surgery simply because it doesn't involve the actual cutting of tissues. However, without proper planning even the best technique in the world will not yield the desired result. A review of the basic understanding of anesthesia (both local and general) as it applies to rhinoplasty is also given. Finally, the basic technique for both the closed and open approach is given. Admittedly the "basic techniques" as given are those of the editors and are not necessarily those shared by other

rhinoplastic surgeons. Nonetheless, they should form the basis for a general approach to the open and closed techniques.

Part II addresses some special problems in aesthetic rhinoplasty. To begin, tip grafting is discussed in great detail. In addition, variations on grafting the tip and dorsum are included, the so-called umbrella graft in particular. To give the reader further options, dorsal bone grafting is discussed. In addition, the boxy tip and alar wedge problems are reviewed.

One of the more challenging problems in rhinoplastic surgery is lengthening a short nose. Hopefully some of the ideas presented here should stimulate the reader to take this challenge whenever it presents itself. Other special problems that are updated for the reader include rhinoplasty in the non-Caucasian nose, the black nose, and the aging nose. The crooked nose is analyzed and many types of techniques are advocated to improve that particular problem.

Two chapters are devoted to the problem of the secondary rhinoplasty; one considers the open approach and one the closed approach. Finally, a chapter is devoted to a few difficult cases. In the last chapter of this section, the aesthetics of the cleft lip nose are reviewed. The reader will get the benefit of more than 30 years of the contributor's experience.

Part III is devoted to airway obstruction. Although concentrating largely on the aesthetics of the rhinoplasty result, functional problems are still foremost. There are times when existing problems need to be corrected at the time of the aesthetic rhinoplasty, but there are also certain problems that must be avoided if airway obstruction is not going to be a problem following the aesthetic rhinoplasty. Two different perspectives toward the airway obstruction problem are provided. Finally, special attention is given to turbinectomy because of its increasing importance in alleviating airway obstruction.

Part IV discusses ancillary procedures. The nose

is strongly influenced by other parts of the facial skeleton, and consequently a chapter is devoted to chin augmentation. In addition, genioplasty is gone into in great detail, since there are a number of times when simply augmenting the chin with an implant is insufficient to produce the desired result. Less commonly known is the fact that the forehead itself and its slope can influence the nasal appearance. Consequently, the latest methods of changing the forehead contour is discussed. To complete the re-view of ancillary procedures, malar augmentation and lipoplasty of the face and neck are discussed. Recently, much more detailed malar analysis and technique options have become available, which we felt the reader would want to be aware of.

We hope the reader finds the material within this text to be provocative and challenging. The con-tributors are all experts within their subspecialized fields. Their combined ideas are what help make this subject matter the state of the art.

RONALD P. GRUBER, M.D.
GEORGE C. PECK, M.D.

# Acknowledgments

We would like to thank a number of people who have contributed to the finalization of this book. Much of the typing was done by Dan Ashby and Beverley Griffitts. Many thanks must also go to some of the staff at Mosby–Year Book, Inc., which includes Anne Patterson, Jim Ryan, and Karyn Fell. Special thanks is also in order to Wendy Jackelow for her beautiful artwork. In addition, her patience in repeated modifications of drawings was most appreciated by all the contributors.

Finally, special thanks is owed to Gloria Gruber for not only suggesting that this book be done, but also for providing invaluable input as to its organization and format.

RONALD P. GRUBER, M.D.
GEORGE C. PECK, M.D.

# Contents

# PART I

# Basic Techniques

# Nasal Anatomy

John W. Siebert, M.D.

Barry M. Zide, D.M.D., M.D.

A thorough understanding of the involved basic anatomy is fundamental to any surgical procedure. To the rhinoplasty surgeon familiarity with the nuances of nasal anatomy is essential to ensure a pleasing, long-term result. Indeed, the ultimate outcome of any nasal surgery reflects the patient's subtle anatomy, the surgeon's recognition of each individual's variations, as well as the ability of the surgeon to deal with them. All components of the patient's nasal anatomy must be assessed beginning with the skin and subcutaneous tissues and how they vary from region to region on the nose; the nasal musculature and its dynamic effects on nasal contour; the relative size, shape, and strength of the cartilaginous and bony structural framework; and the internal components of the nose. With this in mind we will analyze nasal anatomy accordingly.

An immense literature regarding nasal anatomy exists. We will attempt to delineate the anatomic lessons we have learned from both fresh cadaver dissections and clinical practice. Corresponding anatomic drawings are included to further clarify many of the anatomic dissections. An understanding of the most commonly found variations will enable the rhinoplasty surgeon to achieve aesthetically pleasing, natural results.

## TOPOGRAPHIC NASAL ANATOMY

The surface anatomy of the nose is shown in Figure 1–1. The surface anatomy directly reflects the underlying framework. Thus, careful evaluation of sur-

face subtleties is a prerequisite for favorable rhinoplasty.

## SKIN AND SOFT TISSUES

Variability in nasal skin thickness and texture from region to region and from patient to patient will have a marked effect on the final rhinoplasty result.

Thick, sebaceous skin limits the amount of nasal definition possible. These patients tend to have more postoperative edema, more subcutaneous scar formation secondary to prolonged edema, especially in the nasal tip, and slower settling of the nasal skin. Excision of subcutaneous tissue, especially in the black ethnic nose, is sometimes necessary to optimize tip definition. Conversely, patients with thin nasal skin heal more quickly. They exhibit less postoperative edema, and redraping of the skin over the supporting structures is easily achieved. However, subtle irregularities or asymmetry in nasal cartilage or bone are more apparent.

Nasal skin is generally thinner and more mobile in the cephalic one half to three fifths of the nose. A thicker, more glandular skin is present in all patients toward the nasal tip. The amount of subcutaneous tissue also varies. The skin and soft tissues are generally thinnest over the osseocartilaginous junction of the nose and thickest over the nasion and supratip dorsum. This varying thickness of nasal skin and soft tissues must be considered when fine-tuning the nasal profile. This variability is also why many cartilage grafts exhibit palpable irregular bor-

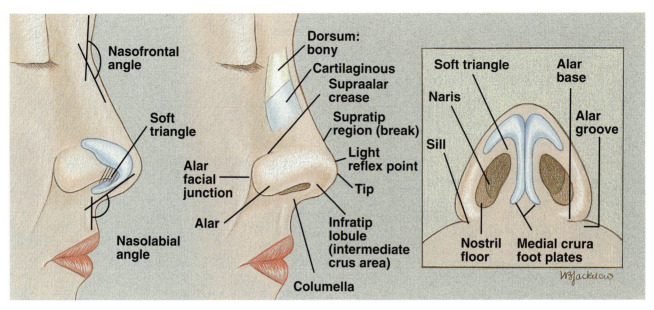

**FIG 1–1.**
Three views of the nasal topographic anatomy.

ders when placed cephalad on the nasal dorsum. Thus, careful contouring and softening of cartilage grafts must be performed to achieve favorable long-term results.

The nasal dome, or area of light reflex of the nasal tip, is separated from the margin of the nostril by a triangular-shaped area known as the soft triangle. This portion of the alar rim consists of two juxtaposed layers of skin, the external skin of the nose and the vestibular lining skin, separated by loose areolar tissue. Incisions in this area should be avoided because notching of the alar rim will occur.

## SENSORY INNERVATION OF THE NOSE

Since local anesthesia is commonly used for nasal surgery, an understanding of the sensory innervation of the nose is mandatory. An easy way to think about the nasal sensation is to divide sensation into external and internal components.

The sensory innervation of the external nose is derived mainly from branches of the anterior ethmoidal nerve, a branch of the nasociliary nerve, as well as contributions from the infraorbital, infratrochlear, and supratrochlear nerves. The terminal branch of the anterior ethmoidal nerve courses beneath the nasal bones and pierces the fibrous connection between the upper lateral cartilages and the nasal bones. It lies in a groove along the underside of the nasal bone. This groove may be mistaken for a

fracture on nasal radiographs. It courses distally and overlies the upper lateral cartilages to the nasal tip (Fig 1–2,A). It is almost always cut by intercartilaginous incisions and results in a hypesthetic nasal tip (Fig 1–2,B and C).

The infraorbital nerve, a terminal branch of the maxillary division of the trigeminal nerve, supplies branches across the external nose, upper lip, nostril sill and floor, columella, as well as the most caudal aspects of the nasal septum. It courses inferomedially within the bony canal before exiting the infraorbital foramen located within the maxilla. The infraorbital foramen is found on a perpendicular line to the medial limbus of the eye, but it opens in a medial and inferiorly directed fashion (Fig 1–3).

The internal vault of the nose receives sensation mainly from branches of the nasociliary nerve and the sphenopalatine ganglion. The nasociliary nerve divides into the infratrochlear nerve and anterior and posterior ethmoidal nerves within the posterior of the orbit. The anterior ethmoidal nerve gives off internal branches to innervate most the internal nasal side wall anterior to the turbinates. It also gives off an internal nasal branch to the nasal septum. The sphenopalatine ganglion is situated at the level of the most posterior aspect of the middle turbinate on each side of the nose, approximately 8 to 10 cm from the nares. The sphenopalatine ganglion gives off all the posterior nasal nerves to both the lateral nasal wall and posterior septum, palatine nerves, and the nasopalatine nerve. This ganglion can be blocked

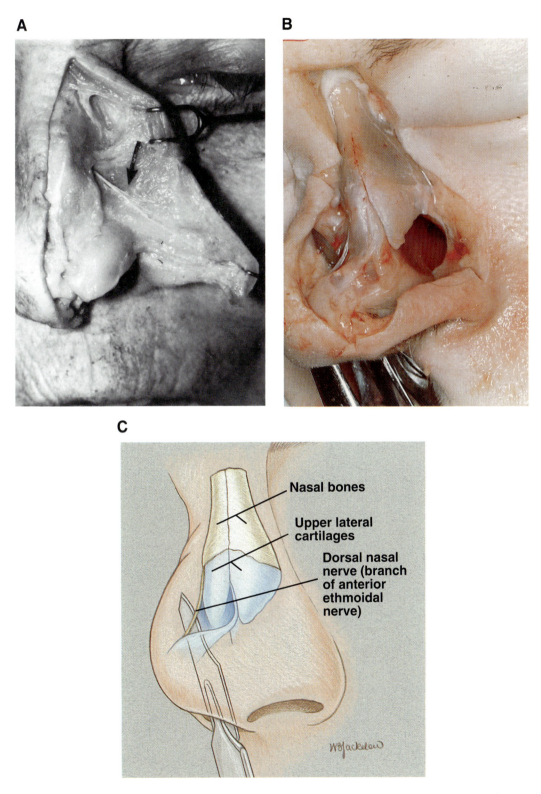

**FIG 1–2.**
**A,** cadaver dissection demonstrating the dorsal nasal nerve *(arrow)*, the terminal branch of the anterior ethmoidal nerve. **B,** the dorsal nasal nerve is almost always transected by an intercartilaginous incision. Notice the scalpel blade about to cut the nerve. **C,** corresponding drawing to **B.** (**A** and **B** courtesy of Barry M. Zide, M.D.)

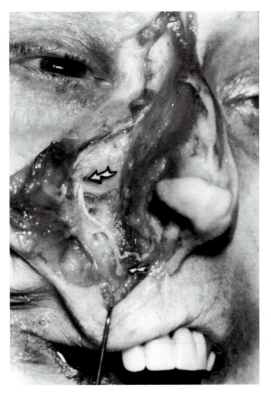

**FIG 1–3.**
Cadaver dissection demonstrating the infraorbital nerve and its foramen *(arrows)*. Notice the branches to the upper lip, columella, and the external lateral aspect of the nose. (Courtesy of Barry M. Zide, M.D.)

topically with cocaine, although its deep posterior location makes this difficult, and it is rarely blocked by most rhinoplasty surgeons using cocaine pludgets. The sphenopalatine ganglion can be blocked directly when posterior septal surgery is required. Placing a needle through the greater palatine foramen in the hard palate located 1 cm medial and 1 cm posterior to the junction of the first and second molars (Fig 1–4,A–C) enables ethmoid and vomerine bone surgery to be easily done under local anesthesia. The ganglion is located about 2 in. from the greater palatine foramen in the hard palate. Thus, a simple 1½-in. needle will not reach. The block is best done by finding the foramen with a 25-gauge needle and then bending a 22-gauge spinal needle to deliver the anesthetic. Obviously, this anesthetic block should be attempted only when complete familiarity with the anatomy has been gained.

## MIMETIC MUSCLES AND SUPERFICIAL MUSCULOAPONEUROTIC SYSTEM

The nose enjoys the luxury of a musculofascial blanket under which all nasal dissections must take place. The medial frontalis muscles coalesce in the lower part of the midforehead to form the procerus muscles. The vertically oriented procerus muscles join by muscle and fascia to the wing-shaped nasalis transversus muscles, which ride up along the nasal sidewalls. These muscles form a "Mercedes symbol" over the nasal dorsum (Fig 1–5,A and B).

On occasion some muscle covers the lateral nasal bones, but frequently this is a muscle-free area which makes any irregularity of lateral nasal bones especially easy to feel.

The nasalis transversus and two other bilateral muscles all arise from the periosteum above the central and lateral incisors and below the piriform aperture. The alar parts of the nasalis muscles pass through the alar bases to lie within the lateral alar lobules (Fig 1–6,A and B). These are the muscles commonly seen to bleed deep within the Weir wedge excisions. Small vascular connections from these muscles may support the overlying skin for V-Y advancement flaps to cover the nasal tip. This muscle, responsible for alar flaring, can be used to test facial nerve function in the comatose patient because airway obstruction will cause the patient to flare the nostrils.

The final nasalis muscle, the depressor septi, arises from the periosteum above the central and lateral incisors as well as from the region of the anterior nasal spine. Additional fibers may originate anterior to the upper fibers of the orbicularis oris as well. The muscle courses cephalad to insert into the membranous septum and the footplates of the medial crura. A few fibers also continue between the medial crura toward the nasal tip (Fig 1–7). Thus, when this muscle contracts, the nasal tip may be pulled downward and the upper lip shortened depending on the extent of muscle fibers continuing into the nasal tip and the upper lip.

The mimetic muscles of the nose are covered, similar to the face, by a fibrous aponeurotic sheet known as the superficial musculoaponeurotic system (SMAS). The SMAS interconnects the nasal musculature so that synergistic activity of several small muscles can produce profound effects on nasal anatomy.

## BONY SKELETON OF THE NOSE

The bony skeleton of the nose is composed of paired nasal bones and the frontal processes of the maxillae (Fig 1–8). The nasal bones are joined in the midline in their cephalad portion and separated only by insinuated periosteum in the internasal suture line at

**A**

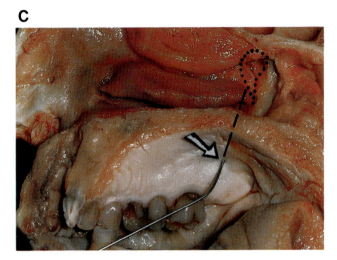

**B**

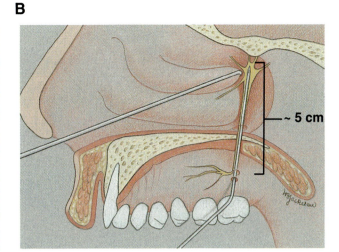

~ 5 cm

**C**

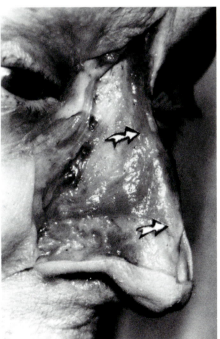

**FIG 1–4.**
**A** and **B,** the sphenopalatine ganglion (outlined with a *stippled line*) can be blocked with local anesthetic via the greater palatine foramen located 1 cm medial and 1 cm posterior to the junction of the first and second molars *(arrow)* with a spinal needle. **C,** the sphenopalatine ganglion being supported by the elevator. IT-inferior turbinate; SS-sphenoid sinus. (**A** and **C** courtesy of Barry M Zide, M.D.)

**A**

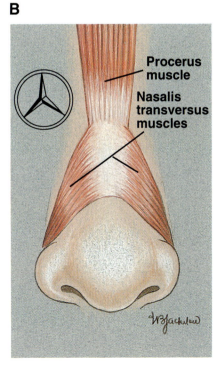

**B**

Procerus muscle

Nasalis transversus muscles

**FIG 1–5.**
**A** and **B,** the superficial muscles of the nose, the procerus muscles and nasalis transversus muscles *(arrows)*, join on the dorsum of the nose to form the internal lines of an equally trisected circle. (**A** courtesy of Barry M. Zide, M.D.)

**A**

**B**

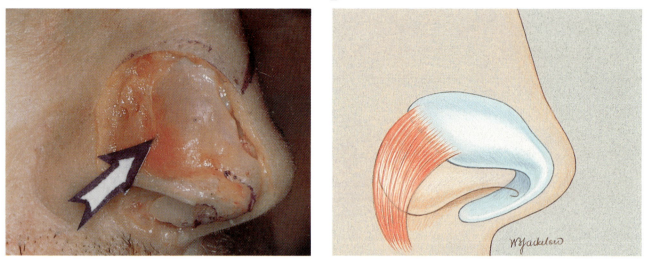

**FIG 1–6.**
**A** and **B,** the nasalis transversus muscles arise from the periosteum above the central and lateral incisors and below the piriform aperture *(arrow)*. The alar parts of the nasalis muscles pass through the alar bases to lie within the lateral alar lobules. (**A** courtesy of Barry M. Zide, M.D.)

their caudal portions. The paired nasal bones are supported laterally by the frontal processes of the maxillae and superoposteriorly by the nasal spine of the frontal bone.

Elevation of the periosteum of the nasal bones

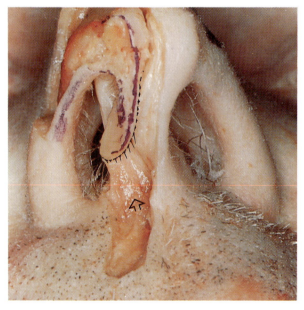

**FIG 1–7.**
The depressor septi *(arrow)* arises from the periosteum above the central and lateral incisors. Additional fibers may originate anterior to the upper fibers of the orbicularis oris as well. The muscle courses cephalad to insert into the membranous septum and the footplates of the medial crura *(stippled line).* (Courtesy of Barry M. Zide, M.D.)

should be limited to maximize soft-tissue adherence laterally. This reduces the chance of collapse of the upper third of the nose, especially if septal work is performed concomitantly. In addition, comminution of the osteotomy fracture lines will be reduced, and palpable bony irregularities will be minimized. Lateral osteotomies should begin low on the maxillary piriform aperture and extend cephalad in a curvilinear fashion up the frontal processes of the maxillae.

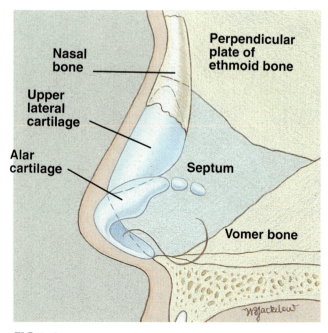

**FIG 1–8.**
The osteocartilaginous framework of the nose.

The "nasal bone infracture" is really a misnomer since this osteotomy is primarily in the frontal process of the maxilla. The delicate nasal bones should be confronted only at the apex of the osteotomy because a back fracture or transverse osteotomy is required to complete the bony infracture.

The lacrimal sac and lacrimal drainage system are theoretically at risk during lateral osteotomy. However, the anterior lacrimal crest, formed by the frontal process of the maxilla, as well as the anterior portion of the medial canthal tendon and associated fascia protect these structures. Lacrimal obstruction is rarely reported.

In patients with unusually short nasal bones, approximately 15 mm or less in length, the cartilaginous structures represent a greater proportion of the nasal skeleton. Lateral osteotomies in such patients tend to overnarrow the middle vault and result in nasal valve collapse. They should be avoided, but when performed, interposition cartilage grafts (spreader grafts) should be placed between the septum and the upper lateral cartilage to compensate for this tendency to collapse.

## CARTILAGINOUS STRUCTURES OF THE NOSE

### Lateral (Upper Lateral) Cartilages

The upper lateral cartilages along with the quadrangular cartilage of the septum constitute the cartilaginous pyramid of the nose (see Fig 1–10). The upper lateral cartilages are paired structures attached to the dorsal septum in the midline, the undersurface of the nasal bones superiorly, and the frontal processes of the maxillae superolaterally. Laterally the upper lateral cartilages attach to the piriform aperture via dense fibroareolar attachments. The caudal quarter of the lateral cartilages diverge from the septum and end in free edges (Fig 1–9). This portion of the lateral cartilages is mobile and moves with respiration. This area between the septal cartilage in the midline and the upper lateral cartilages is covered by mucosa continuous with mucoperichondrium overlying the cartilage and constitutes part of the internal valve of the nose.

Cephalically, the upper lateral cartilages extend to as much as 10 mm beneath the caudal aspect of the nasal bones in the midline (Fig 1–10). Fibrous attachments secure the upper lateral cartilages to the undersurface of the nasal bones. Inadvertent or careless surgical trauma can interrupt this connection and consequently collapse the middle third of the

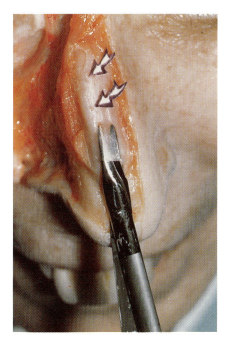

**FIG 1–9.**
The caudal quarter of the lateral cartilages diverge from the septum and end in free edges *(arrows)*. (Courtesy of Barry M. Zide, M.D.)

nose. This deformity is extremely difficult to correct unless recognized at the time of trauma.

The lower portions of each lateral cartilage become thicker and roll to varying degrees onto themselves. Exaggerated rolling of these distal ends can result in excessive width in the middle third of the nose or supratip area. The caudal ends of the upper lateral cartilage extend for a variable distance underneath the cephalic scroll, or margin of the alar cartilages. Fibroareolar attachments between the upper lateral and lower lateral (alar) cartilages gradually stretch with age as drooping of the nasal tip becomes evident. These attachments are routinely cut during intercartilaginous incisions to mobilize the soft-tissue envelope of the nose in rhinoplasties.

### Alar (Lower Lateral) Cartilages

The alar cartilages are paired structures that form a cartilaginous framework for the nasal tip. Each alar cartilage consists of a medial and lateral crus, which join together in a transition zone known as the intermediate crus. Many authors state that the medial and lateral crura join together at the dome of the alar cartilages, which corresponds to the point of light reflex on the nasal tip. However, in most cases the division between the medial and lateral crura is not precise. The alar cartilages are attached to the upper

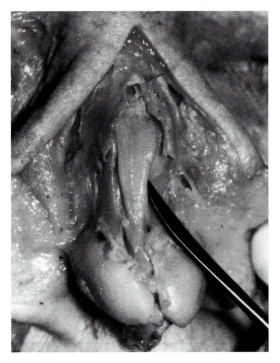

**FIG 1–10.**
The cephalad extent of the upper lateral cartilages extend to as much as 10 mm beneath the caudal aspect of the nasal bones in the midline. The nasal bones have been removed in the midline to demonstrate this. (Courtesy of Barry M. Zide, M.D.)

lateral cartilages, to the septum, to the piriform aperture, to the overlying skin, and to each other by fibrous and muscular attachments. Each medial crus continues toward the base of the columella and these diverge from one another to form the footplates of the medial crura. These footplates are bound to the caudal septum by fibrous attachments, which would be divided by full transfixion incisions. Many fibers of the depressor septi muscles insert directly onto these footplates. Action by these muscles pulls down the nasal tip.

The ultimate shape of the nasal tip is only partly dependent on the shape and consistency of the alar cartilages. Depending on the quality of overlying skin (especially the sebaceous nature) and subcutaneous tissues, the nasal tip may bear little resemblance to the shape of the alar cartilages. Prior surgery or inflammatory conditions all contribute to determining the nasal tip size and shape.

The possible configurations of the alar cartilages are countless, and many authors have attempted to categorize them. The more common varieties and how to surgically deal with them will be dealt with in subsequent chapters.

The generally recognized major mechanisms of

nasal tip support include the medial and lateral crura, the attachment of the footplates of the medial crura to the caudal border of the nasal septum, and the fibrous attachments between the upper lateral cartilages and the alar cartilages (Fig 1–11). Lesser contributions to tip support are the interdomal connections between both alar cartilages, fibrous connections to the anterior septal dorsum at the anterior septal angle known as the suspensory ligament of the nasal tip, and the attachment of the alar cartilages to the overlying skin and musculature.

## Nasal Septum and Septal Cartilage

The nasal septum divides the nasal cavity into two lateral chambers. The anatomic components include both osseous and cartilaginous parts (see Fig 1–8). The bony parts include the perpendicular plate of the ethmoid bone, the vomer, the nasal crest of the maxilla, and the nasal crest of the palatine bone. The quadrangular cartilage is the cartilaginous component. It protrudes anteriorly to the piriform aperture and provides midline support to the nose.

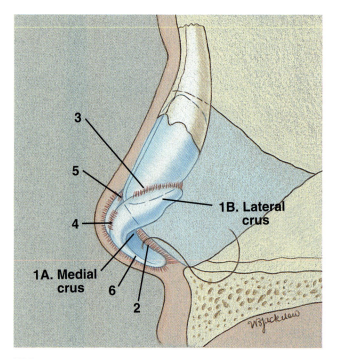

**FIG 1–11.**
The mechanisms of nasal tip support include *1*, the medial and lateral crura; *2*, the attachment of the medial footplates to the caudal border of the nasal septum; *3*, the fibrous attachments between the upper lateral cartilages and the alar cartilages; *4*, the interdomal connections between both alar cartilages; *5*, the suspensory ligament of the nasal tip; and *6*, the attachment of the alar cartilages to the overlying skin and musculature.

The quadrangular cartilage is firmly bound to the vomer posteriorly and inferiorly. The perichondrium is continuous with the periosteum. Anteriorly and caudally the perichondrium of the septal cartilage extends out to join with the periosteum of the anterior nasal spine and maxillary crest. The caudal margin of the septal cartilage is separated from the medial crura of the alar cartilages and columella by the membranous septum, which is formed by juxtaposition of mucosal flaps from each side. The anterior portion of the septal cartilage is flexible. As such, minimal or moderate trauma to the nose may not necessarily fracture the septum or displace the septum from its attachments to the vomer, anterior nasal spine, or maxillary crest. Posteriorly the cartilaginous septum is less pliable and contiguous with the vomer and the perpendicular plate of the ethmoid bone (see Fig 1–8). A tongue of quadrangular cartilage is insinuated between the perpendicular plate and the vomer for a variable distance. When obtaining a cartilage graft from the nasal septum the surgeon must be sure to include this posterior extension if the requirements for the graft are great. By including this posterior extension of the quadrangular cartilage, grafts up to 4 × 2 cm in size can be harvested, even allowing for 1 cm caudal and dorsal remaining struts on the nasal septum for midline support.

All the components of the septum may contribute to nasal obstruction. The perpendicular plate of the ethmoid may be the only component deviated in the patient complaining of difficulty breathing. Thus, this cannot be overlooked in evaluating patients with obstructive symptoms. In fact, following lateral osteotomy nasal obstruction may occur if deviations to the perpendicular plate are not observed and appropriately dealt with.

The dorsal border of the cartilaginous nasal septum varies in width. Where the quadrangular cartilage meets the nasal bones, it flares and sometimes bifurcates into a Y to form a palpable groove on the dorsum of the nose in some patients. Since this part of the septum is fused with the upper lateral cartilages, this flattened Y may actually be due to the upper lateral cartilages (see Fig 1–10).

The caudal septum forms a gentle curve contributing to the shape of the supratip and columella. The anterior septal angle should be assessed by caudally directed digital pressure on the upper lip. Blanching of the nasal skin occurs at the anterior septal angle. To avoid late supratip fullness following rhinoplasty this maneuver must be performed to ensure appropriate trimming at the anterior septal angle. This is especially true when full transfixion (transmembranous septum) incisions are used. The midseptal angle is really a gentle curve at the level of the caudal aspect of the columella. Prominence to the midseptal angle may allow excess columella to be seen; however, excess medial crura or a redundant membranous septum are just as likely to be causatory factors. The posterior septal angle is located just above the nasal spine articulation. Its fullness along with the size of the anterior nasal spine and thickness of the depressor muscles helps to determine the nasolabial angle and the relative length of the upper lip.

### Accessory (Sesamoid) Cartilages of the Nose

Accessory cartilages are found between the lateral and alar cartilages as well as lateral to the alar cartilages. They form a bridge between the alar cartilage and the edge of the piriform aperture. Their contribution to nasal shape is minimal.

### Turbinates (Conchae)

There are four pairs of nasal turbinates located on the internal aspect of the lateral nasal wall (Fig 1–12). The supreme and superior turbinates are small. The middle and inferior turbinates are rich in cavernous sinuses. The inferior turbinate, in particular, is involved in regulation of the nasal airway due to its rich vascular network and size. Vasomotor supply to the inferior turbinate regulates its size and thus its role as an airway valve. Sympathetic innervation results in vasoconstriction and reduction in

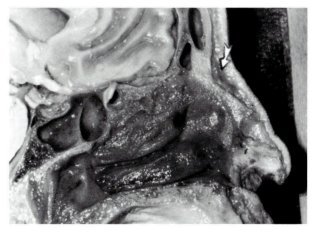

**FIG 1–12.**
The four nasal turbinates are located on the internal aspect of the lateral nasal wall (arrow). (Courtesy of Barry M. Zide, M.D.)

size. Parasympathetic stimulation results in vasodilation and enlargement. Chronic enlargement may lead to hypertrophy or polypoid degeneration requiring surgical intervention to deal with the subsequent nasal obstruction.

Located just below the attachment of the inferior turbinate, in the inferior meatus, the nasolacrimal duct drains tears from the lacrimal sac. The superior meatus is the drainage site of the anterior ethmoid sinus. All other sinuses drain through the middle meatus except the frontal sinus. The nasofrontal duct enters the nose anterior or just below the anterior portion of the middle turbinate.

## BIBLIOGRAPHY

Courtiss EH, Goldwyn RM: Resection of obstructing inferior nasal turbinates: a 10-year follow-up, *Plast Reconstr Surg* 86:152, 1990.

Hollinshead WH: *The head and neck,* New York, 1982, Harper & Row.

Lang: *Clinical anatomy of the head,* New York, 1983, Springer.

Letourneau A, Daniel RK: The superficial musculoaponeurotic system of the nose, *Plast Reconstr Surg* 82:48, 1988.

McCarthy JG, editor: Rhinoplasty. In *Plastic surgery,* Philadelphia, 1990, Saunders.

McKinney P, Johnson P, Walloch J: Anatomy of the nasal hump, *Plast Reconstr Surg* 77:404, 1986.

Zide BM: Nasal anatomy: the muscles and tip sensation, *Aesthetic Plast Surg* 9:193–196, 1985.

# Nasal Proportions

Bahman Guyuron, M.D.

The aesthetic surgeon of the 80s and 90s takes special pride in the achievement of one goal when performing rhinoplasties, and that is a "proportionate nose." For years, however, the definition of a proportionate nose was left to the individual surgeon's discretion. Today, we have formulated a scientific approach of defining a balanced nose that lends itself to transference and teaching.

Proportionality and balance are the main components of beauty. They are used during the planning of orthognathic surgery, craniofacial surgery, or aesthetic surgery. Distortion of balance even between the digits of a hand will take away from its attractiveness and will stand out as an abnormal, unpleasant structure. In fact, everything in nature that looks desirable has some degree of balance and harmony. This might change from time to time with personal taste or fashion, but a proportionate nose and face will remain attractive regardless of color or size. Not only does a balance between the nose and face have to exist, there also has to be harmony between the different units of the nose as well. This is where detection capability and the art of correction come into play. This is what separates a good nose from a bad nose and a good surgeon from a not-so-capable one. Furthermore, this detail orientation will reveal the different standards held by surgeons and patients. A 15-minute rhinoplasty becomes inconceivable at this point if every unit of the nose is put in harmony with the rest of the nose and face.

The goals of this chapter are to describe a scientific approach of analysis of the face and detection of the imperfections and to set the stage for the planning of surgery, which will be described in the next chapter.

## GENERAL FACIAL PROPORTIONS

No experienced surgeon concentrates solely on the nose and ignores other features of the face. It is of utmost importance to analyze each unit of the face before a detailed balance between the different parts of the nose and the rest of the face is put to test. In so doing, a systematic, step-by-step analysis might help avoid missing some critical imperfections of other parts of the face that may interfere with achieving an ideal rhinoplasty result.

The length of the forehead from the hairline to the glabella and the distance from the subnasale (junction of the nose and lip) to the lowermost portion of the chin are usually equidistant and match that of the glabella to the subnasale (Fig 2–1). However, a long or short forehead or lower face and chin (Fig 2–2,A and B) demand a discussion of different procedures with the patient or some minimal alterations in the planning of rhinoplasty to achieve a somewhat more harmonized nose. Making the nose too long or short to compensate for what in reality is a long or short chin or forehead would be a definite mistake. Within an aesthetically desirable range, however, one can choose the size of the nose that would properly match a slightly disproportionate chin without any, or at least not a

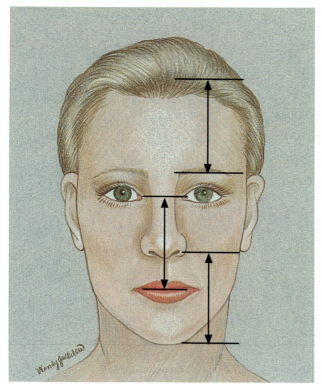

**FIG 2–1.**
Artistic rendering revealing the proportions of the upper, mid, and lower thirds of the face.

significant, compromise in the ultimate surgery outcome.

The forehead is reviewed also for irregularities and asymmetries. In the middle portion of the face, the malar bones play a significant role in the appearance of the nose. If these are hypoplastic, the nose will automatically look more projected. Augmentation of hypoplastic malar bones might require less alteration on the nose (Fig 2–3, A and B). On the front view, critical analysis should be conducted to compare the midlines of the upper, lower, and middle portions of the face to ensure that they are lined properly. It is not unusual to find a deviated chin or lower part of the face (Fig 2–4, A and B). In such a case, the patient should be made aware that unless the asymmetry of the lower aspect of the face is corrected, regardless of what is done to the nose, the chin may not look straight. It is surprising how often patients are unaware of their facial asymmetries. Not discussing this type of imperfection prior to the surgery may result in patient dissatisfaction in spite of an otherwise creditable rhinoplasty outcome.

The intercanthal distance and the eye position are also important in achieving pleasing rhinoplasty results. One must note whether the intercanthal distance is normal, increased, or decreased. Generally, the distance between the medial canthi is equal to the distance from the medial to the lateral canthus. A short intercanthal distance is going to demand a lower bridge in order to give the optical illusion of a wider intercanthal distance. The reverse is also true. If the intercanthal distance is too great, a higher bridge and nasion will give an optical illusion of a decreased intercanthal distance. If these facts are ignored, the ultimate rhinoplasty result might be a deterioration to the appearance of hypotelorism, hypertelorism, or telecanthus. Similarly, a narrow bridge will be better for a patient who has a decreased intercanthal distance, while a wide bridge might be advantageous for a person who has a wider intercanthal distance.

On profile, the degree of forehead projection, particularly in the glabellar area, is important. The position of the glabella dictates how deep the nasion should be (Fig 2–5, A and B); therefore it is critical to ensure that the glabella is in a proper position. Should it be too depressed or projected, it would interfere with the achievement of an aesthetically satisfying result and indeed might set the aesthetic goal in a wrong base.

Similarly, balance of the lower part of the face has a significant role in rhinoplasty. Generally, on a profile, either the upper and lower lips are lined up, or the upper lip is slightly anterior to the lower lip. Distortion of this relationship is often a reflection of a skeletal deformity and, if left undetected, will usually disturb the rhinoplasty result.

Finally, the proper chin position is definitely an important factor in achieving a good rhinoplasty result (Fig 2–6, A and B). If the chin is long, short, overprojected, or underprojected, it will dictate alteration of the chin or modification of the rhinoplasty plans within an aesthetic range. It is not advisable to convince patients who are seeking rhinoplasty to have malar augmentation or genioplasty, particularly when they do not understand or desire to undergo these procedures. However, the advantages of such a complimentary procedure should be clearly stated and emphasized. Fortunately, these imperfections can be corrected at a later time, as long as the aesthetic surgeon has not modified the rhinoplasty plans significantly in an attempt to compensate for the other abnormalities.

**A**

**B**

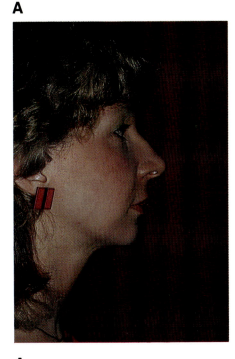

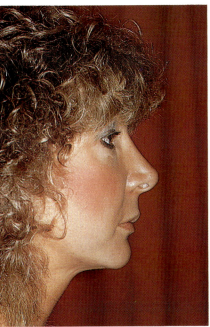

**FIG 2–2.**
Preoperative profile of a patient with a deficiency of the lower portion of her face **(A)** who required an advancement genioplasty and rhinoplasty in order to achieve proper balance **(B)**.

**A**

**B**

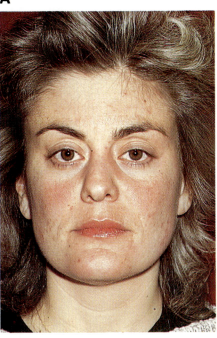

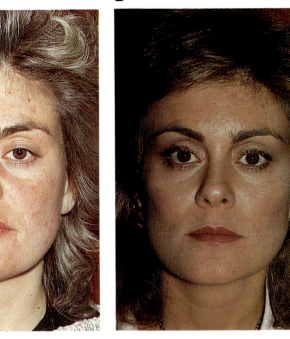

**FIG 2–3.**
Preoperative photograph of a patient with malar hyperplasia, a prominent chin, and a less-than-ideal nose **(A)**. Same patient following rhinoplasty, malar augmentation, and reduction genioplasty **(B)**. Without ancillary procedures, the rhinoplasty result would not have been as pleasing.

## CLINICAL NASAL PROPORTIONS

The nose is examined in five views. Each view will help detect some of the imperfections of the nose that the other views may not. These views include front, profile, right and left quarter, and basilar views.

On the front view, the bridge outlines are seen as two parallel shadows continuing from the eyebrows to the tip of the nose. There is a smooth and continuous transition of the nasal bones to the upper lateral cartilages without any visible depressions or demarcations. Often, this balance is disturbed by the widening of the nasal bones or the presence of a

**A**                    **B**

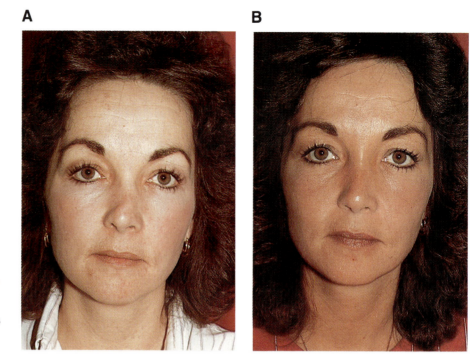

**FIG 2–4.**
Preoperative photograph of a
patient with significant
asymmetry of the lower portion
of her face **(A).** Following
rhinoplasty, however, the
asymmetry persists and detracts
from the end result of the
rhinoplasty **(B).**

discontinuous shadow at the junction of the nasal
bones and upper lateral cartilages, and this might indicate a need for some type of graft at this juncture
(Fig 2–7). The width of the nasal bridge shadow corresponds with the width of the highlights of the tip.
There is, however, a break in the shadow of the
bridge outline before the tip highlights are seen.

On a front view with the head straight, a portion
of the nostrils is seen in a symmetrical fashion. An
imaginary vertical line from the midglabella to the
philtrum dimple that passes through the midline upper incisor will reveal any bridge or tip deviation.
Furthermore, an imaginary line through the medial
canthi on a person with normal intercanthal distance
will pass about 1 mm inside the lateral boundaries of
the alar bases (Fig 2–8).

**A**                    **B**

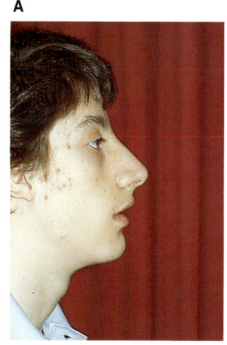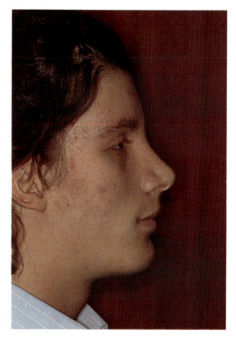

**FIG 2–5.**
Preoperative photograph of a
patient with a receding forehead
**(A).** Same patient following
rhinoplasty and forehead
advancement **(B).** Without a
forehead advancement, the
nasofrontal relationship would
not have been acceptable. (From
Guyuron B: Facial assessment for
aesthetic plastic surgery. In Rollin D,
editor: *Aesthetic Plastic Surgery*, ed 2,
Boston, Little Brown, in press. Used
by permission.)

A

B

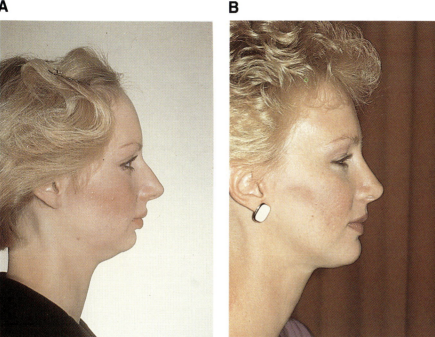

**FIG 2–6.**
Patient with a deep labiomental groove due to a receding chin, preoperative view **(A).** She underwent mandibular advancement and rhinoplasty in order to achieve more facial harmony **(B).**

Not only is it important to notice the deviation of the nasal bones on the front-view analysis of the nose, more critically, the position of the underlying anterior septal cartilage should be noted as well. Removal of the hump that has to some degree camouflaged the deviation of the underlying septum might unveil the abnormally positioned structures. These are the patients who may become extremely un-

happy because their previously perceived straight nose is now deviated. To avoid such an undesirable event, detection and correction of this problem are crucial. At the very least, the patient should know that there is a challenge at hand and that the surgeon's attempts to correct the problem might not always turn out absolutely ideal.

Abnormalities of the upper lateral cartilages can

A

B

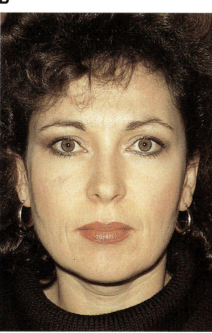

**FIG 2–7.**
**A,** preoperative photograph of a patient reveals a discontinuous nasal outline. **B,** establishment of a graceful nasal shadow and outline postoperatively. (From Guyuron B: Predictive rhinoplasty. In Rollin D, editor: *Aesthetic Plastic Surgery,* ed 2, Boston, Little Brown, in press. Used by permission.)

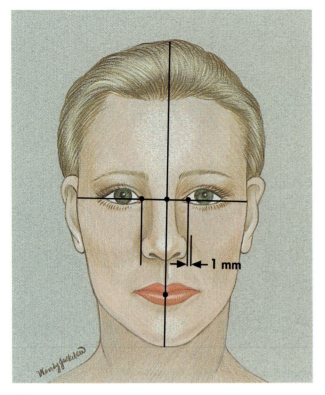

**FIG 2–8.**
Artistic illustration of the proportions of the alar base to the medial canthi. On a balanced nose, the distance between the alar bases is slightly wider than the distance between the medial canthi. This excess width is approximately 1 mm on either side. (From Guyuron B: Predictive rhinoplasty. In Rollin D, editor: *Aesthetic Plastic Surgery*, ed 2, Boston, Little Brown, in press. Used by permission.)

result in an imbalance of the caudal half of the bridge due to asymmetries or excess width. The tip highlights, as was stated earlier, are as wide as the width of the bridge. There are generally two distinct light reflections, as long as the lighting is proper for the observation.

The alar domes are symmetrical and nicely defined (Fig 2–9,A and B). A variety of lower lateral cartilage shapes can be seen that, if undesirable, may require a different approach for appropriate correction. At this view also, the sebaceous gland should be evaluated in terms of activity and quantity. If the skin is thick and sebaceous, achievement of proper definition of the tip and supratip break might be difficult and sometimes impossible.

The columella is slightly visible on the front view. Any excessive caudal projection of the columella should be noted (Fig 2–10,A and B). Furthermore, nostril symmetry, positioning, and width are noted in this view. A short upper lip could be a reflection of an underlying maxillary problem or the result of a long nose. Asking the patient to smile in this view will reveal the degree of tip movement toward the lip, the amount of incisor show, and also lip shape change. Rarely, a horizontal groove appears across the upper lip when the subject smiles. If this goes unnoticed on preoperative evaluation, the rhinoplasty may be blamed for this result.

The patient's chair is then turned 90 degrees so that the proportions of the nasal profile can be examined. The first area to examine is the nasofrontal junction—the deepest part of which is called the na-

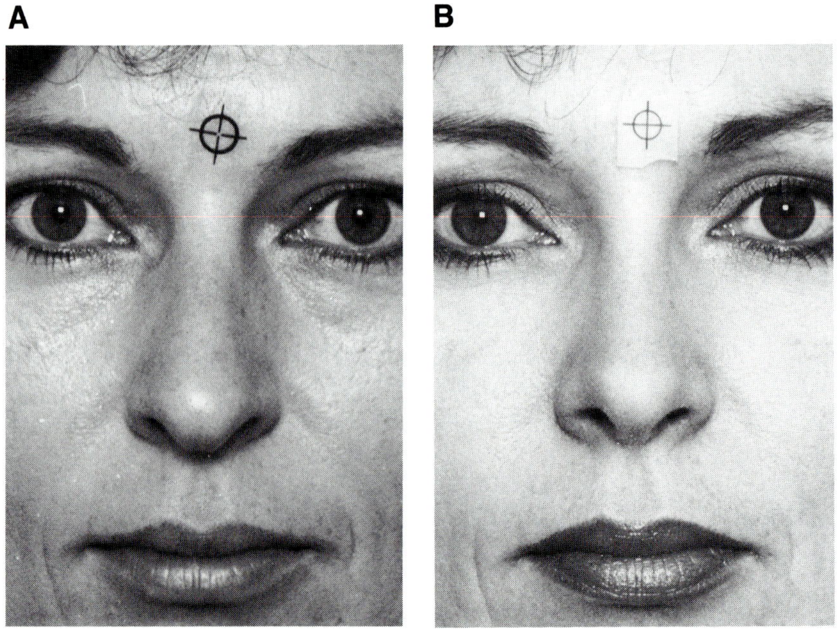

**A**                                                       **B**

**FIG 2–9.**
Preoperative close-up photograph of a patient with unpleasant nasal tip definition **(A).** Following rhinoplasty the patient has a more natural and desirable configuration of the nasal tip **(B).** (Photograph B from Guyuron B: Predictive rhinoplasty. In Rollin D, editor: *Aesthetic Plastic Surgery*, ed 2, Boston, Little Brown, in press.

**A**      **B**

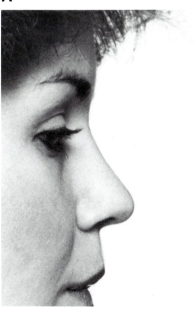

**FIG 2–10.**
Preoperative photograph of a patient with an excessively hanging columella **(A)** and following correction of this undesirable feature and a full rhinoplasty **(B).** (From Guyuron B: Predictive rhinoplasty. In Rollin D, editor: *Aesthetic Plastic Surgery,* ed 2, Boston, Little Brown, in press. Used by permission.)

sion. This is a depression between the forehead and the nose that is generally about 4 to 6 mm deep.[1] The deepest portion of the nasal root is located at the level or slightly above the upper lid margin in a straight gaze. The bridge of the nose has a gentle curve that becomes slightly deeper in the central portion of the nose. If a straight line is drawn to connect the most anterior point of the nasal tip to the nasion on an attractive nose, one will note a curve of about 0.5 to 1 mm deep for a male and 1 to 1.5 mm deep for a female (Fig 2–11). A straight nasal bridge will not look desirable on either a male or female nose.

Next, one needs to compare the nasal length from the medial canthi to the subnasale with the length of the lower portion of the face and upper lip (Fig 2–12). Generally, the length of the nose equals the distance from the stomion (junction of the lips) to the chin. The nasolabial angle is approximately 105 to 108 degrees for a female and 100 to 103 degrees for a male (Fig 2–13,A and B). Generally, the tip is slightly higher than the bridge, and this creates a supratip break. Any inadequacies of this area need to be corrected. Occasionally, one has to deal with an overprojected nose and tip (Fig 2–14,A and B). The alar base is located about 2 mm cephalad to the subnasale, and the columella is approximately 4 mm caudal to the alar rim on the profile (Fig 2–15).

The nasal spine creates a pleasant transition

**A**      **B**

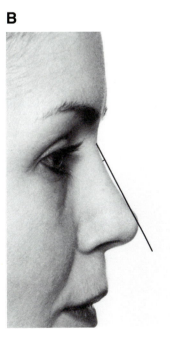

**FIG 2–11.**
The preoperative profile of a nasal bridge **(A)** is compared with the postoperative profile **(B).** A straight line connecting the nasion to the nasal tip demonstrates a definite curve that gives a pleasing dorsum.

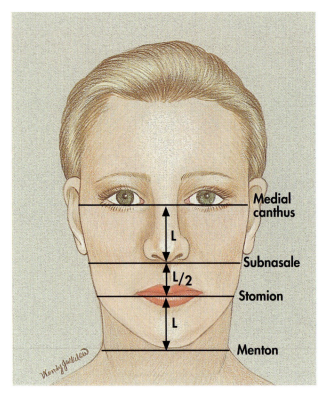

**FIG 2–12.**
An artistic rendering illustrates the proportions of the nose length (from the medial canthus to the subnasale) to the upper lip (from the subnasale to the stomion) and lower portion of the face (the stomion to the menton). Generally, the nose length equals that of the lower portion of the face, and the upper lip length is half the length of the nose. (From Guyuron B: Facial assessment for aesthetic surgery. In Rollin D, editor: *Aesthetic Plastic Surgery*, ed 2, Boston, Little Brown, in press. Used by permission.)

from the nose to the lip. Any excess or deficiency of this nasal element will result in an imbalance of this area. Furthermore, in this view, the alar base distance to the medial canthus should be noted. A shorter-than-usual distance can disturb the harmony of the nose and would require correction in order to achieve a more ideal aesthetic rhinoplasty result (Fig 2–16,A and B).

On the basilar view, the alar dome symmetry can be seen (Fig 2–17,A and B). The highest point of the alar dome should correspond to the highest point of the nostril. The nostrils are oval shaped with a slight widening at the nostril base. A significant difference between the anterior and posterior width of the nostril is a reflection of excessive alar base, which should be noted and corrected. Furthermore, the nostril asymmetry can be easily detected in this view. Right and left quarter-view photographs will reveal bridge contour abnormalities that can be missed on the front view or profile.

## THE ROLE OF LIFE-SIZE PHOTOGRAPHS

An important development in my personal approach to rhinoplasty has been the use of life-size photographs. By obtaining and analyzing these photographs on the basis of the soft-tissue cephalometric principles reported previously,[2, 3] the surgeon can use this blueprint in the operating room and view the imperfections of the nose. This will result in a

|   A   |   B   |

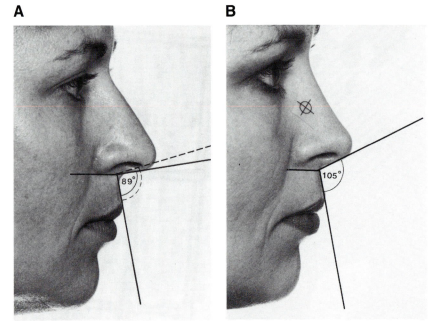

**FIG 2–13.**
A preoperative nasolabial angle **(A)** is compared with the postoperative, desirable relationship between the lip and nose **(B).** This range is from 105 to 108 degrees on a female. (From Guyuron B: *Plast Reconstr Surg* 81:489–498, 1988. Used by permission.)

**A** 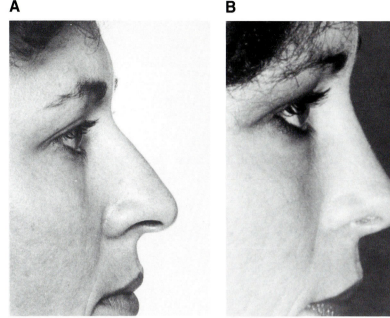 **B**

**FIG 2–14.**
An overprojected nose **(A)** requires lower lateral cartilage reduction in order to achieve a balanced nasal tip projection **(B)**. (From Guyuron B: *Plast Reconstr Surg* 81:489–498, 1988. Used by permission.)

custom-designed rhinoplasty that will provide the patient with a pleasing, balanced nose in harmony with the rest of the face. It avoids a prototype nose that may or may not be appropriate for every patient.

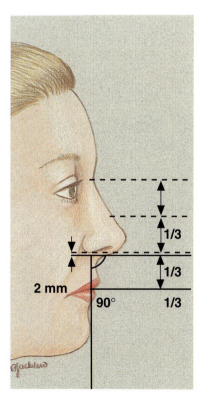

**FIG 2–15.**
Artistic rendering of the relationship of the alar base, subnasale, and columella.

## TECHNIQUE OF LIFE-SIZE PHOTOGRAPHY

In order to achieve an exact life-size enlargement of the photographs, small sticker markers are placed over the glabella and inferior orbital rim, the latter being located by palpation. To further ensure the accuracy of this technique, a ruler is placed on the side of the face at the level of the orbit during front-view photography and at the level of the bridge of the nose during profile photography. These indices are used in the dark room to achieve proper magnification.[2]

## ANALYSIS OF LIFE-SIZE PHOTOGRAPHS

A drafting film (Polydraft, Teledyne National Tracing Paper, Indianapolis) is used as an overlay to analyze the life-size photographs. The ultimate goal of the front-view analysis is to reveal the bridge deviation, tip distortions, and alar base imbalances.[2]

**Front View**

**Step 1.**—The midpoint of the upper portion of the face is located by bisecting the intercanthal distance. This technique is used only if the upper part of the face is symmetrical. When significant asymmetrical features are present, a different approach must be taken (Fig 2–18,A).

**A**    **B**

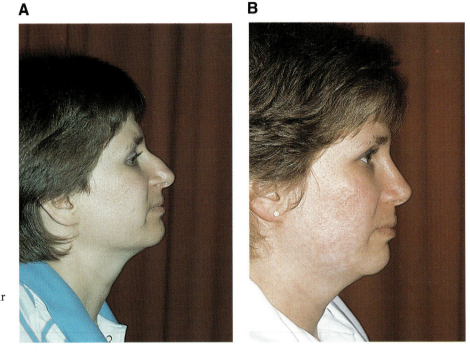

**FIG 2–16.**
The distance from the medial canthus to the alar base can be short, as in this patient preoperatively **(A).** It was lengthened by advancing the alar base caudally **(B).** (From Guyuron B: *Plast Reconstr Surg* 81:489–499, 1988. Used by permission.)

**Step 2.**—The midpoint of the upper lip will be marked at the philtrum dimple if the remainder of the face appears symmetrical. These two midpoints are then connected to define the vertical midfacial plane. The medial intercanthal distance is measured and compared with the width of the eye fissure. If these measurements are equal, two vertical lines are dropped parallel to the midfacial vertical plane from the medial canthi (Fig 2–19).[2] These two lines normally pass 1 to 2 mm medial to the lateral margin of a balanced alar base. However, if the intercanthal distance is not equal to the palpebral fissure width,

**A**    **B**

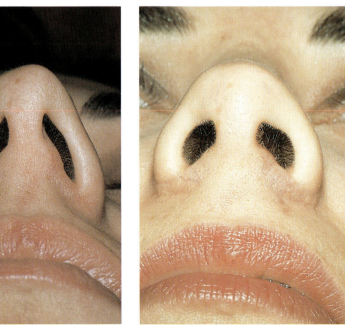

**FIG 2–17.**
On a basilar view, the alar dome asymmetry and alar width difference are apparent preoperatively **(A). B,** following correction.

**A**

**B**

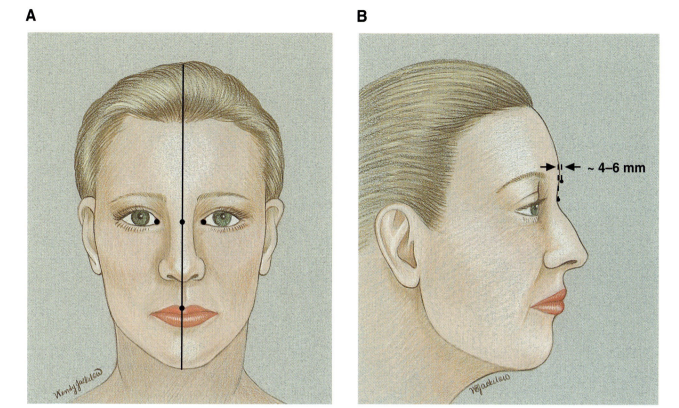

**FIG 2–18.**
**A,** the midpoint between the medial canthi is connected to the midpoint of the upper lip (From Guyuron B: *Predictive rhinoplasty* [in press]. Used by permission.) **B,** the nasion *(N)*, the deepest portion of the nasofrontal groove, is about 4 to 6 mm deep in relation to the glabella. (From Guyuron B: *Plast Reconstr Surg* 81:489–498, 1988. Used by permission.)

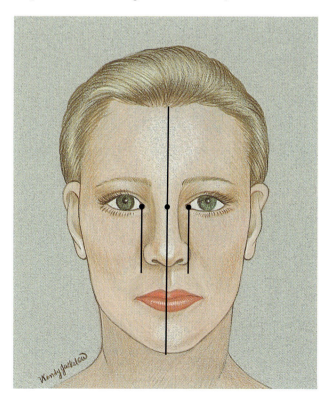

**FIG 2–19.**
A vertical line is dropped from each medial canthus to pass vertically through the alar base. (From Guyuron B: Predictive rhinoplasty. In Daniels R, editor: *Aesthetic Plastic Surgery,* ed 2, Boston, Little Brown, in press. Used by permission.)

then the latter will be used to judge the width of the alar base.

### Profile

A drafting film is placed over the life-size profile photograph.

**Step 1.**—The initial step in analyzing the profile is to define the nasofrontal groove. The nasion (the deepest portion of the nasofrontal groove) is about 4 to 6 mm deep in relation to the glabella. If this groove is too shallow or too deep, the ideal point for the nasion is defined in the horizontal plane 4 to 6 mm deep and vertically at the level of the lower border of the upper lid margin in a straight gaze (Fig 2–18,B).[2]

**Step 2.**—The most prominent portion of the tragus (tragion) is connected to the nasion. According to our study, this line forms an angle of 69 degrees with the vertical facial plane. This line is used to en-

sure proper positioning of the horizontal Frankfurt plane (Fig 2–20).[2]

**Step 3.**—The upper border of the tragus is connected to a point ½ cm below the infraorbital rim and continued past the nasal outline (Frankfurt horizontal plane) as marked before photography on the patient (Fig 2–21).

**Step 4.**—In order to define the vertical facial plane, a line is dropped from the nasion in a 90-degree relation to the Frankfurt horizontal plane (Fig 2–22).

**Step 5.**—From the nasion, the radix direction is drawn in a 34-degree angle for a female and a 36-degree angle for a male in relation to the vertical facial plane.[2]

**Step 6.**—The distance between the nasion and the stomion (upper and lower lip junction) is measured and divided into three equal distances.[2]

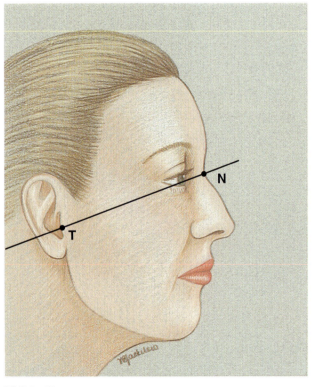

**FIG 2–20.**
To ensure proper positioning of the horizontal Frankfort plane, the most prominent portion of the tragus (tragion [T]) is connected to the nasion (N). (From Guyuron B: Predictive rhinoplasty. In Daniels R, editor: *Aesthetic Plastic Surgery*, ed 2, Boston, Little Brown, in press. Used by permission.)

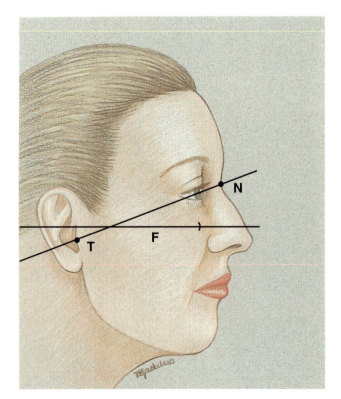

**FIG 2–21.**
The upper border of the tragus is connected to the infraorbital rim as marked before photography on the patient. (From Guyuron B: Predictive rhinoplasty. In Daniels R, editor: *Aesthetic Plastic Surgery*, ed 2, Boston, Little Brown, in press. Used by permission.)

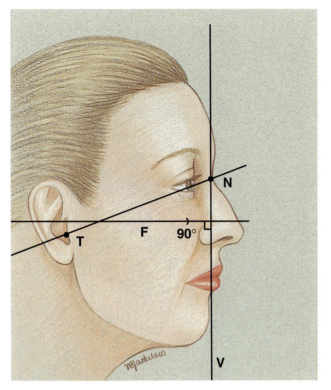

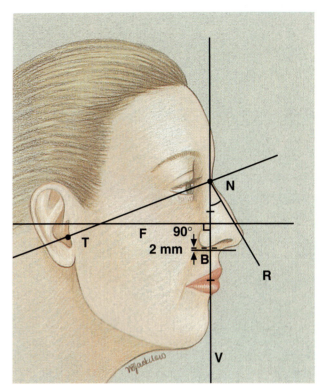

**FIG 2–22.**
A vertical line *(V)* is dropped from the nasion *(N)* to the Frankfort horizontal plane *(F)*. T = tragion. (From Guyuron B: *Plast Reconstr Surg* 81:489–498, 1988. Used by permission.)

**FIG 2–23.**
A line *(B)* is drawn parallel to the Frankfort horizontal facial plane *(F)* at the junction of the upper two thirds with the lower third of the distance from the nasion *(N)* to the stomion. R = radix. (From Guyuron B: *Plast Reconstr Surg* 81:489–498, 1988. Used by permission.)

**Step 7.**—A horizontal line is drawn parallel to the Frankfort horizontal facial plane 2 to 3 mm below the junction of the lower third with the upper two thirds (Fig 2–23).[2] This outlines the horizontal guide for the location of the subnasale.

**Step 8.**—The most projected portion of the upper lip (labrale superius) is marked. A vertical line is drawn 1 to 2 mm behind this point parallel to the vertical facial plane (Fig 2–24).[2] The subnasale is located at the intersection of this line and the previous horizontal line.

**Step 9.**—A line is projected from the subnasale in a 105- to 108-degree angle for a female and a 100- to 103-degree angle for a male in relation to the vertical line drawn to construct the nasolabial angle (Fig 2–25). The nasal profile can now be drawn with pleasing proportions on the triangular nasal frame.

**Step 10.**—The bridge template, which has three different contours, one with a 0.75- to 1-mm-deep curve for a male nasal bridge, 1.5- to 2-mm depth for

a female, and another with a 2- to 2.5-mm depth for a younger female, is used to draw a bridge (Fig 2–26).

**Step 11.**—A double-break tip outline is then drawn (Fig 2–27) by using the multitip template.[2] The proper tip size is chosen for the nose frame by moving the template up and down.

**Step 12.**—A line is dropped posteriorly from the subnasale in a 6-degree angle to the line *(L)* drawn in Step 8. This line generally touches the most prominent portion of the chin (pogonion). If the chin recedes, the reversed template is used to draw a proper labiomental groove and chin prominence (Fig 2–28). The labiomental groove is usually 3 to 4 mm deep on a female and 4 to 5 mm deep on a male.[2] A reliable way to achieve proper chin placement is to draw a line connecting the most anterior margins of the upper and lower lips. This line usually touches the most anterior portion of the chin.

The final analysis will then be highlighted with a

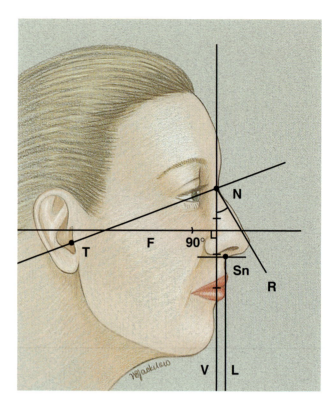

**FIG 2–24.**
A vertical line *(L)* is drawn 1 to 2 mm behind the most prominent portion of the upper lip (labrale superius), parallel to the vertical facial plane *(V)*. *SN* = subnasale. (From Guyuron B: *Plast Reconstr Surg* 81:489–498, 1988. Used by permission.)

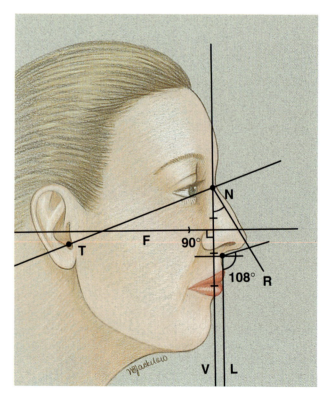

**FIG 2–25.**
A line is projected from the subnasale in a 105- to 108-degree angle for a female and a 100- to 103-degree angle for a male in relation to the vertical line. (From Guyuron B: *Plast Reconstr Surg* 81:489–498, 1988. Used by permission.)

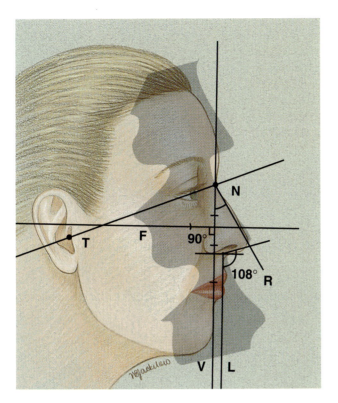

**FIG 2–26.**
A bridge template with three different contours is used to draw the bridge. (From Guyuron B: Predictive rhinoplasty. In Daniels R, editor: *Aesthetic Plastic Surgery*, ed 2, Boston, Little Brown, in press. Used by permission.)

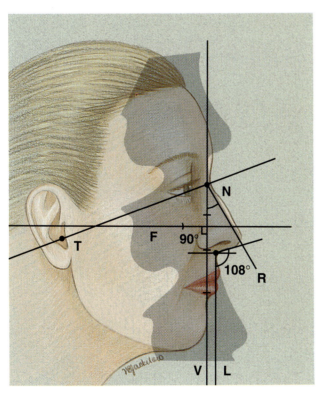

**FIG 2–27.**
A double-break tip outline is drawn by using the multitip template. (From Guyuron B: Predictive rhinoplasty. In Daniels R, editor: *Aesthetic Plastic Surgery*, ed 2, Boston, Little Brown, in press. Used by permission.)

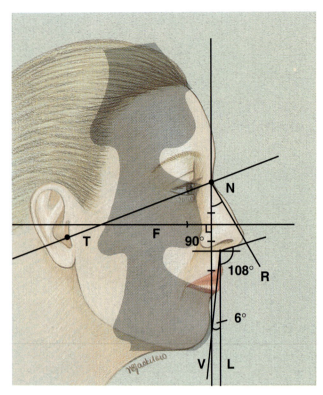

**FIG 2–28.**
The chin contour and labiomental groove are designed by using the template. (From Guyuron B: Predictive rhinoplasty. In Daniels R, editor: *Aesthetic Plastic Surgery*, ed 2, Boston, Little Brown, in press. Used by permission.)

smooth, single-line outline. The difference between the patient's nose and proposed nasal outline will be measured and recorded. These numbers will then be used in the operating room. The measurements are taken over the nasion, proximal part of the bridge, midportion of the bridge, supratip area, tip and columella region, as well as the subnasale. The advantage of this technique is to draw a proportionate nose that is aesthetically pleasing without the surgeon possessing major artistic capabilities. The disadvantages, however, are the need for an experienced photographer who would diligently enlarge the photographs while realizing the importance of their accuracy and having the necessary time to analyze these photographs.

## REFERENCES

1. Guyuron B: Guarded burr for nasofrontal deepening, *Plast Reconstr Surg* 84:513–516, 1989.
2. Guyuron B: Precision rhinoplasty I—Role of life-size photographs and soft tissue cephalometric analysis, *Plast Reconstr Surg* 81:489–498, 1988.
3. Guyuron B: Precision rhinoplasty II—Prediction, *Plast Reconstr Surg* 81:500–505, 1988.
4. Guyuron B: Predictive rhinoplasty. In Daniels R, editor: *Aesthetic Plastic Surgery*, ed 2, Boston, Little Brown, in press.

# Patient Selection in Rhinoplasty: Practical Guidelines

## Mark Gorney, M.D.

The desire to appear normal or aesthetically pleasing is older than plastic surgery. The puritan ethic that has, until recently, dominated our culture and disapproves of narcissism is rapidly breaking down. The growing popularity of rhinoplasty surgery has unfortunately created in our country a carnival-like atmosphere of which advertising by unqualified practitioners is only one aspect. In this climate it becomes imperative to establish clear criteria for patient selection; without these, there will be an inevitable parallel increase in patient dissatisfaction and litigation.

Who, then, is the "ideal" candidate for rhinoplasty? There is no such thing; however, the surgeon should certainly seek those personality factors that will enhance the physical improvements desired. There are, in most cases, clear indications of who will do well and enjoy the results. A person who is obviously intelligent, preferably educated, and who listens (rather than merely hearing) and clearly understands the pros and cons is a good candidate. Individuals who have a clearly discernible physical problem about which they have an understandable but not neurotic concern are good candidates.

Persons whose jobs require them to look attractive or who must compete with younger people are probably good candidates. Someone with a sense of humor is always a better candidate than a dour, anxious individual. Rhinoplasty patients are in a category by themselves and should be evaluated with the utmost care. Generally speaking, men make more difficult patients than women do. They do not tolerate pain as well and are generally more fussy.

There are basically two major categories for rejection of a patient seeking rhinoplasty. One is anatomic unsuitability; the other is emotional inadequacy.[1] Of these, emotional inadequacy is by far the more important. It is reviewed here on a purely pragmatic basis. The inexperienced surgeon must learn early to differentiate between healthy and unhealthy reasons for seeking aesthetic improvement. It becomes absolutely critical to develop a sixth sense regarding motivation because a substantial number of poor results are based on emotional dissatisfaction rather than technical failure.

In our society, there is still a certain stigma attached to seeking aesthetic improvement. This may add a significant element of guilt to a pre-existing distorted body image. Jacobson and others[2] neatly liken the body image to a gyroscope. When it is functioning well, we do not notice it. It does not decide the course or steer the ship. In a storm, however, the ship becomes difficult to steer if the gyroscope is not functioning.

Obviously, every patient seeking rhinoplasty cannot be referred for a psychiatric evaluation, nor is it necessary. Patients seeking plastic surgery believe that they are trying to do something positive about their problems. If they are asked to see a psychiatrist, they might consider themselves failures. In all likelihood they will walk out and never come back to you. Seldom do patients have sufficient self-awareness to realize that their problems lie more in their minds than in the physical parts they wish corrected.

There are no objective criteria in this gray zone. The criteria are not only subjective but also totally different for patient and physician. The patient has an idea of what he wants; the surgeon knows, more or less, what can be done. The problem is for the two to communicate as accurately as possible beforehand. It is much easier to arrive at a prior mutual understanding than to look back retrospectively with regret. In the eyes of the law, however, responsibility of selecting the patient rests squarely on the surgeon's shoulders.

Obviously, there are significant differences in the psychodynamics of the male vs. the female rhinoplasty candidate. Jacobson and others[2] have pointed out that both sexes have positive psychological expectations and a conscious wish for attractiveness; women, however, more frequently wish to change themselves to feel more attractive. Men seem more interested in changing others' attitudes toward them.[2, 3] The male patient, according to Jacobson and others,[2] more often than the female patient shows the following characteristics:

1. A family or cultural background conflicting with his present life.
2. Difficulties in heterosexual adjustment.
3. A self-deprecating attitude and feelings of inadequacy.
4. Familial conflict and either conscious or subconscious shame related to ethnic background.

The characteristics of the individual least likely to be satisfied with his postoperative result can be formed into a useful acronym—SIMON:

- Single
- Immature
- Male
- Overexpectant
- Narcissistic

There are often identifiable, common traits in certain types of aesthetic surgery candidates. Patients with outstanding or "lop" ears often demonstrate a hostile, aggressive, "chip-on-the-shoulder" attitude. Most often, they have inherited their deformity from a parent who also suffered ridicule in childhood. Cleft lip/palate patients tend to have reclusive, involutional personality patterns. Patients seeking rhinoplasty, on the other hand, frequently show a guilt-tinged, second-generation rejection of their ethnic background masked by excuses such as not photographing well. Often it is not so much a desire to abandon the ethnic group as it is to be viewed as individuals, to rid themselves of specific physical attributes associated with their particular ethnic group.[2, 4-6]

Motivation rather than specific psychodynamics should be the plastic surgeon's overriding concern. Is there a pragmatic desire to improve appearance, or is there a pathologic projection of subconscious problems onto a physical fault? Contrast these two commonly heard statements:

- "I don't like my nose. It's too big for my face and I don't photograph well."
- "I've always been terribly self-conscious about my nose. My father's family all have noses like this. I hate it!"

Many patients can say anything convincingly, but the second statement should trip a red flag and invite further inquiries into the patient's real motivation.

Strength of motivation is important and has a startlingly close relationship with patient satisfaction. A strongly motivated patient will have less pain, a better postoperative course, and a significantly higher index of satisfaction, regardless of the result.

## PATIENT SELECTION AND LIABILITY POTENTIAL

Despite all this, it is possible to establish some nearly objective criteria for patient selection and liability potential. These criteria are listed in order of descending importance:

### Objective Deformity Vs. Patient Concern

Figure 3–1 graphically shows a plot of the patient's objective deformity as judged by the surgeon vs. the patient's degree of concern about the deformity. Two extremes of patient selection are as follows:

1. The patient who has a major deformity but demonstrates minimal concern (lower right-hand corner)
2. The patient who has a minor deformity that causes extreme concern (upper right-hand corner)

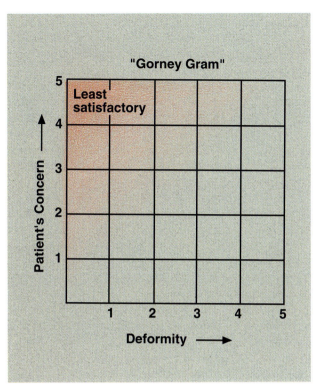

**FIG 3–1.**
"Gorney gram." There is a close relationship between the final outcome of any elective procedure and the patient's "concern ratio." The greater the patient's preoccupation with his problem, the less satisfactory the final outcome, even if the problem is minimal in the surgeon's objective evaluation. The opposite is also true. Most patients fall in a broad band indicated by the *diagonal line.*

The latter represents the poorest candidate. One seldom sees the patient in the lower right-hand corner, but the majority of patients seeking aesthetic surgery fall somewhere on a diagonal band between the contralateral corners. The decision to accept or reject a patient for surgery must be the surgeon's ultimate responsibility. I have found it very useful to note, some time during the initial visit, on a "tic-tac-toe" type of diagram (see Fig 3–1) my coded impression of where the patient falls. Thus when a patient, whom I dimly recall, expresses interest in proceeding with the surgery, a glance at the chart with the X in the appropriate square serves as a reminder about this patient's candidacy.

**Great Expectations.**—Experience invariably teaches the plastic surgeon to avoid the patient who expects surgery to change his whole life. If the surgeon operates on someone who has a large, crooked nose and significant "hang-ups," the result is likely to be someone with a smaller, straighter nose and even greater problems. Certainly, a reasonable degree of positive change is expected and usually occurs; however, aesthetic surgery, regardless of excellence, is dubious therapy for severe personality disturbances.

**The Demanding Patient.**—The individual who brings pictures, drawings, and exact specifications should engender suspicion as a general rule. Such a person has little insight into the realities of reconstructive surgery and, by definition, forces the surgeon to attempt to fulfill expectations that cannot be realized. More than likely, this type of patient is very explicit, very fussy, and very demanding about tiny imperfections and will not understand the fact that you are working with human tissue, not clay.

**The Indecisive Patient.**—We have already discussed the relationship between motivation and result. To the question, "Doctor, do you think I ought to have this done?" the correct answer is something like "This is a decision that I cannot make for you. I will neither encourage nor discourage this operation. I can only tell you what I think we can accomplish. If you have thought about it carefully and feel strongly that you would like to have it done, you will probably be satisfied with the results. If you have any doubts at all, I strongly recommend that you think about it further or not have it done at all."

It is very difficult to dissuade a jury or an arbitration panel when one of the patient's principal complaints is that he was "talked into" the surgery.

**The Immature Patient.**—For reasons other than growth and development, one should carefully evaluate the degree of maturity in the young candidate. There is, of course, no linear relationship between maturity and age. Immature individuals often have excessively romantic and unrealistic expectations regarding the effects of the rhinoplasty. When confronted with a mirror postoperatively, they sometimes exhibit disconcerting shock reactions and alarming behavior. If they have been talked into the surgery by a relative or friend, this only compounds the problem.

**The "Important" Patient.**—Beware of patients who make a conscious effort to impress others by their stature, profession, community standing, peer groups, and the like. Such individuals often suggest that a successful result on them will immediately bring on a flood of referrals and undying fame. They may also likely turn out to be very difficult patients who have weak egos and need constant shoring up.

They are difficult to satisfy and tend to forget their financial obligations.

**The Secretive Patient.**—Some applicants make a fetish of absolute secrecy about their surgery. Besides the fact that such arrangements are difficult to guarantee, exaggerated concern regarding this aspect of the operation indicates a significant degree of guilt about what they are contemplating.

**Familial Disapproval.**—I prefer that the immediate family be in agreement with the proposed operation and may refuse to do it if they are not. Too often failure to communicate or an unsatisfactory result produces an automatic "See, I told you so!" reaction. This only intensifies the patient's feelings of guilt and dissatisfaction and associated difficulties.

**Failure to Establish Rapport.**—An experienced aesthetic surgeon can usually determine within minutes of entering the examining room whether the individual sitting in the chair will become a patient. Within moments of the opening conversation there are often discernible "bad vibes." One of the most significant mistakes in plastic surgery is to take on as a patient someone whom one truly dislikes. A clash of personalities cancels out all other factors, regardless of the "challenge" of the case.

**The Truly Ugly Patient.**—The patient whose deformity borders on the monstrous usually has grave mental or deep psychiatric problems. With the exception of persons who may be helped by the brilliant craniofacial surgery techniques of Tessier, such individuals are rarely candidates for aesthetic surgery in the traditional sense. Once again, the challenge may prove to be too much of a temptation. In the end, the surgeon winds up converting the truly grotesque into the merely ridiculous.

**The "Surgiholic".**—Beware of the patient who has had multiple or repeated aesthetic procedures. Such a patient obviously has a severe and probably incorrigibly distorted body image. Aside from the technical difficulties involved, you will suffer comparison to the other surgeons. If you are more successful, you may be harrassed by requests for "just one more, please."

### An Ounce of Prevention

There should be a frank discussion of fees and costs, if not by the surgeon, then by someone in the sur-

geon's office. Experience has shown that payment in full and in advance for cosmetic surgery tends to diminish subsequent unhappiness with the final results.

One of the most valuable and least expensive investments you can make is a chalkboard in every examining room. All illustrations and diagrams should be on the chalkboard and not on the permanent record. Unless you can duplicate exactly what you have drawn, a permanent record may come back to haunt you.

In counseling the patient, avoid the use of complex medical terminology. Use simple, understandable language, and tailor your explanations to your impression of the patient's capacity to understand. Do not make any promises, stated or implied. Do not patronize your patient, but do encourage questions; an informed patient is a good patient.

The "laying on of hands" is never more important than when talking to an anxious patient. Your reassuring touch during the course of the examination will often give the patient a subconscious impression of the kind of surgeon you are.

It is an ironclad rule in our office never to accept patients at the first visit. I ask them to go home, think about what I have told them, and return (at no fee). I ask them to write down any questions, and at the second visit, I go over the highlights of our original conversation and cover, once again, the most significant complications that may occur. When I am convinced that the patients are well and truly motivated and clearly understand what I have told them, then and only then do I allow them to book the surgery.

At surgery, it is axiomatic that all patients under local anesthesia should be adequately sedated. No permit should be signed after sedation is administered since it may be held to be invalid. All members of the surgical team should clearly understand that the patient, under the influence of narcotics, can misinterpret the most innocent words or jokes and that these can come back to haunt them. Under no circumstances should there be arguments of any kind, even in jest. There should be no swearing for any reason. Assistants and observers should be warned to save expressing any doubts for later. There is no such word as "oops!" in the operating room, whether the surgeon drops a hemostat or comminutes the nasal bones. It helps to talk to the patient and be highly visible at the beginning and end of the procedure. It is extremely therapeutic to have music in the operating room if the surgery is being performed while the patient is under local anesthesia. It not only diffuses the unfamiliar and terrifying atmosphere but also tends to cover up the sounds of the operating room, which of themselves are extremely anxiety producing.

The surgeon should always report to the family immediately after the operation. If they are not present, a telephone call may be the least expensive investment any surgeon can make. A visit on the evening prior to the operation is immensely reassuring to the patient. If the patient is admitted to a hospital, the surgeon should be the last person the patient sees before going under the anesthetic and the first face that the patient focuses on in the recovery room. Discharge instructions should be clear, specific, and in writing. Availability during the first few days is essential. If the surgeon signs out, it should be to someone equally competent, and the patient should be notified of this ahead of time.

When dressings come off, there will be innumerable questions, all of which require simple, reassuring answers. There will be fewer questions and the patient will be less anxious if these questions have been addressed preoperatively.

## SUMMARY

Litigation and misunderstanding between patient and physician in rhinoplastic surgery have as a common denominator not poor results, but poor communication. Underlying all dissatisfaction is a failure to establish or maintain rapport between the patient and surgeon. This vital relationship can be shattered by the surgeon's arrogance, hostility, or indifference (real or imagined), but especially by the patient's feeling that "the surgeon didn't care."

There are only two ways to avoid this debacle. One is to make sure that the patient has no reason to feel this way. The other is to learn to avoid the patient who is going to feel this way no matter what is done.

## REFERENCES

1. Gorney M: Psychiatric and medical-legal implications of rhinoplasty, mentoplasty, and otoplasty, Symposium of Aesthetic Surgery of the Nose, Ears, and Chin, vol 6, Miami, 1973.
2. Jacobson WE et al: Psychiatric evaluation of male patients seeking cosmetic surgery, *Plast Reconstr Surg* 26:356, 1960.
3. MacGregor FC, Shaffner B: Screening patients for nasal plastic operations, *Psychosom Med* 12:277, 1950.
4. Meyer E et al: Motivational patterns in patients seeking elective plastic surgery (women who seek rhinoplasty), *Psychosom Med* 22:193, 1960.
5. Palmer A, Blanton S: Mental factors in relations to reconstructive surgery of nose and ears, *Arch Otolaryngol* 56:148, 1952.
6. Stern K, Fournier G, LaRiviere A: Psychiatric aspects of cosmetic surgery of the nose, *Can Med J* 76:469, 1957.

# Nasal Analysis and Operative Planning

Rollin K. Daniel, M.D.

Nasal analysis has become a critical part of the rhinoplasty operation for two reasons. First, the number of surgical techniques (grafts, sutures) available has increased dramatically, as well as our ability to change critical reference points (nasion, tip, subnasale) and characteristics (projection, rotation). Second, the number of techniques available has increased geometrically, but experience with each technique has decreased significantly—there simply is no opportunity to master through experience every surgical maneuver. The solution to this dilemma is nasal analysis and operative planning.

## METHODS

Three methods of nasal analysis are readily available: clinical examination, surface measurements, and photographic evaluation.

### Clinical Examination

After a minimum of a 1,000 rhinoplasties, a surgeon has sufficient experience to look at a nose and realize both its problems and potential. I routinely ask patients to state three things that they want changed about their nose in order of importance.[5, 15] These desires are extremely important to satisfy, or else the patient will not be happy with the result. Then, I try to determine what is unattractive about the nose. The most common problems are the following: (1) the hump on profile, (2) the round tip, (3) the width

of the nose (usually at the X point of the base bony width), (4) alar flare, (5) deviations/crookedness, and (6) the columella portion relative to the columella labial angle and/or columella/nostril. Once a general impression of the problem is obtained, I begin a systematic nasal examination.

An internal examination is done by evaluating all five of the following areas: (1) caudal septum/anterior nasal septum (ANS)/vestibule; (2) the nasal valve (septum, mucosa, upper lateral cartilage); (3) the attic of the osseocartilaginous vault; (4) the cartilage/vomer/perpendicular plate; and (5) the posterior choanae. Turbinate size and condition are noted. Palpitation of the septum is done, especially if preceding nasal surgery was performed. Once recorded, the nose is sprayed with oxymetazoline (Afrin), and a second postspray examination will be done after the external examination is completed.

The external nose is divided into four components: (1) tip, (2) alar-columella complex, (3) osseocartilaginous vault, and (4) radix. A printed outline is used to record these observations—it also forces me to look at the nose in a systematic, complete manner and avoids any lapses or quick decisions. Visual examination is complimented by palpation of the nasal structures. How thick is the skin envelope? How rigid or flexible are the alar cartilages. Is the subnasale web composed of bone or muscle? Palpation is critical for determining anatomic composition and surgical response, hence the need for experience. As regards intrinsic tip characteristics, I am most concerned about volume (cephalic lateral crura), width (interdomal distance), and definition (tip refinement at the domal segment–lateral crura junction).[6] Next, the extrinsic tip characteristics are evaluated, including (1) position and relative dorsal length (nasion-to-tip) (2) rotation of the tip angle relative to the alar crease; and (3) projection, from the alar crease to the tip, as well as and its three components (premaxilla, columella, infralobule).[7] During this examination the patient is frequently asked to turn her head and smile. Once the tip is analyzed, the alar base–columella complex is evaluated. The factors of concern are the following: (1) columella-labial angle, (2) columella-lobular angle, (3) columella-nostril relationship, (4) caudal septum/ANS deviations, (5) nostril contour/composition, and (6) alar flare vs. interalar width. "Guesstimates" are made of each angle, and relative relationships to intercanthal width are noted.

The radix area and dorsum are "separated" visually by a line drawn on the dorsum at the level of the lateral canthus. The radix characteristics include (1) the nasion (level, depth, width); (2) nasofrontal angle with emphasis on the glabella limb; (3) the nasofacial angle with emphasis on the dorsal limb; and (4) its anatomic composition, bone or soft tissue. In this era of conservative rhinoplasty, setting the height and location of the nasion has become the critical first step in operative planning. The osseocartilaginous vault is analyzed as a combined and single unit: (1) overall deviations/crookedness/asymmetries; (2) radix lines; (3) bridge height (high, normal, low) and shape (convexity, straight); (4) bony vault width along the bridge and at its base width (X point); and (5) cartilage vault, especially its width and relative potential for collapse. Once the clinical examination is done and the deformity recorded, I formulate and detail a preliminary operative plan. Decisions are made regarding approach, tip surgery, types of osteotomies, and alar wedges vs. nostril sill excision. Each step is carefully detailed. This plan will be revised and refined at least four times prior to surgery. The internal examination is then repeated because vasoconstriction will be maximal. Photographs are then taken, and a second consultation is scheduled.

## Surface Measurements

At the second consultation, I look at the patient before opening the chart. What bothers me most about the nose? What would look good in relationship to the face, height, and personality? How much can the nose be changed? How elegant or refined can it be? Then I review the patient's requests and my initial analysis and operative plan. Revision 1 is made in the operative plan. At the end of the second consultation, I record her surface measurements (Fig 4–1,A and B). Dots are placed at key landmarks including the following: (1) glabella (G); (2) nasion (N); (3) base bony width (X point); (4) tip landmarks (right dome [RD], left dome [LD], tip [T], supratip [S'], and columella break point [C']); (5) alar crease (AC); (6) subnasale (SN); and (7) reference points for the Frankfort horizontal plane. Then with a simple ophthalmic calliper the following measurements are recorded: (1) midfacial, lower facial, and submental heights; (2) three nasal lengths (N-T, N-C', N-SN); (3) four widths, including intercanthal (EN-EN), bony (X-X), alar flare (AL-AL), and interalar (AC-AC); (4) tip distances involving the interdomal width (RD-LD), supralobule (T-S'), and infralobule (T-C'); and (5) projection at the radix, keystone, and tip, both AC-T and SN-T. Then by using an acrylic angle measurer from craniofacial surgery the following angles are measured: nasofrontal, columella-labial, and tip angle. Revision 2 may be made in the operative plan as accurate data regarding widths are obtained, especially alar flare vs. interalar width. Also, the actual vs. the initial impression of projection may be affected.

## Photographic Analysis

The key to accurate photographic analysis is photographic excellence.[8] The critical components are as follows: (1) a 35-mm single-lens reflex (SLR) camera with a 105 lens and a reference grid in the viewfinder; (2) slide film, preferably Ecktachrome 100 for rapid processing; (3) a neutral background; (4) a marking pen, ruler, and hair clips; and (5) balanced lighting in a medical configuration.[6] The most difficult attribute to obtain is reproducible lighting. A minimum requirement is two light sources at equidistant height and angulation in front of the patient and a slave light to eliminate shadows behind the patient. As detailed elsewhere, the physical characteristics of the light reflexes is dictated in a large part by the lighting configuration, i.e., a single light gives a single light reflex, and asymmetrical lights can only produce asymmetrical light reflexes.[16]

Once the lightening problem is solved, proper positioning becomes critical. All makeup is removed from the nose, earrings are removed, and the hair is held back with clips. At the minimum, the Frankfurt horizontal plane reference points are marked, in-

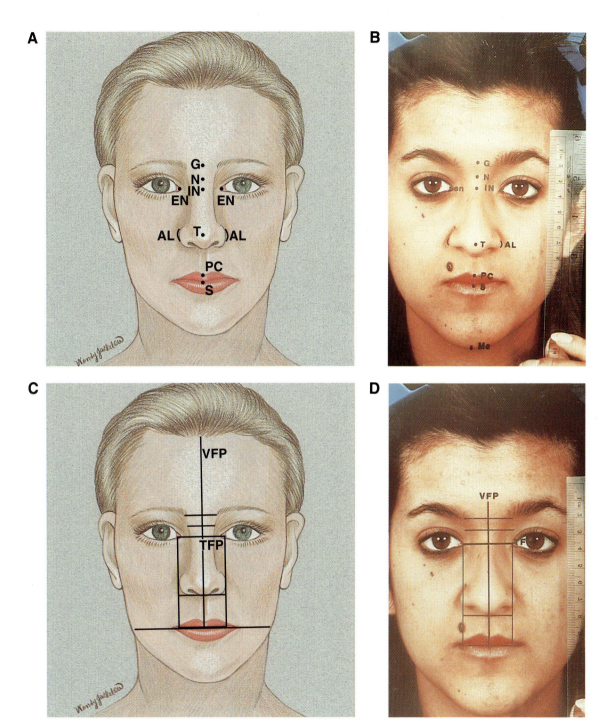

**FIG 4–1.**
Anterior view. **A** and **B**, reference points include the following: glabella *(G)*, nasion *(N)*, endocanthus *(EN)*, intercanthal midline *(IN)*, tip *(T)*, alar flare *(AL)*, philtral column midpoint *(PC)*, and stomion *(S)*. **C** and **D**, the reference lines are the vertical facial plane *(VFP)* from the glabella to the stomion and the transverse facial plane *(TFP)* through the endocanthus. See the text for a step-by-step analysis. (**A** and **C** from Daniel RK, editor: *Aesthetic plastic surgery*, ed 2, Boston, Little Brown, in press. Used by permission.)

cluding the top of the external auditory canal and infraorbital rim. The patient is given a clear plastic ruler to hold. The head is positioned by using the grid in the viewfinder to have the Frankfurt horizontal plane parallel to the floor and the facial midline perpendicular. Four views are taken: anterior, right lateral, right oblique, and basilar. A second identical camera is used for print film, and additional photos are taken including static and dynamic views. The need for instant assessment of minor details from multiple views precludes the use of slides in the operating room.

The anterior and lateral slides are taken to the photo lab where "life-size" 8 × 10-in. prints are made (48-hour turnaround costs $7.50 per print) in which 1 cm on the ruler in the slide equals 1 cm on the print. Then, an orthodontic tracing overlay is taped to the photographs. A four-step procedure is then done: (1) analysis of the nasal deformity, (2) outline of the ideal nose, (3) alternative operative strategies, and (4) a proposed operative plan. Revision 3 occurs when the photographic plan is compared with the clinically derived plan.

## METHODS OF PHOTOGRAPHIC ANALYSIS

The use of photographs for planning a rhinoplasty is not new. Over the years, numerous authors have proposed methods for photoanalysis, including Brown and McDowell,[3] Fomon and Bell,[9] Bernstein,[2] and Anderson.[1] Yet when critically assessed, the goal was the rather simplistic establishment of an ideal profile line to present to the patient.

Renewed interest has occurred from a generation of surgeons trained in craniofacial techniques. Utilizing the data of Farkas et al.[10–12] as background support, Guyuron,[13, 14] Daniel,[7] and Byrd[4] have expanded the role of photographic analysis and paved the way for eventual computerization. These three methodologies will be described briefly.

### The Guyuron Technique

Without question, Guyuron has made the greatest contribution in defining the ideal, determining the requisite surgical excision/grafting, and comparing preoperative plans with postoperative results in a large series of cases.[13, 14] His methodology is based on defining an ideal triangular frame from reference points at the nasion (N) and subnasale (SN) with the interconnecting nasofacial angle. Then templates are

used—a bridge template and a columella/tip double-break template. Thus, a final outline of the ideal nasal profile is drawn to provide a proportionate and balanced nose for each patient. The differences between actual and ideal are measured in seven zones, each with its computed skeletal "response rate." The zones and response rates are as follows: (1) nasion, 25%; (2) proximal portion of the bridge, 66%; (3) midbridge, 75%; (4) supratip, 45%; (5) tip, 45%; (6) columella, 45%; and (7) subnasale, 25%. For example, if tip rotation is desired, then for each millimeter of rotation desired 2 to 2.5 mm of caudal septum must be removed. These response rates were determined from comparing preoperative and postoperative life-size photographs, xenoradiographs, and surgical specimens. The disadvantage of this technique is the templates, which are not as individualistic as one would desire, and the difficulty of measuring excised specimens. From a numbers viewpoint, the entire question of tip projection and position are not sufficiently precise in their determination. For example, tip position/projection only results once the nasion and subnasale are set; next, the nasofacial angle and then the template intersection result in tip position. The primary advantages of the Guyuron system is its linkage between preoperative planning, surgical design, and postoperative result.

### The Byrd System

The Byrd system of "dimensional analysis" has as its principal goal determination of the "ideal nasal length" as derived from the individual's face and then using it to determine both radix and tip projection.[16] The first step is to determine the ideal ($i$) nasal length (NT$i$) for the face: NT$i$ = chin vertical (S-Me) or 0.67 of the midfacial height (G-AC). Then the ideal nasal tip projection (AC-T$i$) = 0.67 NT$i$, and the ideal radix projection from the cornea (C-N$i$) = 0.28 NT$i$. The level of the nasion (N) is set empirically at the supratarsal eyelid fold. Once the height and level of the nasion are set, the ideal tip projection is measured from the alar base plane. Since the ideal nasal length is known, tip position is determined by the intersection of two arcs—one centered at the nasion and the other at the alar crease.

The disadvantages of this system are the relative paucity of information regarding the subnasale/columella/nostril relationships and the assumption that the nasion and alar crease point are in an ideal vertical relationship. If the nasion–alar crease vertical relationship is off or the eyes are deep set, then false

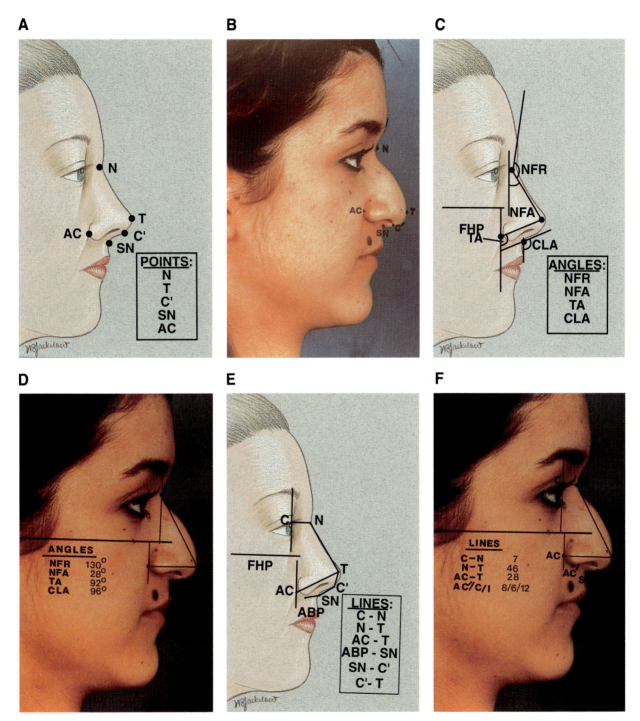

**FIG 4–2.**
Lateral analysis consists of four points, four angles, and four distances. **A** and **B,** important reference points include the nasion *(N)*, tip *(T)*, columella break point *(C')*, and subnasale *(SN)*. **C** and **D,** the four angles are the nasofrontal *(NFR)*, nasofacial *(NFA)*, tip angle *(TA)*, and columella-labial *(CLA)*. **E** and **F,** the four distances are the nasion projection *(C-N)*, dorsal length *(N-T)*, tip projection *(AC-T)*, and subdivided tip projection consisting of three components: maxillary *(AC'-SN)*, columella *(SN-C)*, and infralobule *(C'-T)*. (**A, C,** and **E** from Daniel RK, editor: *Aesthetic plastic surgery,* ed 2, Boston, Little Brown, in press. Used by permission.)

**A**                                **B**

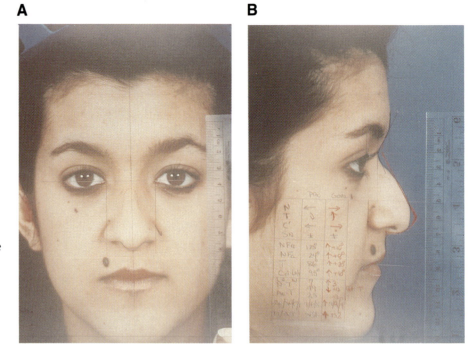

**FIG 4–3.**
**A** and **B,** operative planning using life-size photographs. The first step is to define the deformity, then superimpose the ideal, and finally reconcile the realistic. In addition, one can diagram alternative strategies. (From Daniel RK, editor: *Aesthetic plastic surgery,* ed 2, Boston, Little Brown, in press. Used by permission.)

angles will occur. The tremendous advantage of this system is that it defines the ideal for an individual face without imposition of collective ideals or templates. Also, quantitative linkage of radix projection, tip projection, and dorsal length is extraordinarily valuable. In addition, this system has been successfully computerized and the visuals digitized, which allows extensive preoperative planning with visual assessment of alternatives.

**The Daniel Method**

The author's method began with surface anthropometric measurements using the technique of Farkas.[7] Life-size photographs were added and initial planning done using the Guyuron system. However, the desire to individualize the system led to a reliance on three groups of landmarks: (1) reference points (nasion, tip, columella break point, subna-

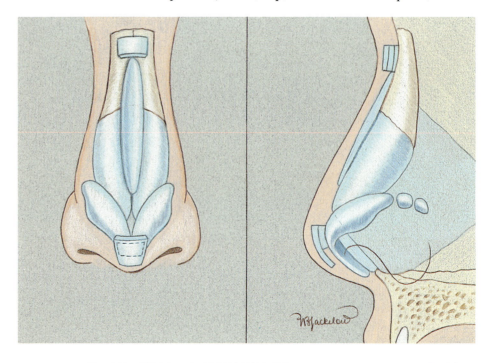

**FIG 4–4.**
The operative approach consisted of minimal hump reduction followed by numerous grafts in the radix area, cartilaginous vault, columella, and tip. No osteotomies were planned.

**A**

**C**

**E**
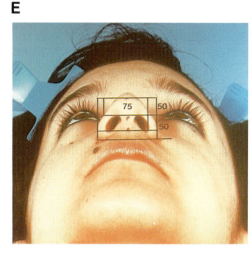

**B**

**D**

**F**
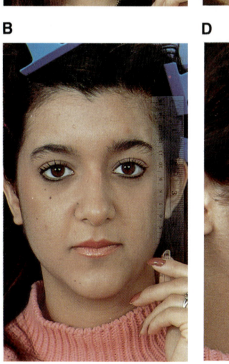
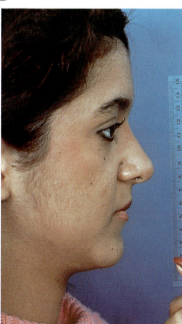
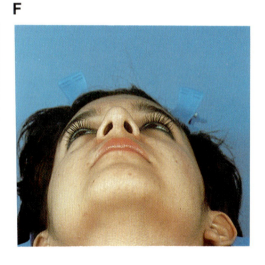

**FIG 4–5.**
Preoperative deformity (**A, C,** and **E**) and postoperative result (**B, D,** and **F**) at 2 years. (From Daniel RK, editor: *Aesthetic plastic surgery*, ed 2, Boston, Little Brown, in press. Used by permission.)

sale); (2) angles (nasofrontal, nasofacial, tip, columella-labial); and (3) distances (radix projection, C-N; dorsal length, N-T; tip projection, AC-T; and segmental tip projection, AC′-SN, SN-C′, C′-T) (Fig 4–2). The first step is to define the existing nasal de-

formity, which involves measuring and recording each of these 12 variables. The second step is superimposition of the ideal beginning with the nasion, both level and projection, then the tip angle and its projection, followed by each aspect of the nose (Fig

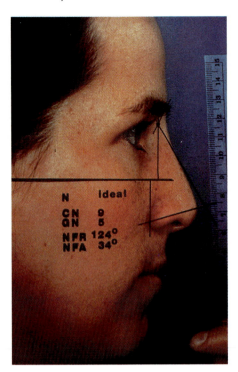

**FIG 4–6.**
Operative planning in a secondary rhinoplasty patient. The goal is to lower the level and decrease the position of the nasion. Once the ideal nasion is defined, then achieving an ideal nasofacial angle of 34 degrees results in significant improvement in tip projection. (From Daniel RK, editor: *Aesthetic plastic surgery*, ed 2, Boston, Little Brown, in press. Used by permission.)

4–3). At this point, the ideal nasal profile is defined, and one can determine what changes have to be made. Again, realistic goals have to be defined, especially as regards each of the cardinal landmarks (Figs 4–4 and 4–5). For example, given the combination of a prominent forehead and deep-set eyes, one may not be able to alter the radix significantly.

The disadvantage of this system is its reliance on angles, which can be significantly off in poor-quality photographs. Also, a knowledge of what is ideal and how to determine it are essential for each of the 12 factors. Although the method can be time-consuming initially, it requires only 7 to 8 minutes once mastered. The advantage of this technique is its flexibility and totality. Virtually every landmark can be cross-checked and adjusted (Figs 4–6 through 4–8). The height of the nasion has the ideal radix projection from the cornea as determined by Byrd but is cross-checked by the Guyuron method, which relates it to depth from the glabella and alternatively as a determinant from the ideal tip position. Virtually every component of the nasal profile is assessed with emphasis on aesthetic angles, not draconian numbers or templates.

With any of these three methods, it is important to assess various operative strategies. For example, draw the consequences of tip projection when it is kept constant, reduced, or increased. Will a radix graft reduce the amount of hump reduction but cause a catastrophic increase in tip projection to

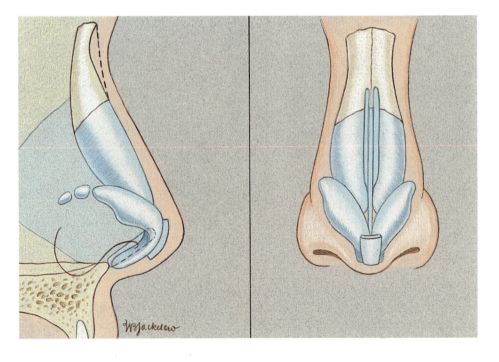

**FIG 4–7.**
The operative approach consisted of radix reduction followed by asymmetrical spreader grafts and an open-structure tip.

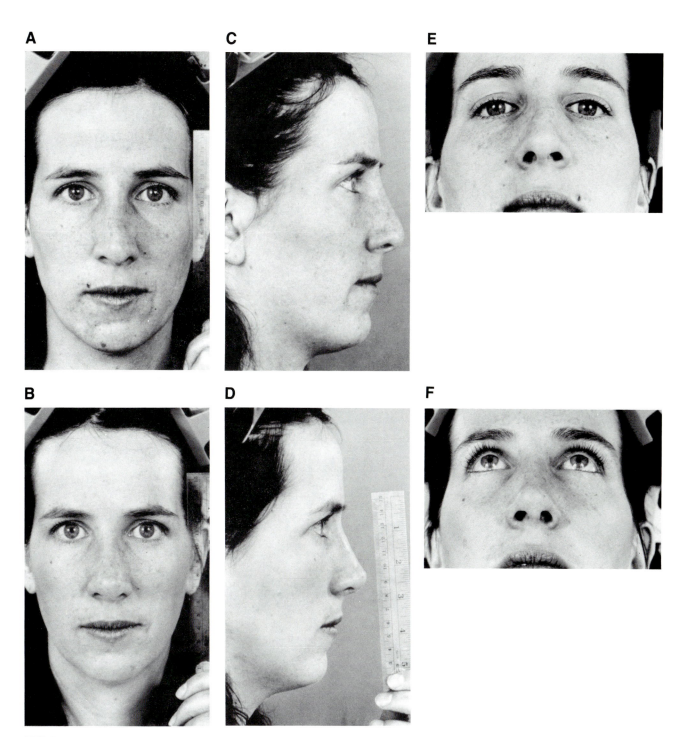

**FIG 4–8.**
Preoperative deformity (**A, C,** and **E**) and postoperative result (**B, D,** and **F**). Both deformity and crookedness have been improved. (From Daniel RK: *Aesthetic plastic surgery,* ed 2, Boston, Little Brown. Used by permission.)

achieve the desired nasofacial angle. If a radix graft is considered, assess the consequences of doing a graft vs. leaving the radix the same. The value of photographic analysis is the ability to assess various surgical strategies without detrimental consequences for the patient.

## OPERATIVE PLAN

At the final preoperative visit, the surgeon reconciles photographic analysis with the previous operative plan and tissue realities. One assesses each operative step. Is the obtuse columella segment composed of modifiable caudal septum/ANS or noncompliant soft tissue with a retrussive dentation? Can the desired tip projection be achieved? Will the soft tissue respond? Revision 4 is completed, and an operative sequence is defined. This in-depth plan serves as a "road map" rather than a "blueprint." There is neither uncertainty as to the goals nor hesitation as to the methods. Intraoperatively, nasal anatomy and consequential changes may require alterations in the plan. Most often it is a quantitative alteration rather than abandonment of a step, i.e., a nostril sill excision rather than a type II alar excision or the addition of a tip graft to a domal definition suture. The goal remains the same; only the technique is increased or decreased as the situation dictates.

## REFERENCES

1. Anderson JR: Personal techniques of rhinoplasty, *Otolaryngol Clin North Am* 8:399, 1975.
2. Bernstein L: Esthetics and rhinoplasty, *Otolaryngol Clin North Am* 8:547, 1975.
3. Brown JB, McDowell F: *Plastic surgery of the nose*, rev ed, Springfield, Ill, 1965, Charles C Thomas.
4. Byrd S: Dimensional rhinoplasty, *Plast Reconstr Surg* (in press).
5. Daniel RK: Primary rhinoplasty: emphasis on approach. In Vistnes L, editor: *Procedures in plastic and reconstructive surgery: how they do it*, Boston, 1991, Little Brown, p 120.
6. Daniel RK: The nasal tip: anatomy and aesthetics, *Plast Reconstr Surg*, Feb 1992.
7. Daniel RK, Farkas LG: Rhinoplasty: image and reality, *Clin Plast Surg* 15:1, 1988.
8. Daniel RK, Hodgson J, Lambros VS: Rhinoplasty: the light reflexes, *Plast Reconstr Surg* 85:859, 1990.
9. Fomon S, Bell JW: *Rhinoplasty—new concepts: evaluation and application*, Springfield, Ill, 1970, Charles C Thomas.
10. Farkas LG: Is photogrammetry of the face reliable, *Plast Reconstr Surg* 66:436, 1980.
11. Farkas LG, Kolar JC, Munro IR: Geography of the nose: a morphometric study, *Aesthetic Plast Surg* 10:191, 1986.
12. Farkas LG, Munro IR: *Anthropometric facial proportions in medicine*, Springfield, Ill, 1970, Charles C Thomas.
13. Guyuron B: Precision rhinoplasty. Part I: the role of life-size photographs and soft-tissue cephalometric analysis, *Plast Reconstr Surg* 81:489, 1988.
14. Guyuron B: Precision rhinoplasty. Part II: prediction, *Plast Reconstr Surg* 81:500, 1988.
15. Regnault P, Daniel RK: Septorhinoplasty. In *Aesthetic plastic surgery*, Boston, 1984, Little Brown, pp 101–171.
16. Zarem HA: Standards of photography, *Plast Reconstr Surg* 74:137, 1984.

# Considerations in Anesthesia for Rhinosurgery

William A. Mathews, M.D., F.C.C.P.

One more step had now to be taken. We trickled the solution under each others' lifted eyelids. Then placed a mirror before us, took pins, and with the head tried to touch the cornea. Almost simultaneously we are able to state jubilantly; "I can't feel anything."

Written by Karl Koller a very short time after he had found that cocaine possessed local anesthetic properties, these words pique one's imagination as to whether or not indeed they did feel jubilant from cocaine intoxication. This is extremely unlikely from the small dose, but a bemusing thought. Just as this quotation raises questions, the considerations of anesthesia for rhinosurgery raise questions. Three questions will be addressed in this chapter.

1. Shall I use local anesthesia?
2. Shall I use general anesthesia?
3. What is the role of cocaine in the management of rhinosurgery today?

In a survey of our community, we found that 80% of our plastic surgeons utilized general anesthesia for nasal reconstructive procedures. Interestingly enough, 80% also used cocaine. The statistics on the use of cocaine as a topical anesthetic in nasal surgery were no different in 1976 when Feehan and Mancusi-Ungaro[3] reported in a survey of 839 plastic surgeons that 80% used cocaine during rhinoplasty.

## ANATOMIC CONSIDERATIONS

The entire sensory innervation of the nose is provided by the ophthalmic and the maxillary divisions of the trigeminal nerve. Near the superior orbital fissure the ophthalmic nerve divides into its three main branches—lacrimal, frontal, and nasociliary. The frontal nerve enters the orbital cavity through the superior orbital fissure, travels above the ocular muscles, and terminates in its two branches, a large supraorbital branch and a small supratrochlear nerve. The supraorbital nerve passes directly forward, leaves the orbit through the supraorbital groove to reach the forehead, where it contributes to the sensory innervation of the upper eyelid and the frontal sinus, and then passes over the glabella at the base of the nose. The supratrochlear nerve leaves the orbit and is distributed to the skin and fascia of the medial parts of the forehead and upper eyelid. The more important nasociliary nerve enters the orbit through the superior orbital fissure and eventually reaches the anterior ethmoidal foramen. From here, it continues as the anterior ethmoidal nerve through the foramen into the cranial cavity, where it lies embedded in the dura on the cribriform plate. It enters the nasal cavity through the nasal slit and terminates in the medial and lateral internal nasal branches. The medial division supplies the mucous membrane of the upper and anterior portion of the nasal septum. The lateral branch supplies the lateral wall of the nasal cavity and finally appears on the face as the external nasal branch between the nasal bone and the upper nasal cartilage and supplies branches to the skin and fascia of the lower part of the dorsum and the tip of the nose.

The maxillary nerve courses forward from the trigeminal ganglion through the middle fossa and in relation to the lower portion of the cavernous sinus. It traverses the pterygopalatine fossa and enters the orbit as the infraorbital nerve through the inferior orbital fissure. In the pterygopalatine fossa, the maxillary division gives off two short thick ganglionic branches that are closely related to the sphenopalatine ganglion. These nerves have only a relationship of contiguity with the ganglion, for the fibers pass either close by it or through it without having any synaptic relationship with the cells of the ganglion, which is a parasympathetic station of the facial nerve. From the ganglionic area, numerous so-called branches of the ganglion pass forward to the pharynx downward to the palate and medially to the nasal cavity and upward to the orbit, thus contributing a great deal to the sensory innervation of the interior of the nose.

An absolute essential to regional anesthesia is an appreciation of the exact course and distribution of the nerves that must be anesthetized. Line drawings will aid in getting a spatial relationship firmly fixed in mind before undertaking regional anesthesia of the nose (Fig 5–1,A–D).

## REGIONAL ANESTHESIA OF THE NOSE

Whether regional or general anesthesia is chosen, a proper evaluation of the patient's general physical and mental condition must first be carried out. In addition to this, the necessary laboratory work will have been done and should be reviewed once again immediately before the procedure. We feel strongly that no local anesthetic procedure of any magnitude should be undertaken without an intravenous catheter in place, and for this reason, with the exception of flurazepam (Dalmane) and on occasion ranitidine (Zantac), we give all of our preoperative medication intravenously. Flurazepam is administered the night before for patients who may desire evening sedation, and ranitidine is given to patients with a history of peptic disease or hiatal hernia to decrease the danger of acid aspiration.

In the holding room before intravenous sedation is administered, the operative consents are reviewed and any pertinent questions concerning medications and food and fluid intake discussed before sedation is given. At this time, everything that will happen to the patient in the operating room is explained and discussed in such a manner that the patient will feel at ease and confident.

The basic anesthetic triad of (1) an automatic blood pressure device, (2) a continuous electrocardiogram, and (3) a pulse oximeter is always used regardless of the magnitude of the procedure. At this point the patient is given 1 to 3 mg of midazolam (Versed) and transported to the operating room where the appropriate monitoring devices are affixed. If the procedure is to be done with the patient locally anesthetized and sedated, we usually place a foam rubber mattress over the operating table so that the patient experiences less discomfort; also at this time a pillow is usually placed under the knees to flex them. Incremental injections of 250 $\mu$g of alfentanil are administered until the patient is drowsy. Each incremental injection is carefully evaluated in terms of depression of respiration and blood pressure. Most patients will receive from 500 to 750 $\mu$g before becoming well sedated.

The surgeon now begins to achieve anesthesia of the interior of the nose by inserting either pledgets or flossy cotton applicators into the nose. The first one is placed superiorly under the dorsum of the root of the nose so as to anesthetize the branches of the anterior ethmoidal nerve, and other applicators are placed in the area posterior to the middle meatus and over the sphenopalatine ganglion so as to anesthetize the branches of the short sphenopalatine nerve and that portion of the greater palatine nerve distributed to the nasal cavity.

The choice of agents for topical anesthesia is clearly limited to the use of either cocaine or lidocaine. There is absolutely no evidence to support the use of cocaine in other than 4% concentration. We do not ever allow higher concentrations in the operating room.

Systemic absorption of cocaine does occur when it is applied to mucosal surfaces. It is absorbed more rapidly from the trachea and alveoli and next most rapidly from the pharynx, followed by the internal nose. There is great individual variation in serum levels achieved after intranasal application of cocaine in doses of 1.5 to 2 mg/kg. This may be influenced by the circulatory status, the pH of the nasal mucosa, and the presence or absence of inflammation, which may increase the rate of absorption. Blood levels of topically applied local anesthetic agents simulate those of rapid intravenous injection in

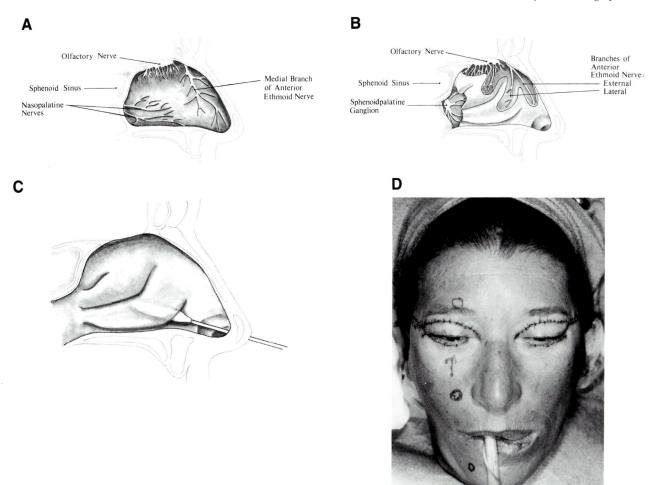

**FIG 5–1.**
**A,** medial wall of the nose showing septal innervation. **B,** lateral wall showing innervation and the sphenopalatine ganglion posterior and position in relation to the middle turbinate. **C,** swab placed in the nose and advanced posteriorly to anesthetize the sphenopalatine ganglion and nerves. **D,** anatomic relationship of the supraorbital notch, pupil, infraorbital foramen, and mental foramen along the same vertical line.

form; however, the peaks are lower, take longer to develop, and after 6 to 10 minutes reach approximately a third to half of what would have been achieved with a rapid intravenous injection.[2] Blood levels are a function of the total dose and not related to the concentration of the solution used, so 5 mL of 4% cocaine will give the same end blood levels as 2 ml of a 10% solution. The addition of vasoconstrictors, because they are effective in preventing high blood levels with infiltration anesthesia, is commonly thought to also decrease the rate and the final achieved level of topically applied local anesthetic drugs. This is distinctly not the case, and the addition of epinephrine in no way adds to the safety or reduces the absorption of cocaine when applied topically. Another common misconception is that the

10% solution causes such intense vasoconstriction that fewer reactions occur than with the 4% or 5% solution. This is a fallacy, and the same degree of vasoconstriction will be achieved with a 4% solution as with more highly concentrated solutions and pastes, which are inviting toxic levels and disaster. One cannot with certainty state what the maximum safe total dosage of cocaine for topical application is in a healthy adult. In fact, the oft-quoted 200 mg in a 70-kg human is a figure arrived at in a 1924 study analyzing reports of 43 deaths following the use of cocaine in tonsillectomy.[8]

In 1977, Miller et al. measured blood levels with gas-liquid chromatography to demonstrate the absorption from the mucosa following the application of cocaine in 5% and 10% concentrations to the nasal mucosa in patients undergoing rhinoplasty and also in unoperated controls.[9] This study demonstrated that there was no discernible difference between 5% and 10% solutions as to the degree of vasoconstriction. Blood levels very closely correlated with the total milligrams of cocaine used. The apparent half-life of cocaine is considerably longer than generally believed and can vary from 60 to 110 minutes. One explanation for the presence of cocaine in plasma for 4 to 6 hours is conceivably that cocaine persists on the nasal mucosa for as much as 3 to 4 hours, thus resulting in prolonged absorption. The absorption may be delayed because of its inherent vasoconstrictive action, although this is doubtful.[13]

The mechanism by which cocaine produces vasoconstriction and also the side effect of cardiovascular stimulation is inhibition of post–ganglionic nerve, norepinephrine reuptake. Not only are endogenous epinephrine and norepinephrine subjected to a decrease in reuptake, but also exogenous epinephrine administered in the form of topical solutions or injection has a greater opportunity to achieve a blood level that in combination with cocaine and other agents can increase cardiac toxicity. For this reason, we do not allow the use of epinephrine in concentrations exceeding 1:200,000 in our adjuvant local anesthesia for injection. In the only study where hemodynamic parameters were measured by the presence of a Swan-Ganz catheter, Barash et al. demonstrated that 1.5 mg/kg applied topically to the nasal mucosa before intubation had no significant effect on blood pressure, pulse rate, cardiac index, left ventricular stroke work index, and total peripheral vascular resistance.[1] While we feel that certain aspects of the study are flawed, this would seem to indicate that up to 1.5 mg/kg can be safely applied topically to patients without untoward cardiovascular effect. The administration of cocaine to patients who are under therapy with monoamine oxidase inhibitors is absolutely contraindicated. We totally disagree with the statement by Hirshman and Lindeman that we should reevaluate the discontinuation of monoamine oxidase inhibitors before anesthesia when this anesthesia includes topical cocaine.[6] When vasoconstriction of the nasal mucosa is desired and one does not want to use cocaine, we have had limited experience with the use of a mixture of 4% lidocaine and phenylephrine (Neo-Synephrine). This is made by taking the 5-mL, 4% lidocaine ampule for a retrobulbar block, discarding 2 mL of this, and combining the remaining 3 mL with 1 ampule of 1% injectible Neo-Synephrine. This is then used as a topical solution that now has a con-

centration of 3% topical lidocaine with 0.25% Neo-Synephrine. Another alternative is to add 0.1 mL of 1% epinephrine to 5 cc of 4% lidocaine.

While waiting for proper topical anesthesia, one can now proceed with the regional block. There are several approaches to this. In many instances, the patient will be administered a small dose of methohexital (Brevital) combined with an equal volume of 1% lidocaine. In our practice, we frequently administer approximately 40 mg of Brevital combined with 40 mg of lidocaine by intravenous push. This will eliminate the coughing and sneezing frequently seen with rapid administration of Brevital and also eliminates burning on injection. When the patient has lost lid reflex, one can then proceed to infiltrate, starting at the lateral aspect of the nose and carrying it superiorly along the lateral structures of the nose up to the orbit. Following this, one can block the external nasal nerve, and the infiltration can then be carried from one side across the midline inferior to the nose to include the inferior aspect of the columnella. At this point, if hydrodissection of the septum and of the nasal bulb is desired, infiltration can be carried out there also. It is essential that careful aspiration be made and the injection staged. It is frequently our practice when the rhinoplasty is going to be performed with local anesthesia and sedation to do a bilateral infraorbital block in the holding room with a 30-gauge needle and buffered lidocaine.

The addition of 1 mEq of sodium bicarbonate per milliliter of local anesthetic when it is combined with epinephrine will elevate the pH so as to eliminate burning and stinging on injection. With a bilateral infraorbital block in place preoperatively by the anesthesiologist, the surgeon can in the operating room introduce his needle into an already anesthetized field and produce his field block with minimal discomfort to the patient. It is important to remember to always inject from a previously anesthetized area and carry the needle forward into a nonanesthetized area. The salient features in preventing pain on local injection are needle size, proper pH adjustment of the solution, and speed of injection. It is our policy to do the field block by using 1% lidocaine with 1:200,000 epinephrine. There is no reason why the procedure cannot be safely done with other longer-acting agents such as bupivacaine if so desired.

It is imperative to *keep in mind that eventually every milligram of injected local anesthetic reaches the bloodstream.* While we initially deposit the drugs into the vicinity of tissues we wish to anesthetize, there are secondary effects beyond neural blockade that involve the central nervous system (CNS), cardiovascular system, respiratory system, and other organs. It is these secondary effects that produce dangerous reactions. The final common denominator in an *adverse reaction is a toxic concentration of drug perfusing the affected organ system.* The common practice of proscribing limits on amounts of drugs to be injected is useful but fallacious. The amount of drug that can be tolerated will depend upon the pharmacokinetic scenario present in a given patient at a given time. Just as it requires less anesthetic to give general anesthesia to a metabolically or physiologically disturbed patient, it also requires *less local anesthetic to produce a toxic reaction.* It is very common to see a reaction to local anesthetic agents at a half to two thirds the usual dosage in patients with congestive failure due to their inability to rapidly clear the vascular compartment of the pharmacokinetic model.

The ability to prevent local anesthetic reactions due to inadvertent intravascular administration and overdosage will depend upon a knowledge of the factors predisposing to overdosage and scrupulous attention to detail.

Local anesthetic agents may exert pharmacologic actions other than peripheral nerve blockade. The CNS and cardiovascular system are particularly susceptible.

As the dosage and blood level of local anesthetic agents are progressively increased, an initial excitatory CNS effect occurs and is followed by a state of generalized CNS depression. The convulsive action of local anesthetic agents is related to an inhibition of inhibitory cortical neurons such that facilitory pathways act in an unopposed fashion and lead to seizure activity. At higher anesthetic dose levels an inhibition of both inhibitory and facilitory neurons causes generalized CNS depression.

Local anesthetic–induced changes in the cardiovascular system are characterized initially by an increase in peripheral vascular resistance due to a direct effect on peripheral vascular smooth muscle and an increase in cardiac output due indirectly to action on the CNS.[10]

The predominant cardiovascular effects of high doses of local anesthetic agents include systemic hypotension due to a generalized vasodilation and a decrease in myocardial contractility leading to a fall in cardiac output. Sinus bradycardia and, ultimately, cardiac arrest can occur. There is great hope for the new agent ropivacaine as a substitute for bupivacaine with less cardiac toxicity.[4,12]

Respiration is unaffected by local anesthetic agents until doses causing overt CNS toxicity are achieved.

True allergic reactions to local anesthetic agents are extremely rare and are mainly related to the use of the procaine-like ester compounds. Certain preservatives in local anesthetic solutions such as methylparaben and propylparaben may also cause allergic reactions.

The local tissue toxicity of regional anesthetic agents is limited primarily to skeletal muscle and is spontaneously reversible. No cytotoxic effects have been observed in nerves exposed to the normal concentrations of clinically available agents.[11]

Systemic toxicity is usually due to an inadvertent intravascular injection, administration into highly vascular sites, or the use of an excessive dose. Treatment consists of maintenance of a patent airway, adequate ventilation with 100% oxygen, use of anticonvulsant agents such as midazolam or barbiturates to control seizures, vasopressor drugs, and fluid loading to support the circulation if hypotension should occur. Inasmuch as the reaction is a continuum that may be mild or proceed rapidly to cardiovascular collapse, small doses of barbiturates and benzodiazepines are used so as not to compound the depressant effect of the local anesthetic drug.

## GENERAL ANESTHESIA

After being properly sedated in the preanesthesia room the patient is brought to the operating room where the usual required anesthesia monitoring triad of continuous electrocardiogram, automated blood pressure device, and pulse oximeter is further supplemented by the availability of expired carbon dioxide determination. We are adamant in requiring this for all general anesthesia and feel also that this should display a waveform rather than give an analog readout. One hour before the scheduled time of operation, the patient is orally administered 150 mg of ranitidine and 15 mL of chilled Bicitra. If the patient has a history of peptic disease, reflux, or repeated episodes of postoperative nausea and vomiting, metoclopramide (Reglan) is administered. At this time the preoperative physical examination is done and pertinent laboratory data reviewed. Particular attention is paid to the airway, how far the mouth can be opened, and the distance from the mandible to the thyroid cartilage. In addition to this, a Mallampatti classification is performed (Table 5–1).[7] The Mallampati classification is carried out by asking the patient to open his mouth as wide as he

tion produces a less anxious and better sedated patient. In our experience patients without preoperative medication are more difficult to manage and have more intraoperative bleeding.

### Anesthesia

The anesthesiologist monitors the patient with the appropriate equipment and begins the intravenous medications. We have found that the best protocol includes a narcotive and a sedative. The patient may receive fentanyl or morphine depending on the anesthesiologist's choice. After the narcotic is administered intravenously in small doses, diazepan (Valium) or Midazalam (Versed) is titrated to the patient's clinical status. When slurring of speech and loss of ocular muscle coordination occurs, the patient is ready for local infiltration. The local anesthetic that we use is a fresh mixture of 1 cc of epinephrine (1:1000) in 50 cc of 1% lidocaine (Xylocaine). Using a 5-cc syringe with a 25-gauge needle, we proceed with local infiltration to create a circumferential block around the nose (Fig 6–1). Never inject local anesthetic into the dorsum or the nasal tip. This will avoid any distortion of the areas

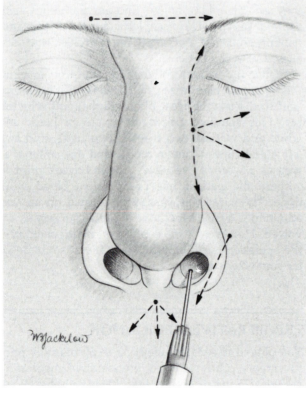

**FIG 6–1.**
Circumferential block with local anesthesia.

to be sculptured. After the circumferential block, the local anesthetic is infiltrated into the nasal valve region and along each side of the lateral nasal bones. Infiltration of the septum is then performed. In all, a total of only 10 to 15 cc of local anesthesia is injected. One must wait a minimum of 10 minutes for blanching of the skin, nose, and surrounding facial area to occur before beginning surgery.

In our practice we never use the topical application of any form of cocaine to anesthetize the nasal mucosa. The use of topical cocaine can cause serious cardiac arrythmias and increase the morbidity of this procedure. In the majority of patients we can achieve adequate anesthesia with preoperative intramuscular medication, intravenous sedation, and local anesthesia. In certain patients, general anesthesia is an appropriate option that permits uncomplicated and safe surgery.

## PREOPERATIVE MARKINGS

We always mark the patient preoperatively. Using a purple felt-tipped pen, we outline the caudal borders of the lower lateral cartilage and the intracartilaginous incision, which resembles gull wings. In general we try to retain about 5 mm of lower lateral cartilage. We mark the caudal border of the nasal bone, the inner canthal line, and the level of hump reduction.

## NASAL TIP SURGERY

Prior to nasal tip surgery, we pack the posterior of the nasopharynx with moist gauze. We use a double-hook retractor to evert the lower lateral cartilage. An intracartilaginous incision is made to preserve about 5 mm of caudal lower lateral cartilage (Fig 6–2). Peck-Josephs scissors are introduced through this incision to mobilize the fibroadipose tissue from the dermis of the nasal dorsum (Fig 6–3). The vestibular lining is then separated from the underside of the lower lateral cartilage (Fig 6–4). The surgeon incises the medial aspect of the cephalad portion of the lower lateral cartilage and then peels this cartilage laterally to the return of the lower lateral cartilage. We resect at the return of the lower lateral cartilage and retain the lateral-most portion (Fig 6–5). This avoids producing a depression. The resected portion of lower lateral cartilage is then placed on a sterile Telfa pad to be preserved for possible graft-

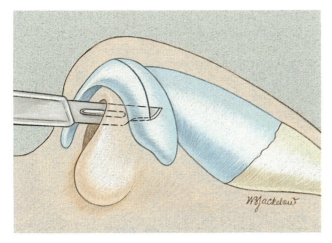

**FIG 6–2.**
Intracartilaginous incision.

ing. Sculpturing of the opposite lower lateral cartilage is performed by using the same technique.
Once this area has been sculptured, the surgeon will
notice a discrepancy in level between the caudal
lower lateral cartilage and the area of the excised cartilage. The definition is in the shape of gull wings.

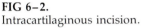

## ELEVATION AND ROTATION OF THE TIP

A transfixion incision is made at the caudal end of
the septum. If the patient has a long nose or a hang-

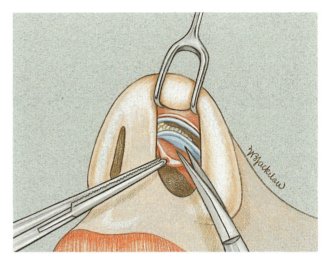

**FIG 6–4.**
Separating the vestibular lining from the cephalad lower
lateral cartilage.

ing columella, the surgeon uses a scalpel with a no.
15 blade to resect about 2 mm of the posterior two
thirds of the columella since this part of the columella directly affects the length of the nose and the
nasal lobule angle (Fig 6–6). Overcorrection of the
posterior two thirds of the columella causes a retro-
see columella. The nasal spine should never be resected because this will also cause a retracted columella.

The anterior third of the columella affects tip
rotation. By obtusely resecting 1 to 2 mm of the
anterior third of the columella, one produces tip
rotation and a more natural angle of the anterior
lobule. Overresection of the anterior third of the
columella causes an overly rotated nasal tip.

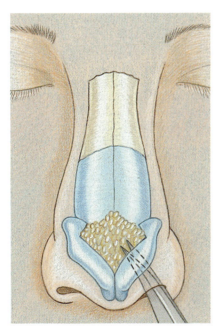

**FIG 6–3.**
Dissecting the fibroadipose tissue from the dermis.

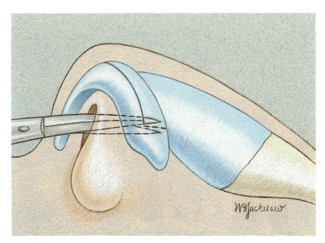

**FIG 6–5.**
Resection of cephalic lower lateral cartilage.

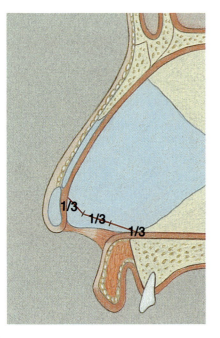

**FIG 6–6.**
Technique for elevating the posterior two thirds of the columella and rotation of the tip.

## HUMP REDUCTION

Peck-Joseph scissors are introduced through the intracartilaginous incision again, and the skin over the dorsum of the nose is mobilized from the dorsal nasal bone and dorsal septal cartilage (Fig 6–7). A no. 8 carbide tungsten rasp is used to lower the dorsal nasal bone (Fig 6–8). An osteotome should never be used to lower the nasal dorsum due to its lack of precision and control. A scalpel with a no. 15 blade is then introduced through the same intracartilaginous incision to the level of the lowered nasal bone. With this scalpel, the surgeon then incises the dorsal septal cartilage at the appropriate level of cartilaginous hump reduction (Fig 6–9). A hemostat is placed into this region and the incised portion of dorsal cartilaginous septum removed. With one finger, the surgeon then pushes down on the nasal tip while looking at the lateral profile to note any irregularity or unevenness in the dorsum.

## NASAL BRIDGE SURGERY

Nasal bridge surgery is necessary in a patient with a wide nasal bridge or an open roof requiring lateral infracturing of the nasal bones. A 4-mm osteotome is placed at the piriform fossa and the vestibular lining punctured. The osteotome is oriented at the level of the maxilla and nasal bone, as low on the maxilla as possible. Starting from the caudal border of the nasal bone, the surgeon proceeds to infracture to the level of the inner canthal line. Just before the inner canthal line, the surgeon begins the vertical component of the lateral infracture (Fig 6–10). In this area the lateral nasal bone is fragile, and less power is needed to infracture it. Once the vertical component of the infracture is complete, the surgeon places gauze over the lateral aspect of the nasal bone and uses manual pressure to reduce the bone and to narrow one side of the nasal bridge. The same procedure is applied to the opposite lateral nasal bone to produce reduction in the same manner. After appropriate infracture the superior aspect of the nasal bone may have a rough edge and usually requires rasping.

The most common complications after lateral infracturing of the nasal bones are inadequate infracture, an asymmetrical nasal bridge, and a stair-step deformity caused by infracturing at a high level.

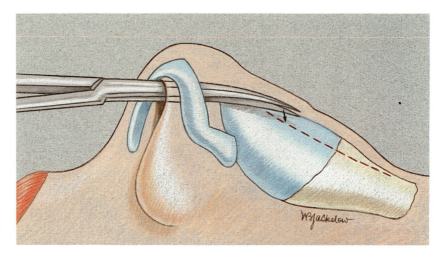

**FIG 6–7.**
Separation of soft tissue from the nasal dorsum.

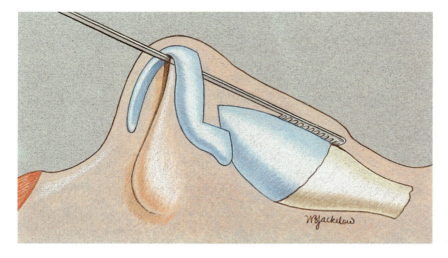

**FIG 6–8.**
Rasping the nasal bone.

## TRIMMING THE UPPER LATERAL CARTILAGES

The surgeon now evaluates the middle vault at the level of the upper lateral cartilage. The surgeon rarely needs to trim the caudal borders of the upper lateral cartilages since this would cause a narrowing or a depression in the middle vault. In a patient with a wide middle vault we recommend separating the upper lateral cartilages from the midline septum by using a scalpel with a no. 15 blade. If dorsal hump reduction was performed, the upper lateral cartilages may have already been separated. If not, separating the upper lateral cartilages from the midline septum will cause appropriate narrowing in this area without causing a depression or nasal obstruction.

## SUTURING THE TRANSFIXION INCISION

After hump reduction the surgeon proceeds with septal surgery. The sequence of surgery in basic rhi-noplasty is important. Septal surgery should never precede hump reduction because a tremendous amount of force is applied to the dorsum of the nose during this procedure. A surgeon could dislocate the osteocartilaginous junction and produce a saddle deformity if the septum is weak. Thus it is much safer to perform septal surgery after hump reduction. Once septal surgery is complete, the surgeon closes the transfixion incision with a heavy chromic suture. Only one suture is usually needed.

## ALAR BASE RESECTION

Alar rim surgery is necessary in the patient with a wide alar base caused by nasal flaring, a wide floor, or a combination of both. Alar rim sculpturing is performed at the end of the basic rhinoplasty. By sculpturing the lower lateral cartilages, the surgeon lowers tip projection. The decrease in tip projection may produce nasal flaring that was unnoticed on the previous evaluation.

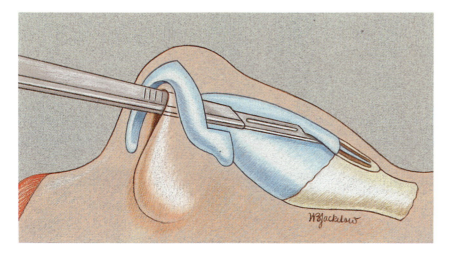

**FIG 6–9.**
Lowering the dorsal aspect of the septum with a scalpel.

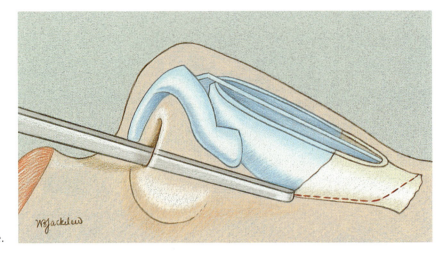

**FIG 6–10.**
Osteotomy technique.

We perform the modified Weir technique. A scalpel with a no. 15 blade is used to make the inferior incision in the nasal crease. This incision should never be carried farther than the midpoint of the alar crease. The perpendicular incision is then made into the alar rim at the level of the necessary resection. Usually 2 to 3 mm of alar rim is resected. The superior incision is carried out to meet the inferior incision at the midway point of the alar crease (Fig 6–11). This tissue is then freed from the underlying muscle and excised with Peck-Joseph scissors, with care taken to avoid removing any vestibular lining. Removal of vestibular lining would cause notching in the alar base. Hemostasis is obtained with electrocautery, and the incision is closed by using meticulously placed 5–0 nylon sutures. Usually three sutures are necessary to approximate the skin of the alar rim. The same procedure is performed on the opposite alar rim.

The basic rhinoplasty is now complete, and the surgeon should reevaluate tip projection. The most common complication after basic rhinoplasty is inadequate tip projection. By sculpturing the lower lateral cartilage the surgeon reduces its volume and lowers the nasal tip pyramid, which in turn reduces nasal tip projection. The surgeon treats inadequate tip projection with either an onlay graft or an umbrella graft, depending on septal support (see Chapter 9).

## DRESSING

After packing the nasal passageways we apply half-inch plastic sterile strips bandages on the dorsum of the nasal tip leading to the nasal bridge. A quarter-inch plastic strip bandage is used in the area of the anterior lobule. The tape splinting immediately reveals any irregularity of the nasal dorsum; this helps the surgeon to evaluate tip projection and serves as a final check on the relationship between the projection of the nasal tip pyramid and the bridge. An aluminum splint is placed over the nasal bridge and secured with half-inch silk tape. A mustache gauze is secured with tape and collects any oozing or drainage.

The nasal packing is removed in 24 hours. The nasal splint and other plastic strip bandages remain in place for 5 to 6 days. After removal of the splint and plastic strips, no further dressing is placed on the nose. If a radical submucosal resection of the septum is performed, the nasal packing is not removed before 48 to 72 hours.

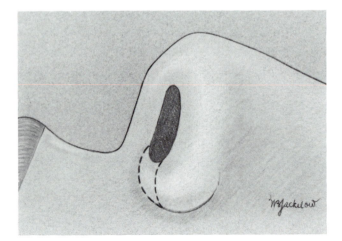

**FIG 6–11.**
Modified Weir resection.

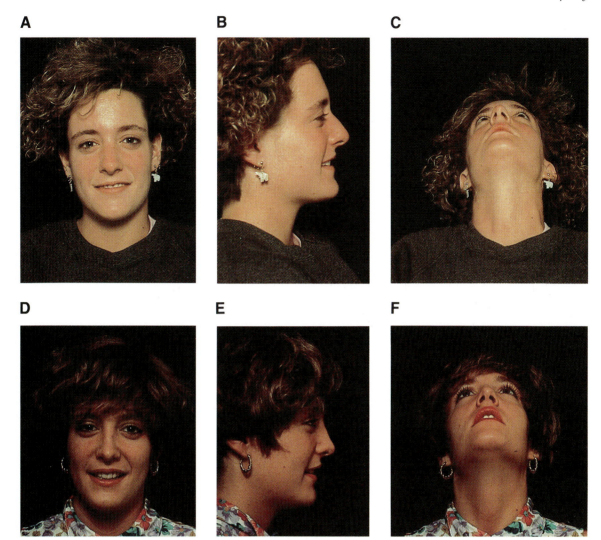

**FIG 6–12.**
**A,** preoperative frontal view: wide nasal bridge, bulbous nasal tip. **B,** preoperative lateral view: mild dorsal hump, long nose, adequate tip projection. **C,** preoperative worm's eye view: rounded and wide nasal tip. **D,** postoperative frontal view: narrow nasal bridge, gull-wing highlighting in the nasal tip. **E,** postoperative lateral view: nice dorsal line and adequate tip projection without grafts. **F,** postoperative worm's eye view: defined nasal tip.

## CLINICAL CASE

This patient came to our office for a primary rhinoplasty. The patient has a wide bridge and bulbous, ill-defined nasal tip. On evaluating her profile, we note a mild dorsal hump, a long nose, and a slightly drooping nasal tip (Fig 6–12,A–C).

Intraoperatively we sculptured the patient's bilateral lower lateral cartilages, rasped the dorsal bone, lowered the dorsal end of the septum, and infractured the nasal bones. The caudal end of the septum was shortened, and the nasal tip was rotated about 2 mm. A modified Weir resection was performed to narrow the alar base. No cartilage grafts were required.

Postoperatively, the patient has a narrower nasal bridge, a more defined nasal tip, and a natural dorsal line (Fig 6–12,D–F).

# Primary Open Rhinoplasty

Ronald P. Gruber, M.D.

This chapter will deal with primary open rhinoplasty. It will be divided up into the following sections:

1. Fundamental problems facing primary rhinoplasty
2. Rationale for the open technique
3. Indications and contraindications for the open approach
4. Preoperative consultation
5. Preoperative planning
6. Basic technique (including anesthesia)
7. Adjunctive procedures
8. Postoperative care
9. Case examples
10. Unsatisfactory results
11. Complications
12. Summary

## FUNDAMENTAL PROBLEMS FACING PRIMARY RHINOPLASTY

There are two fundamental problems facing the field of rhinoplasty surgery: (1) there is little if any training in sculpturing or art, and (2) traditional rhinoplasty techniques make it difficult to evaluate the result, i.e., one simply cannot see what is being sculptured. When an outstanding result is seen following a rhinoplasty, especially that presented by an expert in the field, it is commonly assumed that it is the technique itself that is primarily responsible for the result. I would argue that at least 50% of the result is due to the surgeon's aesthetic sense and ability to

sculpture and reshape the cartilages and bone of the nose to make the result that he desires. It is not enough to know that a tip graft is a solution to a particular patient's problem. It is just as important to know how thick and wide that graft should be, as well as where it should be placed. Without that sense of judgment, the technique of tip grafting itself is no better than a totally different technique that aims to achieve tip projection. Another surgeon who chooses to make the tip more prominent by inserting a cartilage graft between the medial crura and anterior nasal spine may achieve a very similar result. But there, too, the aesthetic sense must be keen if one is to obtain the same objective. The second surgeon must also make a critical decision. In this case, it is whether or not the graft causes the tip cartilages to be overprojected or underprojected. Thus we come right back to the problem of the aesthetic sense of the surgeon and the judgment that is required in aesthetic decisions irrespective of the technique that is employed. This is not to say that some techniques are not superior to others; it is just to emphasize that aesthetic judgment is usually overlooked as the prominent reason why some surgeons achieve results that are so much better than others. In no other aspect of plastic surgery is aesthetic judgment quite so important.

By being able to see what is sculptured (when the nose is opened) and where the cartilages end up, aesthetic judgments are easier to make. Those rhinoplastic surgeons who have already developed that special sense do not have to see the cartilages themselves to appreciate the result. They have done enough rhinoplasties and can extrapolate from their experience what the anticipated result will be. Most plastic surgeons, however, will not have a vast experience of rhinoplasty to draw upon. Seeing what they sculpture simply makes it easier to obtain the desired result.

## RATIONALE FOR THE OPEN TECHNIQUE

The rationale for the technique of open rhinoplasty is based upon the following principles: the amount of extra dissection is less than one half of a square centimeter (Fig 7–1). Most techniques nowadays involve a rim incision with delivery of the tip cartilages. By extending the rim incisions caudally somewhat and connecting them with a transcolumella incision, it becomes apparent that the extra dissection is actually quite small indeed. This extra dissection does not significantly increase the length of the operation. The length of the operation for the open approach, however, is greater simply due to the fact that there are many more maneuvers that can be accomplished through the open approach than through the closed approach. There are a few blood vessels that course the columella in the vertical direction, and they are in fact disrupted. The initial concern was that so doing would not only impose a potential problem for columella-flap survival but would increase postoperative edema as well. At this time, no significant sequelae relating to these extra few vessels in the columella have been seen. There is some suggestion that there is a tendency for more telangiectasia or redness of the nose in some patients who have had the open approach. As time passes it will be more apparent whether or not this is in fact the case. No good comparative studies have been done to indicate that there is any significant long-term sequelae from interruption of the small branches of the columella.

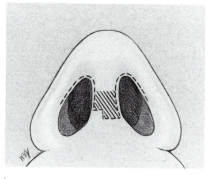

**FIG 7–1.**
The amount of extra dissection (*stippled area*) is less than one half of a square centimeter.

Local anesthesia is a significant cause of distortion (Fig 7–2) and is one of the reasons why the open approach is favored. This problem is especially true when correcting small and subtle problems. After the local anesthesia is injected, the anatomic deformity is often lost, thus making it difficult to judge the result of the corrective maneuver, whether it be removal of a small piece of redundant cartilage or the addition of a small graft. However, when the nasal skin is fully retracted, one can see the cartilaginous framework. After performing several open rhinoplasty procedures, one gets an appreciation of what the normal anatomy should be, and one orients himself to that normal anatomy and attempts to reconstruct the framework according to what the normal cartilaginous anatomy should be. Decisions are made on what the cartilaginous anatomy should look like, first. Immediately thereafter the skin flap is replaced. At that point a second and different judgement (i.e., the external appearance of the nose) can be made, which is also extremely helpful in determining the final result. By having two separate means of judging the final result (the internal and the external) one is more likely to get a better long-term result. The external result is simply not enough of a guideline as to what the nose will ultimately look like.

Some of the distortion problems due to local anesthesia can be minimized by adding hyaluronidase (Wydase) (150 units/30 cc of local anesthesia). The local anesthesia tends to dissipate and spread out much better with the addition of this agent. It is less important in the distal part of the nose as it is in the area of the anterior nasal spine and nasion. This is the area where little or no undermining is done. Without undermining, the local anesthesia tends to stay and gives a very artificial fullness in the area of the glabella and columella-lip junction where judgments must be made. The shape and appearance of the glabella and forehead (see Chapter 25) significantly affect our judgement as to what the shape and size of the nose should be. Anything that can be done to minimize the swelling in this region is therefore helpful. Wydase accomplishes that purpose very well. One of the disadvantages of Wydase, however, is that because the local anesthesia tends to disperse, there is a loss of anesthesia after 2 hours of surgery.

For my colleagues who question the need to use the external approach in such a high percentage of patients, I simply remind them of the reasons so many surgeons use an external approach for chin augmentation. I remind them that the transaxillary approach to the breast would in principle be an ideal

**A**

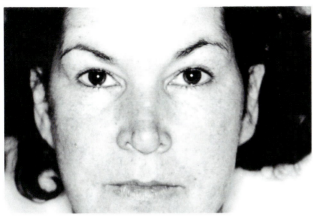

**B**

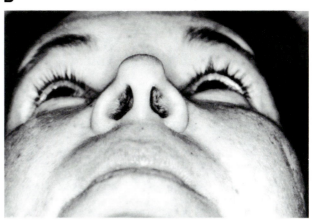

**C**

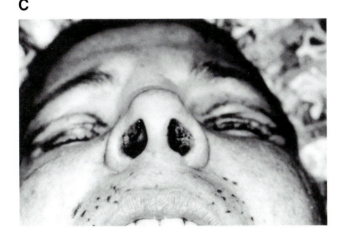

**FIG 7–2.**
Local anesthesia is a significant cause of distortion. The preoperative deformity (in this case a pinched ala) **(A** and **B)** may not be seen after the local anesthetic is put in **(C).** That is why it is an advantage to be able to open the nose and see the deformity. (**B** and **C** from Gruber RP: Primary rhinoplasty. In Vistnes L, editor: *Procedures in plastic and reconstructive surgery*, New York, 1991, Little Brown, p 98. Used with permission.)

method to augment every breast. And yet, the inframammary and periareolar approach are found to be necessary by many surgeons who feel they cannot reach the same goal otherwise.

## INDICATIONS AND CONTRAINDICATIONS

Indications for the open approach are (1) virtually all primary rhinoplasty cases and (2) whenever any significant quantity of work needs to be done. If the deformity is minor and requires little work, there is no need to open the nose (e.g., a small dorsal hump). If the patient is not willing to accept the very small risk of a significant columella scar, the external approach is contraindicated. As a result of these indications and contraindications, over 90% of my cases are done by the open approach.

## PREOPERATIVE CONSULTATION

Preoperative consultation for the open approach is not significantly different from what would be used for the closed approach. It is imperative, of course, to discuss the use of the columella incision and discuss its advantages and disadvantages. I make it perfectly clear to patients that they have a choice of having either approach. I also make it perfectly clear that in my hands, the open approach has yielded much better overall results. I also explain that if the columella scar allows me to give just a small increment of improvement in the dorsal profile or the width of the nasal tip, it is well worth the price. Other people, the patient's friends and family, readily see the tip of the nose. But they seldom see the columella. At some point in the preoperative discussion, however, particularly when the patient's skin (and ala) are thick, the limitations of what can be done for the patient are discussed. Patients readily appreciate the fact that any nose cannot be made by the surgeon. They appreciate the fact that skin cannot drape to any desired shape. By discussing all these things with the patient, the informed consent process is greatly enhanced. Finally, the fact that a "touch-up" or "corrective" surgery may be necessary is emphasized to the patient. Patients are very uncomfortable with the idea that the entire operation may have to be redone. However, they appreciate the fact that "adjustments" may be required, e.g., rasping the dorsum or adding a small graft.

Preoperative planning also includes discussing the patient's needs and desires. This is taken into account in a very serious fashion. For example, some patients want the dorsum of the nose to be concave, and others would prefer a more natural appearance. Others want the nasal width to be unusually narrow, perhaps even narrower than that of the surgeon's desires. Since the nose is ultimately the property of the patient, it behooves a surgeon to adhere to the patient's desires as much as possible, short of giving a result that otherwise might look ridiculous.

## PREOPERATIVE PLANNING

For a detailed discussion of preoperative planning, see Chapters 2 and 4. A brief description of my personal approach will be given here.

Physical examination for aesthetic rhinoplasty concentrates in large part on the thickness of the skin. Whereas we surgeons have control to a large extent over the bony and cartilaginous framework, we have little control over the draping of the skin. Subcutaneous scar formation is a factor that we have little control over. The size of the ala cannot be changed very much, and therefore the remainder of

**A**     **B**     **C**

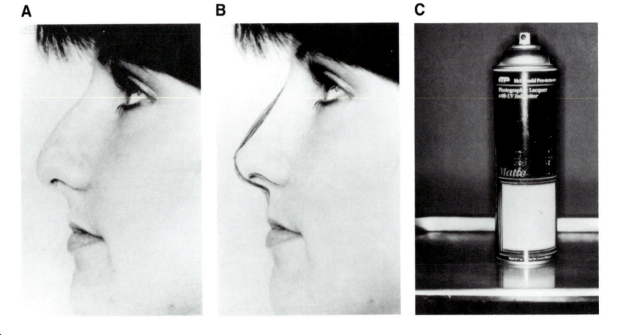

**D**

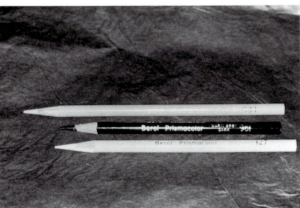

FIG 7–3.
To draw on photos **(A and B)** one can use McDonald's lacquer **(C)** and Berol Prismacolor pencils **(D)**. (From Gruber RP: Primary rhinoplasty: the open approach. In Vistnes L, editor: *Procedures in Plastic and Reconstructive Surgery.* Boston, 1991, Little Brown, p 98. Used with permission.)

the nose including the dorsal length and the vertical height have to be designed around the existing ala. The thicker and bigger the ala is, the larger the nose will have to be. One also has to take into consideration the size of the patient's face. All these judgements are part of the aesthetic plan.

Drawing the anticipated result for the patient helps solidify the communication process between the patient and physician (Fig 7–3, A and B), not to mention solidifying the issue of informed consent. I personally use the computerized video imaging system and find it very helpful. However, I am still more comfortable with drawing on the patient's photographs, simply because I can be more accurate. Ideally the photograph of the patient should be a one-to-one ratio so that the final product can be taken to the operating room and one can get direct measurements from the photograph as to what should be added or subtracted from the patient's nose to give the final result. Since there is time involved in getting prints back from the photographer and since one usually wants to do the photograph drawing right then and there with the patient during the first consultation, the standard Polaroid print is used. The close-up with a conventional Polaroid camera takes a 1:2 ratio. When this Polaroid is sprayed with a lacquer (made by McDonald Company), it is ready to be drawn upon (Fig 7–3, C). Too much spraying of lacquer makes it difficult to dry and difficult to draw upon. The lightest possible coating with the lacquer (which leaves a granular surface) gives the best result. The odor from the spray is often offensive, and therefore the spraying process is done near a window or a door. After that a blow-dryer is used to hasten the drying process. Berol Prismacolor pencils (Fig 7–3, D) are used to draw on the Polaroids. They come in various colors. The only ones really required are black and a light flesh tone. The pencils are obtained from any art store, and the lacquer is obtained from any photography store. Should Prismacolor pencils not be available, an ordinary lead pencil will work.

Drawing on the patient's prints (Polaroids) or on the video screen is perhaps one of the best ways to develop the aesthetic judgement that is not provided in most plastic surgery residencies. A learning curve is involved in the drawing on these Polaroids. With time it becomes easier and faster. It also becomes apparent that it is not always easy to change the profile into something that is pleasing. You might know that a particular nasal profile is not aesthetically acceptable, and yet you may not be able to change it by drawing on it. This is the exact problem that faces the novice surgeon in the operating room. After performing a few maneuvers he knows that he has improved the nose, but it still does not "look right." And yet he does not know what should be done to make it "look better." Drawing on the Polaroids preoperatively helps determine what does make it "look better." Several drawings may be required before one finds the one that looks the best. It is also amazing how very small changes in the length or vertical height or angle of the tip result in that improved result.

One other benefit that results from drawing on the patient's Polaroids (or on the video screen) is that the patient gets to appreciate the surgeon. Another benefit is that the surgeon gets to appreciate the patient better. Once in a while after completing what appears to be a nice-looking profile on the Polaroid, a patient tells you that it is in fact not to his liking. This too is extremely important feedback. Some patients simply do not know what they want and are not able to express it. Some patients request a somewhat shorter nose than you might draw or one with a more concave dorsum than you might draw. A few patients will be unhappy with anything you draw, which suggests that they are not candidates for surgery. And if you cannot draw it, you probably will not be able to surgically produce it.

Patients are given the drawings when they are completed so that when they come back for the second office examination they have time to think about exactly what it is they want. They are also told, of course, that the drawing is not a warranty or guarantee of the result. It is simply the goal that we are setting for ourselves and hope to come as close to it as possible. One final bit of advice regards the use of Silly Putty (Fig 7–4). When a patient obviously needs grafting, it is helpful to simply apply Silly Putty to those areas where grafts are anticipated. The Silly Putty sticks to the skin of the nose, and one can see the change in shape of the nose. One gets a good idea as to the dimensions that the graft should be by doing this. On occasion I even take the Silly Putty to the operating room and use it as a template for cutting the grafts to size.

## BASIC TECHNIQUE

### Local Anesthesia

As soon as patients are brought into the operating room, they are given a small dose of midazolam (Versed) intravenously to make them more relaxed

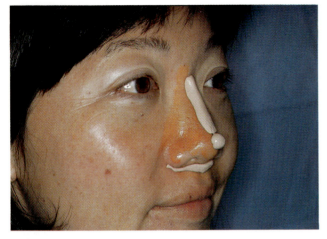

**FIG 7–4.**
Silly Putty is applied to the patient's nose where grafts
are anticipated. So doing gives a better appreciation of
the dimensions that the graft should be. Benzoin keeps
the Silly Putty in place.

and comfortable. Local anesthesia is utilized for the
overwhelming majority of patients. General anesthesia is reserved for those who are unusually appre-
hensive, or request it, or have unusually difficult
problems such as major obstruction of the posterior
aspect of the septum where local anesthesia is often
difficult to achieve. Otherwise all patients receive local anesthesia with sedation. During the course of
the procedure 100 mg of hydrocortisone is given for
the purposes of reducing edema and because it also
gives a certain sense of euphoria in the early postoperative period. The local anesthetic is injected with a
3-cc syringe and no. 27 needle. A certain amount of
hyperinflation is done to maximize hemostasis. As
mentioned previously, Wydase is included with the
local to enhance dissipation of the local anesthetic.
When the septum is injected, however, no Wydase
is used in the mixture because it is easier to elevate
the mucoperichondrium off the septal cartilage if
there is hyperinflation. Cocaine is not used until it is
time to perform the osteotomy. The effect of the cocaine will wear off if it is inserted too soon.

## Columella Incision

There are many types of columellar incisions that
have been employed over the years (Fig 7–5). They
include the slightly curvilinear incision, a chevron
incision, an inverted chevron incision, a W incision,
and a stair-step incision. At this time my preferred
incision is the stair-step incision. Should there be
any slight notching on both sides of the columella,
as does occur occasionally, it will be offset. Thus

from the profile view the notching simply will not be
seen. In addition, it is much easier to line up the
wound edges for repair.

The external columellar incision is connected to
the rim incision (Fig 7–6). By rim incision it is meant
the rim of the cartilage, not the vestibule. This is the
same rim incision that is used for cartilage delivery
techniques. In this case it is simply a more posterior
extension of the usual rim incision until it reaches
the columellar incision. By inserting a small pair of
scissors (Littler or tenotomy) the columellar flap is
elevated. By inserting these same scissors through
the rim incision of the vestibule, the rest of the dorsal skin can be elevated just as is done during the
standard cartilage delivery technique. By placing a
hook on the columellar flap and continuing the dissection from the flap to the dorsal area that has been
undermined, the two areas of undermining are connected.

Inevitably one will on occasion accidentally
transect or nick the rim cartilage and will even make
the rim incision in such a way that a piece of lateral
crus cartilage has been left in the vestibular skin of
the nasal flap. However, this is not usually a problem. The area that has been nicked can be repaired
with a single 6–0 nylon suture, and the piece of cartilage that was left in the dorsal flap can be dissected
out and returned to the tip cartilages and sutured directly back into place. The great advantage of the
open approach is that errors of technique can usually be corrected with ease.

## Skeletonization

Skeletonization of the remaining portion of dorsal
flap is done with the same scissors until the flap is
completely elevated. Then one can insert the small
finger under the dorsal flap until it reaches the nasal
bones. This is the so-called finger insertion test.
There is a tendency for the novice not to want to elevate the skin flap adequately. By not doing so,
however, the exposure that one really needs may
not be obtained. Spreading laterally with the scissors
(without cutting) facilitates the flap elevation process. Hemostasis may be required at this point, although if the local anesthesia was hyperinflated, the
only area that will require cautery is at the external
columella incision. Oftentimes, however, there are
two small vessels in the dorsal flap (one on either
side) that require cautery. These vessels sometimes
will bleed toward the end of the procedure if the
epinephrine effect has worn off. Hemostasis is one
of the benefits of the open approach in that the pro-

**A**

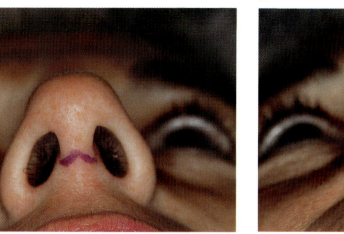

**B**

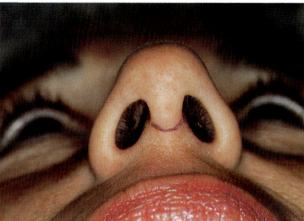

**C**

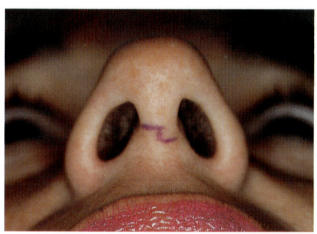

FIG 7–5.
There are many types of columellar incisions, e.g., chevron **(A)**, curved **(B)**, and stair step **(C)**. The latter is the preferred incision because any notching that should occur on one side is camouflaged by normal skin on the other side (on a profile view).

cedure can be dry from beginning to end. Not only can one cauterize vessels along the dorsum where the hump is being moved, but one can also deal with the problem of bleeding if the surgery should happen to go beyond 2 or 2½ hours and the epinephrine has worn off. In the closed approach, this is not possible and has led to a number of cases where there is considerable swelling, discomfort, and ecchymosis, all as a result of inadequate hemostasis.

**Defatting**

Defatting (Fig 7–7) is performed on the surface of the upper lateral cartilage and lower lateral cartilages only. The skin flap itself seldom if ever needs to be defatted. So doing would only jeopardize its circulation. Meticulous defatting of the cartilages, however, makes it so much easier to manipulate their shape.

**Dorsal Modification**

The dorsum is usually the first modification made. Most of the patients require some hump removal. This is done by passing a scalpel with a no. 15 blade through the cartilaginous dorsum at a level that was determined preoperatively (Fig 7–8). For example, if 3 mm of dorsum was planned to be removed on the preoperative photograph, then the scalpel is placed 3 mm below the dorsum and pierces the dorsal-septal cartilage as well as the upper lateral cartilage. Usually no attempt is made on a routine basis to use the so-called extramucosal technique prior to resecting the dorsum. For complicated cases where subsequent septal work will be done and where breathing is a significant potential or actual problem, the extramucosal technique is used. However, for small or moderate hump removals, the mucoperichondrium lining will still be intact after the dorsum is removed. For the larger humps it will not be intact,

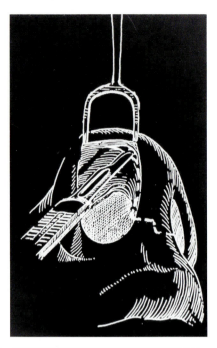

**FIG 7–6.**
The columellar incision is connected to a "rim" incision that runs along the caudal edge of the lower lateral cartilage.

but the tissues will be carefully approximated where necessary to prevent problems at the valve.

The bony hump is then removed with the rasp and not the osteotome. Better control and finer detail can be obtained with a rasp. In those cases where dorsal augmentation is required, the har-

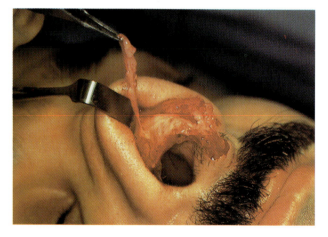

**FIG 7–7.**
The cartilages should be defatted to provide better visualization. The flap itself, however, should seldom if ever be defatted. (From Gruber RP: Primary rhinoplasty: the open approach. In Vistnes L, editor: *Procedures in plastic and reconstructive surgery,* Boston, 1991, Little Brown, p 103. Used with permission.)

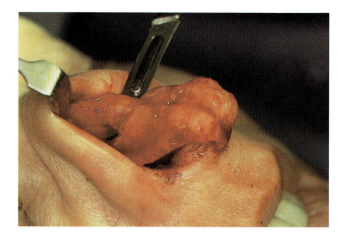

**FIG 7–8.**
Modification of the dorsum can be done precisely by a stab wound incision with a scalpel at the level of hump removal that has been determined preoperatively. (From Gruber RP: Primary rhinoplasty: the open approach. In Vistnes L, editor: *Procedures in plastic and reconstructive surgery,* Boston, 1991; Little Brown, p 101. Used with permission.)

vested graft material is cut to the desired length and width, inserted along the dorsum, and held there with a pair of forceps to judge what the internal appearance is. By retracting the skin flap with a Senz retractor one can appreciate the relationship of the dorsal graft to the existing nasal bones.

One can see enough of the nasal bones to judge what the width of the dorsal graft should be. Without such a visual appreciation, there is a tendency to make the dorsal grafts either too narrow or too wide. Toward the end of the procedure the dorsal graft will be sutured internally at its caudal-most aspect by using nonabsorbable 4–0 or 5–0 nylon sutures. If the harvested specimens are simply not long enough because of the technical difficulties involved, the open approach allows one to put in dorsal grafts in tandem and suture them directly in place (Fig 7–9).

If there is any question about the stability and security of the graft, external sutures can be placed at the end of the surgery. These consist of 5–0 or 6–0 nylon that pierces both the skin and the dorsal cartilage graft and helps to secure it prior to application of the splint. To prevent the cartilaginous graft from slipping, small holes are made with a scalpel (no. 11 blade). The holes should be 1 to 2 mm in diameter. They allow for the ingrowth of fibrous tissue and minimize graft instability. If one has a small, 2-mm hair-plug punch, that can be used instead. When double-layer cartilaginous grafts are used, they are sutured together with mattress sutures

**A** **B**

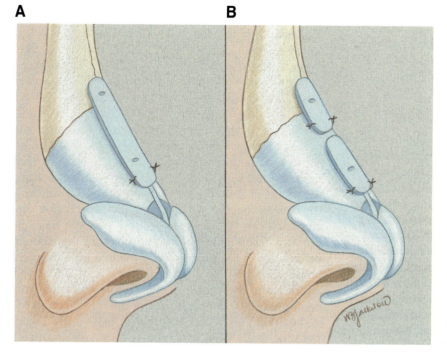

FIG 7–9.
The open approach allows suturing of dorsal grafts in place **(A)**. If the length of the donor material is insufficient, the grafts can be placed in tandem along the dorsum **(B)**. If possible, grafts should be perforated in one or two places with a no. 11 blade to allow ingrowth of scar tissue.

rather than wraparound sutures. Should any trimming of the graft be necessary after inserting it, it can be done when mattress sutures are used but cannot be done as well if wraparound sutures are used. This is because the wraparound sutures would be cut in the process of trimming the edges of the graft.

### Length Modification

Nasal length modification is done by combining the transfixion incision with an intercartilaginous incision. This allows excellent exposure (Fig 7–10) of the cartilage of the septum because the tip cartilages are brought well out of the way. The caudal edge of the septum can be shortened to the length that was determined preoperatively on the patient's prints or Polaroids. The actual technique of intercartilaginous incision is done with a stab-wound incision made with a scalpel and connecting it with another stab-wound incision made in the transfixion incision. It is at this time that one appreciates the loss of existing tip support by making these incisions. However, correcting that support (by suture repair) will be dealt with later. It simply needs to be fully appreciated when making the transfixion and intercartilaginous incision. It also serves to reemphasize the need for suture repair of these structures prior to completing the rhinoplasty.

Modification of the nasal tip involves a wide variety of techniques, many of which will be given here. It should be emphasized that there is not one sole technique to accomplish the intended goal. Whatever the surgeon can do to manipulate and modify the cartilages to the desired shape is what counts. The important concept is that (1) the changes desired are much more easily made through the open approach, (2) errors that occur during the process of making those changes can be

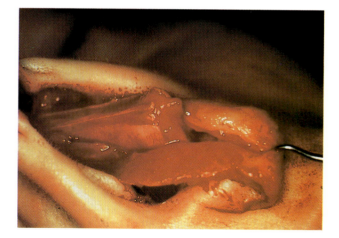

FIG 7–10.
After making a transfixion and intercartilaginous incision, a hook on the tip cartilage gets the tip out of the way for excellent exposure. (From Gruber RP: Open rhinoplasty. In Russell RC, editor: *Instructional courses,* St Louis, 1989, Mosby–Year Book, p 10. Used with permission.)

**A**

**B**

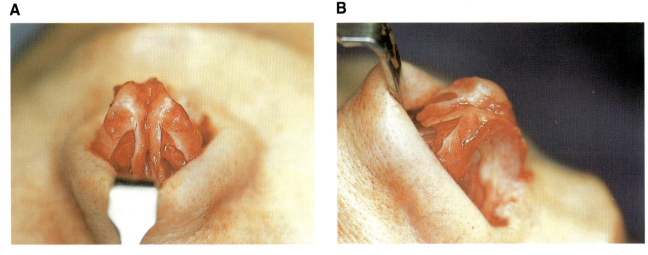

**FIG 7–15.**
When resecting the cephalic part of the lateral crus, a "tail" (**A** and **B**) is often left at the medial aspect. These "tails of the dome" are sutured to the dorsal edge of the septum so as to prevent dropping of the tip.

fore final securing is done, however, one should check the position of the tip cartilages because it is easy to pull them too far up. By returning the dorsal skin flap and evaluating the nose one can see whether they are being held at the right level.

On occasion the patient requires a substantial cephalic crus resection that leaves a cartilaginous void in which only vestibular skin fills the area. Inasmuch as this void may simply contract and distort the final result, it has been found helpful to return some of the resected cephalic crus (upside down) to the area from which it was returned. Before returning it, however, it is reduced in size. Surprisingly, in the process of resecting the cephalic lateral crus with a scalpel, a lot of the convexity is lost, and therefore

when the cartilage is returned, it is essentially a flat (not concave) specimen. Nonetheless, it can fill the gap created by cephalic resection. To emphasize this point once again, it is only necessary when there is a large void in this area.

**Transecting the Lateral Crus as Needed**

Despite having scored the domes and having sutured the posterior aspect of the domes to obtain tip cartilage narrowness, one often finds that the nose is still too broad (Fig 7–16). This is because the lateral crus is basically an arch that has two fixed end points. One end is fixed near the ala; the other is fixed at the dome. Removing more and more of the

**A**

**B**

**FIG 7–16.**
The convex latent crura is often corrected by single transection at its most convex part (**A**). The two elements will automatically overlay one another. Further undermining may be needed in very convex cases to obtain a 2- to 3-mm overlap (**B**). Suture repair may be required to prevent shifting of the two elements.

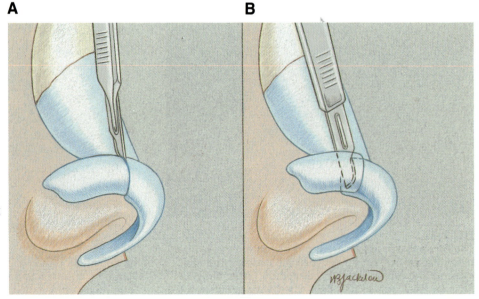

cephalic portion does not necessarily change the actual arch itself until some point is reached when the arch collapses.

There is a much better way of changing the arch of the lateral crus. That is by simply transecting it at its most concave point. A simple transection with a scalpel will result in an improvement in the arch. The two elements of the transection will simply overlap one another, and nothing further will have to be done. In some cases even more of the convexity needs to be removed (particularly in the patient with a boxy tip), and it will be necessary to undermine one side and allow even further overlapping of the elements. Originally when this procedure was done, a small section was routinely removed and the two elements sutured with figure-of-8 nylon sutures. This took additional time during surgery and has since been found to be seldom necessary. The vestibular skin will actually hold the two elements in juxtaposition more often than not, particularly if very little undermining of the cartilages is done. Should a significant overlap be required such that the cartilages become misaligned, sutures are used. At this point 5-0 or 6-0 nylon sutures are used to hold the cartilages in proper alignment.

### Suturing the Lateral Crura

Another method of correcting the convex lateral crus is to suture them together as suggested by Tebbetts. A 4-0 nylon mattress "spanning" suture that may incorporate the dorsal portion of the septum (Fig 7–17) is used. The lateral crura can also be sutured with a single suture directly to the upper lateral cartilage. This will help improve the convexity, too.

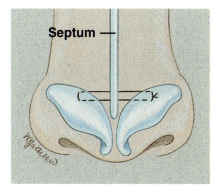

**FIG 7–17.**
Convexity of the lateral crura can sometimes be corrected by a "spanning suture." This nonabsorbable suture will narrow the nose and correct the lateral crus convexity.

### Tip Grafting

The need for tip grafting is usually determined preoperatively (by the drawings). A nasal tip that is deficient will obviously require it. Most of the Oriental and black patients require tip augmentation. The angle at which the tip graft is placed against the existing tip cartilages is a matter of aesthetic judgment, as are so many of the maneuvers discussed previously. The preoperative drawing helps determine what that particular angle will be. In some patients it will be more vertical as the Sheen tip-grafting procedure has usually done. In other cases it will be less vertical and more at the dome of the existing tip cartilages as is recommended by Peck. The judgment as to where the graft goes ultimately depends on what was drawn on the patient's preoperative prints and will be reinforced by what the internal and external nose looks like intraoperatively . To make a quick estimate of what is required, the cartilage graft is cut to the width of the existing middle crura and tip. It is simply held there with a no. 27 needle passed through the graft and the tip cartilages (Fig 7–18). The graft is then sutured in place with 6-0 nylon. The length of the tip graft can be temporarily left longer than needed. One can always trim it off the cephalic end of the graft should it be necessary.

If a double-layer tip graft is necessary, the second one can be simply sutured to the first one. The position, size, and shape of tip grafts are of critical importance to the final appearance of the tip of the

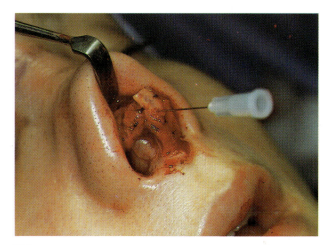

**FIG 7–18.**
A tip graft is held to the tip with a no. 30 needle. Interrupted 6–0 nylon is then used to suture it in place. The location of the graft is dictated by the observed profile that is desired. In some cases it works in the location suggested by Sheen. In other cases it works best in the location suggested by Peck. On occasion it works best in both locations.

nose. Therefore it is advisable to stand at the head of the bed and check the symmetry from that vantage point. If the graft is tilted to one side or lopsided, small pieces of cartilage can be put under one side or the other of the tip graft to prop it up and hold it in a more symmetrical position. On occasion one will want the tip graft to go up and over the dome and actually enter into the supratip region. On occasion, transverse scoring of the tip graft will facilitate contouring it to the existing tip cartilages. This technique is particularly useful for generalized enlargements of a small nose (Fig 7–19).

## Upper Lateral Cartilage Treatment

The middle third of the nose often requires modification either in the form of augmentation or reduction. Occasionally there is a very convex bowing of the upper lateral cartilage, particularly at the bony junction. Direct visualization allows modification of this portion of the upper lateral cartilage that might not be easy to correct any other way. In other cases augmentation is required to prevent a collapsed look of the middle third of the nose. Direct onlay grafts are easily performed with sutures. In some patients, however, it may be necessary to actually insert "spreader" grafts between the upper lateral cartilage and the septum. These grafts can be laid directly between the upper lateral cartilage and the septum (and then sutured), or one can simply develop a tunnel at the septal angle (Fig 7–20). This should be done, of course, prior to dorsal hump removal. I do not find it necessary to insert spreader grafts very

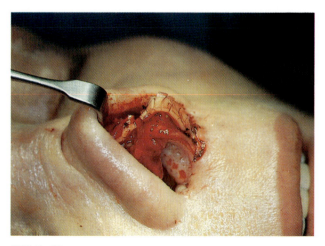

**FIG 7–19.**
Transverse scoring of the graft allows it to contour to the existing tip shape if simple enlargement is all that is required.

often. Part of this may be due to the fact that I tend to leave the nasal bones on the wider side rather than on the narrower side. Narrow nasal bones cause the tip to appear broader. Conversely, slightly broader nasal bones let the tip appear relatively narrow. Since the width of the tip cartilages is the limiting factor, I let that dictate the width of the nasal bones. If the nasal bones are not overnarrowed, the upper lateral cartilages will not fall in, and consequently there will be less need for spreader grafts to separate them away from the septal cartilage.

## Osteotomies

Lateral osteotomy is performed from the buccal-sulcus approach (Fig 7–21). Ten minutes prior to doing so, however, cocaine (4 cc at 5%) is applied to cotton and inserted on either side of the septum up against the medial aspect of the nasal bone. This will provide both anesthesia and hemostasis in this region. A small stab-wound incision is made just above the cuspid tooth in the buccal sulcus. A small separation of a mucous membrane is made with a clamp for a distance of about one-half centimeter. Then the Joseph elevator is inserted and the periosteum elevated until the piriform aperture is reached. A single-guarded, slightly curved chisel is inserted, and the osteotomy is performed. If the nasal bones are very narrow near the radix, the osteotomy begins very low near the piriform aperture, and it extends to the dorsum, but somewhat caudal of the actual nasion. If the bones are broad at the actual nasion, the osteotomy is done from a low position laterally to the dorsum of the nose at the actual nasion. Once the position for the osteotome is determined, the tapping is continued without trying to make too many adjustments in the osteotome. So doing can lead to fracturing of the bone into multiple fragments. Tapping is stopped when a change in the sound is heard as the osteotome reaches the area of the nasion. At this point an upward prying motion of the osteotome handle is performed in order to retrieve the osteotome. That simple maneuver alone usually results in an inward migration of the lateral nasal bones without having to perform any digital manipulation.

Should the patient actually have broadening of the nasal bones near the dorsum, a medial osteotomy is performed prior to the lateral osteotomy for the purposes of removing a small channel of bone and to allow the bones to be closed to one another. This is done by inserting a saw between the upper

**A**

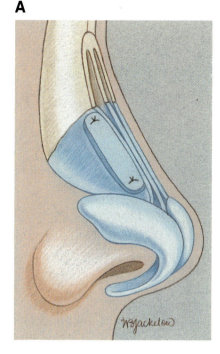

**B**

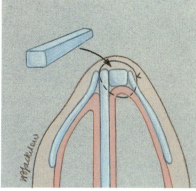

**FIG 7–20.**
When there is a depression in the upper lateral cartilage area, direct onlay grafts can be sutured directly to the upper lateral cartilage **(A).** Alternatively, a spreader graft can be inserted between the upper lateral cartilage and the septum and held there with sutures **(B).**

lateral cartilage and the cartilaginous septum (Fig 7–22). A small groove of bone is thereby removed that equals the width of the saw. Usually no more than a 1- and at most 2-mm-wide saw should be used. With the open technique, however, the actual groove that was made can be seen. After digital pressure on the nasal bones they can be seen to collapse on one another, and the groove should close. If the groove cannot actually be seen to close, then it is an indication that further manipulation, sawing,

or osteotomy needs to be performed. The point is that direct visualization of the nasal bones here gives one an appreciation of the actual width of the nose along the dorsum. Minor adjustments of the bony and cartilaginous material at the junction of the lateral nasal bone and upper lateral cartilage can also be made at this time. Although the procedure of osteotomy has been described here after the tip grafting maneuvers, it is actually best to perform this more gross procedure prior to the more delicate

**A**

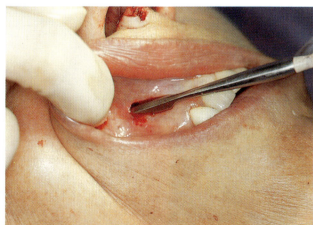

**B**

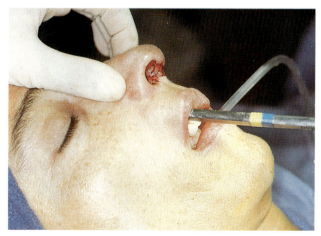

**FIG 7–21.**
A lateral osteotomy is done via the intraoral approach. A small incision is made at the cuspid tooth area **(A).** The periosteum is elevated with a Joseph periosteal elevator before the osteotome is inserted to the level of the piriform aperture **(B).**

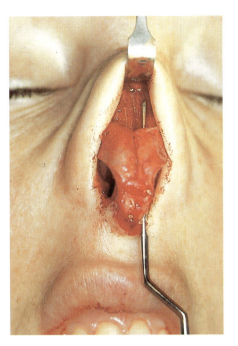

**FIG 7–22.**
When the dorsal nasal bone is broad, a medial osteotomy is done by inserting a saw between the upper lateral cartilage and septum. The groove that results will be seen to collapse after a lateral osteotomy when digital pressure is applied to the lateral bones.

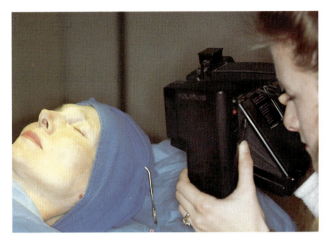

**FIG 7–23.**
Taking a Polaroid picture at the end of the procedure gives one a different perspective of the final result. The Polaroid often suggests that small adjustments should be made.

ones. Using the osteotome and saw tends to cause the sutures that have been placed in the tip cartilages to disrupt.

### Evaluating the Intraoperative Result

At this point an evaluation of the patient's result is made by returning the dorsal nasal skin. One can evaluate the length and vertical height of the nose. One can feel for irregularities externally or internally by sliding the small finger beneath the skin flap. The highest point on the nose is the tip-defining point, which is the cephalic-most edge of the dome cartilages. This point usually lies in a line that is a continuation of the light reflex along the midportion of the ala. There should be a nice, gentle break just superior to the tip-defining point. It is very helpful to take a Polaroid picture of the patient (profile view) because there are often errors in the judgement of length and height that are better appreciated in a two-dimensional view (i.e., a Polaroid) of the patient than a three-dimensional view (Fig 7–23). Small adjustments are also made to the dorsum and its angle with respect to the forehead. Minor adjustments in the length of the nose may also have to be made, which means taking down some of the sutures hold-ing the tip cartilages to the septum. Whatever it takes to give the ideal sculptured result should be done. So doing causes the operation to take longer, but it will save much time in terms of not having to come back for secondary corrections. Needless to say it will make patients much happier.

### Closing

Wounds are closed by using absorbable 5–0 and 4–0 suture for the mucoperichondrium transfixion incision, intercartilaginous incision, and rim incision wherever there is a gap seen. The external columella is closed with interrupted 6–0 nylon suture. Benzoin and half-inch adhesive tape are applied to the nose followed by a four-layer superfast plaster splint that has an extension to the forehead.

## ADJUNCTIVE PROCEDURES

### Alar Base Surgery

Alar base excisions are described in more detail in Chapter 12 and consequently will not be treated in any great detail here. Whatever specific alar base excision is performed, however, is often deferred at the time of primary open rhinoplasty. The reason for this is that in many of the cases where the nostril appears large, resection of the alar base will not be necessary when the lateral crus is transected. Reducing the lateral crus reduces the perimeter of the vestibule. This is actually evident during the rhinoplasty and eliminates the need for an alar base excision that was otherwise planned. In addition, there is often a small degree of scar contracture along the inside of the vestibule where the rim incision was made. This contributes to reduction of the perimeter of the vestibule also. In those cases, however, where a genuine width reduction is desirable (such as a flared ala), alar base resection is performed. This maneuver is performed immediately following completion of the primary open rhinoplasty. If a large resection (that extends laterally around the ala) is planned, it is deferred until the early postoperative period. That way there will not be any question as to the interference of the blood supply to the columella flap. In general, a conservative attitude to alar base resection is taken.

## Graft Materials

Cartilage grafts are harvested from either the septum, the concha, or the rib. The septum is the preferred location. The concha is the second preferred area and is removed through either the anterior or posterior approach. When neither septum or concha are available, a rib is a third choice. Either a floating rib or the leading edge of the costal margin is used. In the latter case, exposure and entry to the costal margin can be obtained by an inframammary incision (in females). If there is any question as to the location of cartilaginous rib material, an x-ray film helps to make that determination. Bone is not my personal preference for reconstructing the nose. Harvesting it is invariably more difficult, especially since most of the procedures are performed with local anesthesia. Furthermore, unless the bone has very good contact with other bone, it has a much greater chance of absorption. When it should be necessary to use bone, particularly when there are no cartilaginous sources, either a cranial bone graft is obtained, or bone from the iliac crest is used.

## Septal Surgery

Septoplasty is often performed at the time of rhinoplasty. For a more detailed discussion see Chapters 22 and 24. When a transfixion incision is made, it is certainly relatively easy to elevate the mucoperichondrium from the caudal approach. However, there is another approach that is even easier, particularly in difficult cases. The approach I am referring to is of course the dorsal approach. After the dorsal hump is removed, the mucoperichondrium can be elevated off of one if not both sides of the septal cartilage. Beginning with the septal angle, the mucoperichondrium is elevated with a relatively sharp dissector. The ordinary Freer elevator is often too blunt. This is because the dorsal 1-cm and caudal 1-cm attachments of the mucoperichondrium to the septum are quite adherent. It is actually easier to use a sharper instrument such as a Beaver knife (no. 44). The Gorney suction elevator is also quite useful. Because the exposure is so much easier from the dorsal approach, elevation of the mucoperichondrium can be done bilaterally with relative impunity. One does not have to be as concerned about mutilating the mucoperichondrial flaps or causing an overt perforation. After the flaps are elevated (Fig 7–24), one is free to score and manipulate the cartilage almost at will. Usually the central portion is removed with either a swivel knife or a button knife and an L-shaped septum is left. If the septum is crooked, a single vertical partial incision is made on one side of the horizontal limb of the L-shaped septum. In addition, the floor of the L-shaped septum is released from the vomerine groove with a button knife. The result of these two maneuvers is to allow the entire L-shaped septum to swing to a more midline position. It can be held there with a suture passed from the frenulum to the caudal edge of the L-shaped septum. The suture is then brought back out to the buccal sulcus (at the frenulum) and tied . It is the exposure that the open approach provides that makes it possible to perform septoplasty of this nature with relative ease (Fig 7–25). After completing the septoplasty, however, it is imperative to return the mucoperichondrial flaps up against the sides of the septal

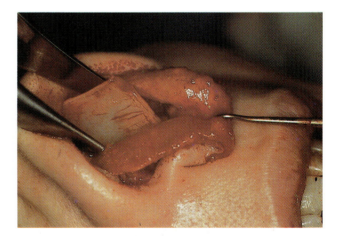

**FIG 7–24.**
Performing a septoplasty from the dorsal approach is often very helpful. The mucoperichondrium is easier to elevate from this approach, and visualization of the septum is usually superb.

**A**

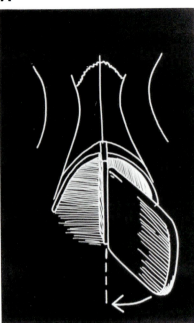

**B**

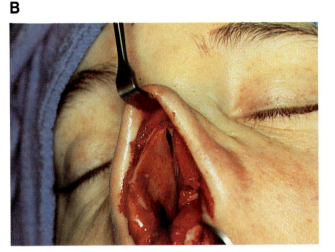

**FIG 7–25.**
After scoring the septum so that it will swing to a more midline position (**A**), it is held in its new position by passing a suture from the frenulum to the caudal part of the septum and back to the frenulum (**B**). (From Gruber RP: Open rhinoplasty. In Russell RC, editor: *Instructional courses,* St Louis, 1989, Mosby–Year Book, p 29. Used with permission.)

cartilage. Interrupted 4–0 mattress absorbable suture is used to keep the mucoperichondrial flaps in proper position. In some cases it is necessary to attach half-millimeter silicone sheeting on either side of the septum; 4–0 nylon mattress sutures will in turn hold the silicone sheeting up against the mucoperichondrium flaps. Only in exceptional cases where the maximum airway is imperative will packing be used. Patients dislike packing so much that it is avoided whenever possible. Another alternative of course is to use magnetized silicone splints.

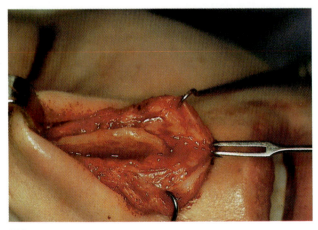

**FIG 7–26.**
Another approach to the septum is to split the medial crura. So doing avoids having to make a transfixion incision.

There is an optional method of performing the septoplasty from the open approach. This involves splitting the medial crura (Fig 7–26). This technique is also best performed with a sharp instrument such as a Beaver knife. The dissection continues by elevating the mucoperichondrium bilaterally. Thus the medial crura and mucoperichondrium are left intact as one unit. However, they are separated off the cartilaginous septum. The advantage of this technique of course is that it avoids the transfixion incision and the scar associated with it. The disadvantages to this approach are that (1) it is not possible to get the tip cartilages as far out of the way and (2) hemostasis in the region of the anterior nasal spine is a bit more difficult. Therefore, the crura-splitting technique is not my preferred approach to the septum.

## POSTOPERATIVE CARE

Each patient is seen on the first day after surgery. It is important to check the columellar flap for possible discoloration. If any is seen, the tape that goes around the nasal tip is released. This is seldom going to be the case but is more likely to occur for the beginning surgeon. A more important reason for seeing the patient early postoperatively is to reassure the patient that he is doing well and to remind him of the things that he needs to do to help wound healing. This involves (1) the application of

Neosporin or Polysporin to the nostrils twice daily; (2) continued application of ice, cold compresses, or witch hazel to the eyes; (3) reminding the patient to take his antibiotics (e.g. cephalexin [Keflex]); and (4) general instructions regarding postoperative management.

On postoperative day 6 the patient is seen again for removal of the external columellar sutures and the splint. Since the taping process was done with benzoin, it can be somewhat uncomfortable, and the patient is advised to take an analgesic 1 hour prior to the splint removal. The nose is cleaned very carefully after the splint is removed and made as presentable as possible. This is the moment when the patient gets an impression of the new nose. It can be a favorable or unfavorable impression. If it should be a favorable one, the patient will remember this experience for a long time to come. If it is an unfavorable one and the patient does not like what he sees, that too will remain for a long time to come.

The patient is presented with a mirror and given positive reassurance that the nose is doing well and will continue to do even better. In the overwhelming majority of cases that is in fact the case, and one can be quite confident in presenting the result to the patient. Since the result is usually approximately 85% of what is anticipated, that result is better than what the patient began with preoperatively. Therefore the patient usually likes what he sees. Patients are usually understanding of the fact that there is some swelling. They are usually able to extrapolate the final result. The patient is seen again a few days later to see whether any unusual swelling occurred, particularly in the supratip area. Should that be the

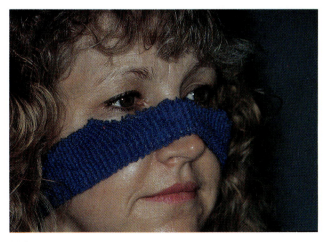

**FIG 7–27.**
A sweatband is occasionally used to reduce dorsal and supratip swelling. It should fit comfortably and be worn for 1 to 2 hours per night. Two weeks of this treatment usually suffices.

case, a sweatband (Fig 7–27) is applied. It is worn by the patient for only 1 or 2 hours in the evenings and applied only to the radix or supratip area where needed. Quite obviously it should not be so tight as to cause discomfort. One out of ten patients requires the sweatband.

At 6 weeks after surgery the patient is again evaluated. If there is persistent edema that has not resolved as fast as anticipated, corticosteroid (K-10) is injected. A dose of no more than 2.5 mg of K-10 is injected into areas such as the supratip. Usually only 1.0 mg is necessary. The solution is actually a mixture of corticosteroid and local anesthesia. Since it does cause a patient a fair amount of discomfort, it is avoided whenever possible. With patients who have thick skin or who are prone to edema, K-10 use is encouraged. These injections can be repeated every 6 weeks for several sessions, although usually not more than two or three are required in those few patients whom I so treat.

## CASE EXAMPLES

### Drooping Tip

The middle-aged male patient in Figure 7–28 had a combination of problems, one involving the airway and the other involving the appearance of his nose. In anticipation that there would be a skin draping problem and in view of the fact that a larger nose would be desirable in a male, care was taken to not overreduce the size of this nose. Preoperative drawing on the Polaroids indicated that a modest amount of dorsal reduction was necessary in addition to shortening of the nose. However, some of the shortening would be accomplished by simply rotating the tip cartilages back up into a more cephalic position. In fact, the drooping tip cartilages were in part responsible for some of the airway obstruction the patient complained of.

At surgery an external columellar incision was made. An intercartilaginous incision was made in conjunction with the transfixion incision so as to allow complete mobility of the tip cartilages. Only a small amount of cephalic lateral crus was resected and the domes were scored. The tip cartilages were secured to the caudal edge of the cartilaginous septum with a pair of 4–0 nylon sutures that went from between the medial crura to the caudal edge of the septum. In addition, dome tails were left after the cephalic portion of the lateral crus was resected. These tails were then used to secure the tip cartilages to the septum to prevent postoperative drop-

**A**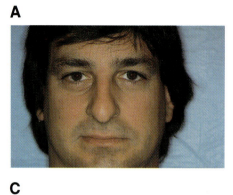

**B**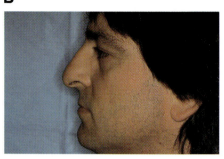

**C**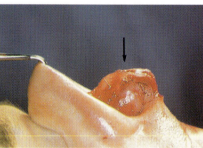

**D**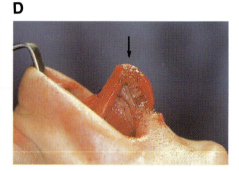

**E**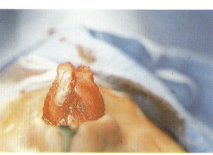

**F**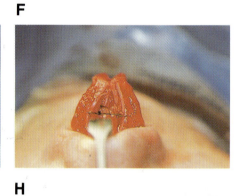

**G**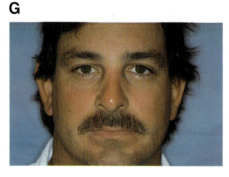

**H**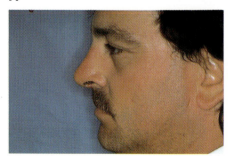

**FIG 7–28.**
This patient with a large nose also exhibited a drooping tip (**A** and **B**). A small amount of dorsum was resected. By rotating the tip cartilages (**C** and **D**) back up onto the septum and holding them in place with nylon sutures, tip projection was achieved. Note how much the dome (*arrow*) has moved as a result of this procedure. No grafting was done. "Dome tails" were preserved and sutured to the dorsal aspect of the septum to prevent recurrence of the drooped tip. A small amount of cephalic lateral crus was resected and the domes were scored. A spanning suture helped reduce the lateral crus convexity (**E** and **F**). Thirteen months postoperatively one sees an improved size of the nose without making it too small (**G** and **H**).

ping. A "spanning" suture (described by Tebbetts) that held the lateral crura to the dorsal edge of the septum also helped to secure the tip cartilages. Only a small amount of dorsum was resected, and a very small amount of the caudal edge of the septum was resected.

Septoplasty from the dorsal approach was done whereby bilateral mucoperichondrial flaps were elevated. The central portion of the septum was resected, and the resultant L-shaped septum was straightened by a single vertical scoring incision. The septum was set in the midline and held there through a single absorbable suture passed from the buccal sulcus to the caudal edge of the septum. At 13 months postoperatively one can see that the nose has not been overreduced in size but rather fits the patient's face rather well. The nasal tip no longer droops and is slightly narrower.

## Boxy Tip

The boxy tip lends itself best to the open approach because the tip cartilages are so accessible for carving and remodeling. The patient in Figure 7–29 complained of a large, bulky nasal tip. As can be seen on the preoperative view, the tip cartilages are indeed extremely broad. Through an open approach the cephalic portion of the lateral crus was resected to leave an approximately 4-mm-wide lateral crus. The lateral crus was completely transected at the most convex portion. The two elements of the lateral crus were allowed to overlap for a distance of approximately 2 to 3 mm. In this case the overlapped crus was resected and the edges repaired with nonabsorbable nylon sutures. In most patients the redundancy does not have to be resected. Because such a large segment of cephalic crus was resected, a

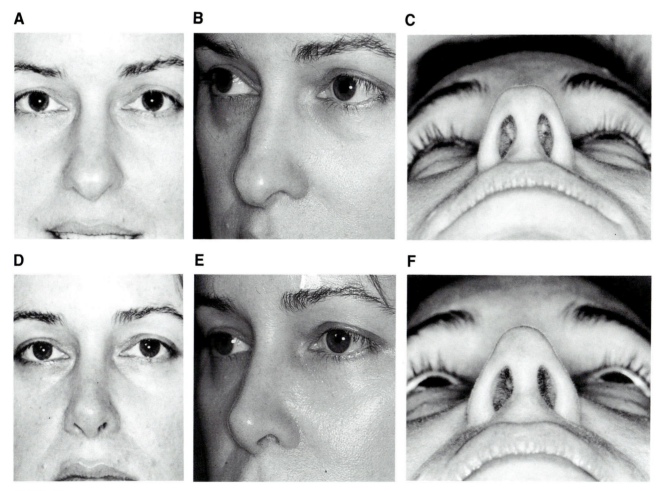

**FIG 7–29.**
This patient exhibited a boxy tip (**A –C**). At surgery the lateral crus was resected. The elements of the lateral crus were allowed to overlap, and the redundancy was resected. The elements were then suture-repaired. The resected cephalic lateral crus was trimmed, turned upside down, and put back in place. At 15 months a distinct improvement is seen (**D–F**). (From Gruber RP: Primary rhinoplasty: the open approach. In Vistnes L, editor: *Procedures in plastic and reconstructive surgery*, Boston, 1991, Little Brown, p 112. Used with permission.)

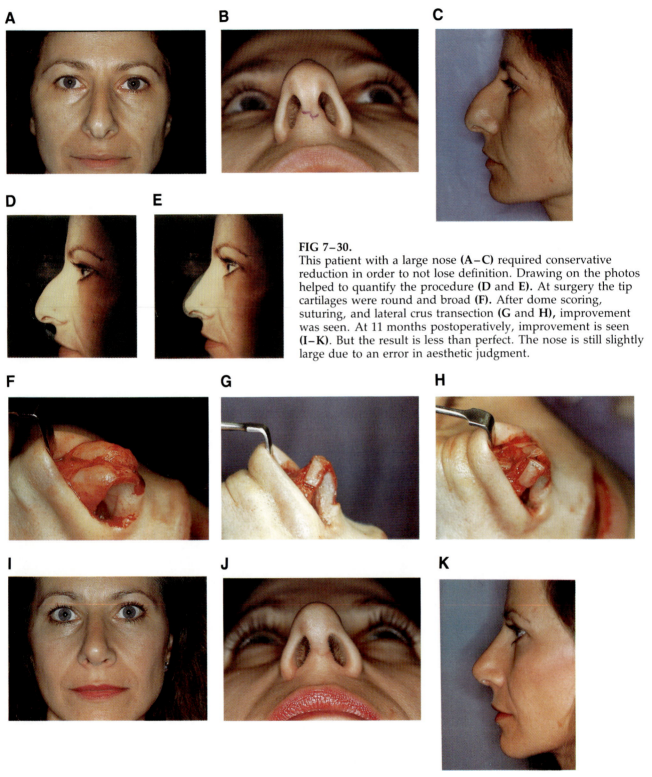

**FIG 7–30.**
This patient with a large nose **(A–C)** required conservative reduction in order to not lose definition. Drawing on the photos helped to quantify the procedure **(D and E).** At surgery the tip cartilages were round and broad **(F).** After dome scoring, suturing, and lateral crus transection **(G and H),** improvement was seen. At 11 months postoperatively, improvement is seen **(I–K).** But the result is less than perfect. The nose is still slightly large due to an error in aesthetic judgment.

small portion of it was returned to cover the area from which it had been removed. This was done by turning over the resected portion and suturing it back into place from whence it came. Through-and-through absorbable sutures to the vestibular skin were used. The usual maneuvers were performed, including scoring the dome and suturing the domes to one another as well as to the cartilaginous septum. At 14 months postoperatively one sees significant improvement in the appearance of the boxy tip. On basal view the columellar scar is barely noticeable.

## UNSATISFACTORY RESULTS

Not all results can be excellent. The patient in Figure 7–30 complained of a large nose. Preoperative drawings helped determine the amount of reduction required. At surgery the tip cartilages were round and broad. The patient received hump removal, shortening, and lateral osteotomies. The lateral crus was cephacillically trimmed and transected. The domes were scored. The tips were sutured to each other (in the cephalic aspect). The improvement is seen postoperatively at 11 months. By keeping it on the large side of the normal range it was possible to maintain some definition. Unfortunately, the nose was simply not made small enough. It was an error in aesthetic judgment.

### Lack of Definition

One of the problems with any approach, particularly the open approach, is a lack of definition at the cartilaginous tip. Part of this is due to the fact that there is extra surgery that is followed by scar tissue. Despite the fact that care is taken to carve the cartilages to the best possible shape, scar tissue can obliterate some of the final result.

A lack of definition (loss of faceting) is particularly noticeable in the patient in Figure 7–31. This is due to the scar tissue filling in the area between the rim of the lower lateral cartilages and the nasal skin. Of interest is the fact that the vestibule is much smaller postoperatively than it was preoperatively despite the fact that alar base excision was not performed. This is due in large part to the transection of the lateral crus at its most convex point, and also due to the fact that the rim incision itself leaves a scar that contracts slightly. Prevention of the problem of definition and faceting loss might have been accomplished by not making the nose as small. The skin sleeve would have been able to accommodate better to a larger cartilaginous-bony framework. No treatment was rendered because the patient was in fact pleased, the problem relatively minor and not very correctable.

### Asymmetry

Even when great care is taken to achieve symmetry of the tip cartilages intraoperatively, asymmetry can develop. In Figure 7–32 we see an example of a patient who underwent a primary open rhinoplasty.

**A**

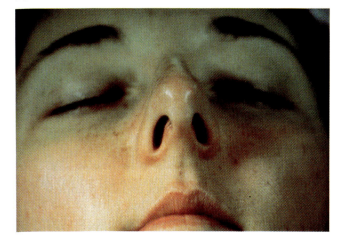

**B**

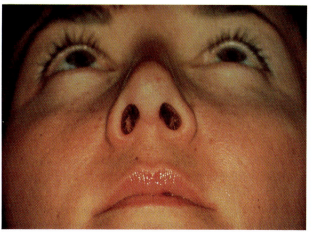

**FIG 7–31.**
Despite the best of sculpturing, scar tissue can blunt the facets of the nasal tip. **A,** preoperatively; **B,** postoperatively. (**B** from Gruber RP: Rhinoplasty and open rhinoplasty. In Peck GC, editor: *Complications and problems in aesthetic plastic surgery,* New York, 1992, Gower, p 2.26. Used with permission.)

ten required for proper support and contour. Two primary types of tip grafts have been proposed, the triangular or shield-shaped graft, based at the level of the nostril-lobular junction and extending to the proper level of tip projection,[10, 15] and the rectangular graft, placed transversely at the level of proper tip projection.[11, 12] In the triangular or shield design, contour is determined by the graft length and support by the graft thickness (or a number of grafts stacked one in front of another). In the rectangular design, contour is provided by the position and number of transverse grafts; support must be provided by a so-called "umbrella graft"[12] composed of a columellar strut for support and a transverse piece for tip contour.

Too much fuss is made, I believe, by surgeons who profess loyalty to one design or another as if the issue were really loyalty to political party or country. Each graft design accomplishes the same ends. Whether a surgeon uses triangular grafts and controls support by graft number and contour by graft pliability and placement, or prefers a rectangular graft and controls support by umbrella struts and contour by lobular underfill is unimportant. What is important is to select a graft design and learn to employ it skillfully.

I prefer the shield-shaped graft,[15] as taught to me by Jack Sheen, which I use essentially without modifications. Over the years, I have learned how to solve an increasing range of nasal tip problems with these grafts by altering either graft number, size, or

consistency, but tip grafting is not an easy technique and requires much patience and practice. It is not for the surgeon who wishes to perform a 20-minute rhinoplasty.

The specifics of graft design and placement in each patient depend upon the circumstances: preoperative tip lobular configuration, soft-tissue volume and thickness, the number of prior surgeries, the resiliency and expandability of the lobular pocket, and most importantly, the patient's preferred tip configuration. At one extreme is the hypoplastic tip lobule or the lobule scarred by multiple prior rhinoplasties. Regardless of the details of the patient's preferred tip configuration, this type of tip requires some solid grafts to expand the lobule and support the tip; other grafts can be placed anterior to the original grafts for additional support and contour. Depending upon the patient's desires and the pliancy of the soft tissues, these additional grafts may need to be crushed or solid (Fig 8–6).

At the other end of the spectrum is the preoperative lobule in a thin-skinned patient that requires grafting for contour but little or no additional support; this circumstance requires mostly crushed cartilage grafts because solid grafts will appear artificially visible and provide too much support. However, crushed grafts alone are very difficult to place and require much patience on the surgeon's part; each subsequent graft tends to displace its predecessors (Fig 8–7).

The surgeon learning to place tip grafts will find

**A**    **B**

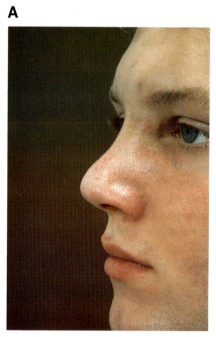
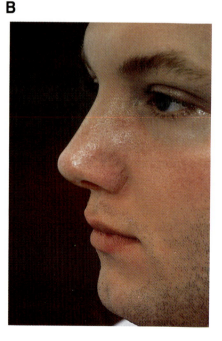

**FIG 8–6.**
Following three operations, this tertiary rhinoplasty patient had bilateral airway obstruction from septal deflection and internal valvular collapse, columellar retraction, and supratip deformity. Reconstruction involved septoplasty for airway and graft material, dorsal grafts of septal cartilage and bone, columellar grafts, and multiple solid and crushed cartilage tip grafts with an ethmoid buttress. **A,** preoperative oblique view. **B,** postoperative oblique view.

**A**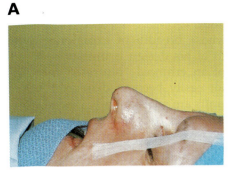

**B**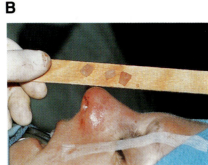

**C**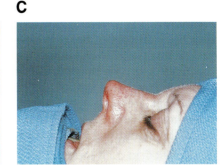

**D**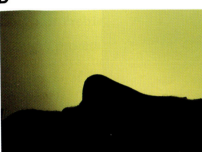

**E**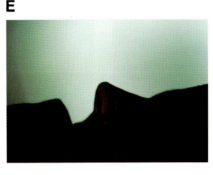

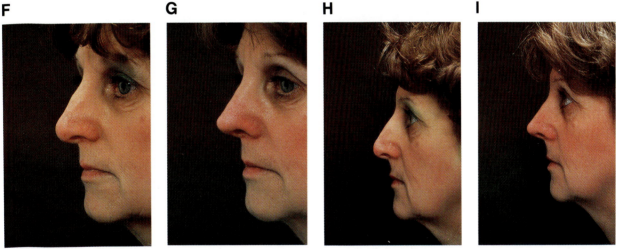

**FIG 8–7.**
Effect of tip grafts on nasal base size. **A,** immediate preoperative view. **B,** following dorsal reduction. Crushed tip grafts are shown. **C,** immediate postoperative view. **D,** preoperative silhouette. **E,** immediate postoperative silhouette showing the effect on nasal balance. **F,** preoperative right oblique view. **G,** 14-month postoperative right oblique view. **H,** preoperative lateral view. **I,** 14-month postoperative lateral view.

it easiest to place one, uncrushed trial graft to help judge graft length and the necessity for other grafts anteriorly or posteriorly. Like many techniques in plastic surgery, exact dimensions cannot be given because they depend upon the circumstances and the peculiarities of the individual anatomy. Essentially, the longest graft should extend from the level of the nostril-lobular junction to the proper level of the most projecting part of the tip (i.e., where it

should be, not necessarily where it is preoperatively). The cephalic edge of the graft should not be visible or blanch the skin, but it must not be so short that the graft does not provide proper tip support or tends to rotate and slip. Once this graft is sized and placed, additional grafts, either thinner or lightly crushed, can be placed anteriorly to round the tip lobule, or other pieces (cartilage or even bone) can be placed posterior to the main graft for additional

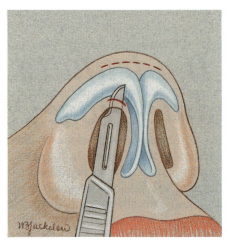

**FIG 9–1.**
Infracartilaginous incision for an onlay graft.

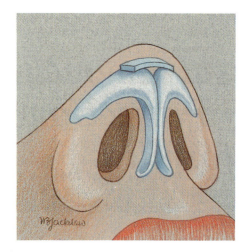

**FIG 9–3.**
The onlay graft.

graft is secured in a straight clamp and placed in the horizontal pocket (Fig 9–3). After augmenting the nasal tip with at least two grafts of lower lateral cartilage or conchal cartilage graft, the surgeon should then reevaluate tip projection. Further augmentation of the nasal tip can be accomplished with more cartilage grafts (Fig 9–4).

The horizontal pocket over the alar domes maintains the position of the cartilage graft(s). The pocket should be only as large as the graft to prevent its movement or displacement. In position, the graft will add projection to the nasal tip and rest on the alar domes with little stress or tension. Suturing the cartilage grafts in the pocket is rarely required.

The surgeon has easily accessible autogenous cartilage to augment and enhance the nasal tip, with very little morbidity. Complications of cartilage

grafting to the nasal tip are infrequent. Extrusion, infection, and graft loss due to absorption are rare. The most common problems we see in our practice are hyperemia and cartilage exposure. Hyperemia may occur in the nasal skin overlying a cartilage graft; it may last up to 2 years but usually resolves with time. Camouflage cosmetics temporarily solve the problem. Cartilage grafts showing through the nasal skin are more common in patients with thin skin. The surgeon can reduce the incidence of this problem by meticulously beveling the edges of the cartilage graft. If necessary, a small secondary procedure may be performed to shave the problem area of the graft. Malposition of the cartilage graft can occur with an improperly designed pocket, movement of the graft, and cartilage graft warp. These problems can be minimized by making a pocket the exact size of the graft and securing the position of the graft

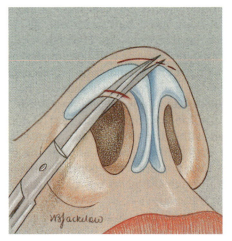

**FIG 9–2.**
Dissection of horizontal pocket.

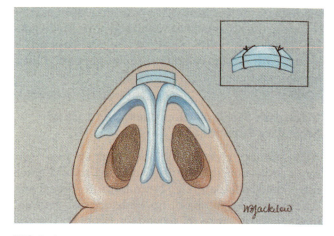

**FIG 9–4.**
Placement of two onlay grafts for nasal tip projection.

with plastic strip bandages for 5 days postoperatively. In general, the benefits gained by nasal augmentation with cartilage grafts significantly outweigh any disadvantages.

## Clinical Case: Onlay Graft

This patient presented to our office for a primary rhinoplasty. She has a wide nasal bridge, an undefined nasal tip, and a wide alar base. In profile she has a slight dorsal hump and inadequate tip projec-

tion. She has a long nose, mild microgenia, and neck lipodystrophy (Fig 9–5,A–C).

Intraoperatively we sculptured the patient's bilateral lower lateral cartilages, rasped the dorsum, and lowered the dorsal aspect of the septum. The nasal bones were infractured and the caudal edge of the septum lowered. A modified Weir resection of the alar bone was performed as well as chin augmentation and suction-assisted lipectomy of the neck. Two onlay grafts of lower lateral cartilage were placed to enhance tip projection.

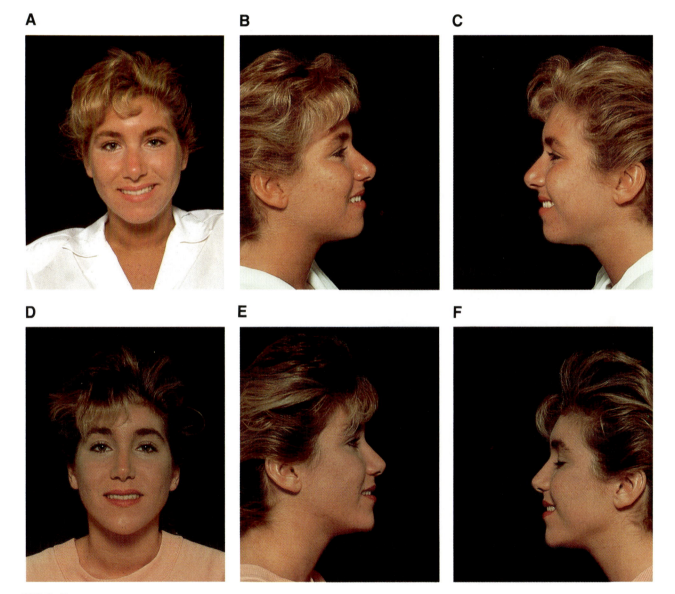

**FIG 9–5.**
Onlay graft. **A,** preoperative frontal view: wide nasal bridge, undefined nasal tip. **B,** preoperative lateral: long nose. **C,** preoperative lateral: slightly drooping tip. **D,** postoperative frontal: narrower bridge and more defined nasal tip. **E,** postoperative lateral: appropriate nasal length and nasolabial angle. **F,** postoperative lateral: adequate tip projection with two onlay grafts.

Postoperatively the patient has improved definition of the nasal bridge and nasal tip. Her profile is more balanced with an appropriate dorsal line, a small chin augmentation, and a better jawline and neckline (Fig 9–5,D–F).

## UMBRELLA GRAFT FOR AUGMENTATION OF NASAL TIP PROJECTION

The umbrella graft is an outstanding technique to augment nasal tip projection. The umbrella graft is composed of a vertical strut of cartilage placed between the medial crura, combined with a horizontal onlay graft (Fig 9–6). The main indication for an umbrella graft is inadequate tip projection with inadequate septal support. Other indications include a drooping nasal tip and a thick-skinned nasal tip.

### Surgical Technique

To harvest conchal cartilage grafts, a posterior auricular incision is made in the right ear. The conchal cartilage is then exposed by using sharp dissection. The straightest segment of the cartilage, approximately 3 cm × 6 mm, is selected as the donor site for the strut of the umbrella graft. The onlay graft measuring approximately 4 × 9 mm is also taken from the conchal cartilage but from an area that has a convex shape needed to simulate the shape of the nasal tip. After harvesting the grafts, the surgeon obtains hemostasis with electrocautery and closes the incision with a running 3–0 plain gut suture. The umbrella graft is now ready for insertion; however, each graft will be placed into a separate and distinct pocket.

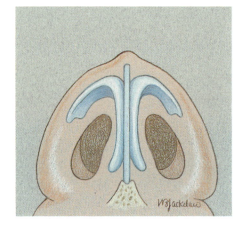

**FIG 9–7.**
Vertical strut between the medial crura.

An infracartilaginous incision is made in the right side of the columella. Using Peck-Joseph scissors, the surgeon develops a vertical pocket between the medial crura from the nasal spine to the nasal tip. The strut of conchal cartilage (3 cm × 6 mm) is placed into this vertical pocket and extended beyond the alar domes (Fig 9–7). The incision is closed with interrupted 5–0 nylon sutures.

A second infracartilaginous incision is made on the right side of the alar dome. This is a stab incision. Peck-Joseph Scissors are used to develop a horizontal pocket over the alar domes. The convex onlay graft (4 × 9 mm) is then placed in this horizontal pocket (see Fig 9–6). If the strut were to stand alone under the skin, it would create a very sharp-pointed nasal tip. For this reason, the vertical strut is covered by an onlay tip graft (Fig 9–8). Multiple onlay grafts may be placed in this horizontal pocket to obtain the appropriate tip projection. The stab incision

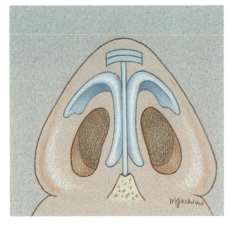

**FIG 9–6.**
The umbrella graft.

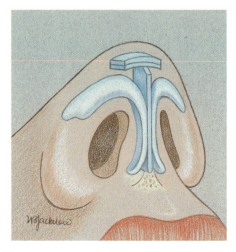

**FIG 9–8.**
Oblique view of the umbrella graft.

does not need to be sutured. Instead, the surgeon places packing intranasally to maintain the coadaptation of the vestibular skin. This packing is removed after 24 hours. A standard rhinoplasty dressing is applied by using plastic strip bandages to secure graft position. A splint is applied only if nasal infracturing is performed. The nasal dressing is removed in 5 days.

### Clinical Case: Nasal Reconstruction

This patient presented to our office for a secondary rhinoplasty. She has a nasal tip deformity, a mild saddle deformity, inadequate tip projection, and a retracted columella (Fig 9–9,A–D).

Intraoperatively we reconstructed the patient's nose with an umbrella graft, three onlay grafts, and a dorsal hull-shaped graft from conchal cartilage. The columella was reconstructed with two rectangular grafts to the posterior two thirds and a triangular graft to the anterior third of the columella.

The patient has a satisfactory result with a more natural appearance. Her profile has an appropriate dorsal line and better tip projection. The reconstructed columella enhances the balance of her profile (Fig 9–9,E–H).

## SADDLE-NOSE DEFORMITY

The most common cause of a saddle deformity is iatrogenic. Other common causes are trauma and

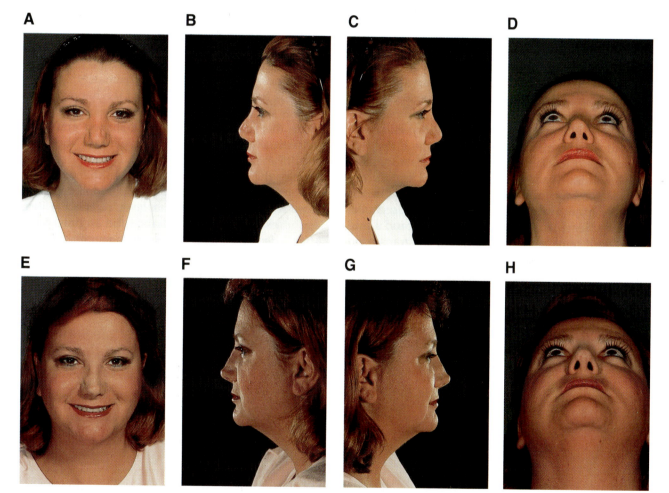

**FIG 9–9.**
Nasal reconstruction. **A,** preoperative frontal view: nasal tip deformity. **B,** preoperative lateral: slight saddle deformity, inadequate tip projection. **C,** preoperative lateral: supratip fullness, short nasal length. **D,** preoperative worm's eye: inadequate tip projection. **E,** postoperative frontal: nasal tip reconstruction with an umbrella graft. **F,** postoperative lateral: reconstruction of the dorsum with a dorsal hull-shaped conchal cartilage graft. **G,** postoperative lateral: reconstruction of the nasal tip with an umbrella graft and two rectangular cartilage grafts. **H,** postoperative worm's eye: appropriate tip projection.

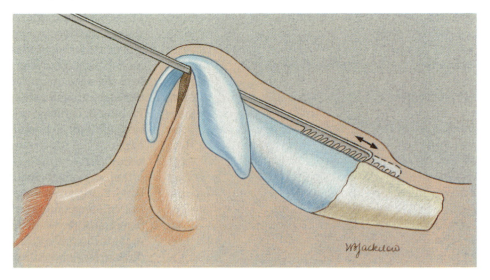

**FIG 9–14.**
Placement of the bone graft.

The graft should be long enough to provide a cantilevering effect to the nasal tip pyramid complex (Fig 9–14). We usually take a graft 4 cm in length. The graft should not project into the nasal tip.

Very small dorsal irregularities or depressions may develop postoperatively. If necessary, the depressions can easily be corrected with very thin shavings of conchal cartilage. An external excision is made in a skin crease in proximity to the depression. The shavings are placed in a small pocket. This incision rarely leaves a noticeable scar. Another complication after iliac bone grafting is pain over the affected hip and difficulty walking. In our experience, the postoperative morbidity does not preclude the use of an iliac bone graft.

## Clinical Case: Saddle Deformity

This patient presented for a secondary rhinoplasty with a moderate saddle deformity and a pinched nasal tip (Fig 9–15,A–C). We used an iliac bone graft to reconstruct the nasal dorsum. An onlay graft to the nasal tip and a triangular graft to the anterior third of the columella was also performed. Postoperatively the patient has a more natural dorsal line and nasal tip (Fig 9–15,D–F).

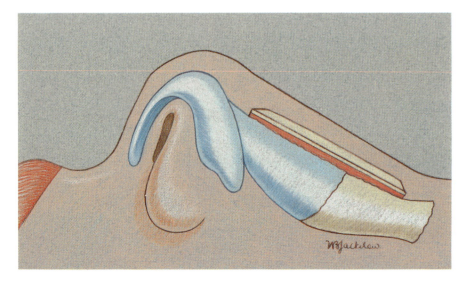

**FIG 9–13.**
Rasping the nasal bone to create a raw surface.

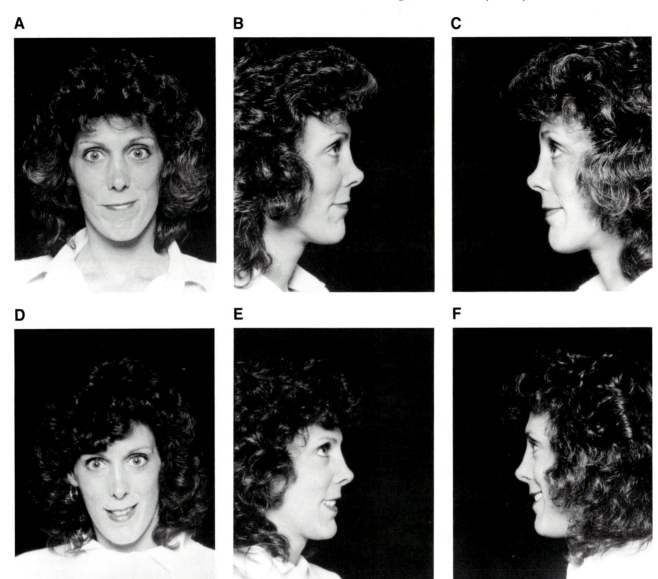

**FIG 9–15.**
Saddle deformity. **A,** preoperative frontal view: pinched nasal tip. **B** and **C,** preoperative lateral: saddle deformity. **D,** postoperative lateral: reconstruction of the nasal tip with cartilage grafts. **E,** postoperative lateral: reconstruction of the dorsum with an iliac bone graft. **F,** postoperative lateral.

## REFERENCES

1. Meyer R: *Secondary and functional rhinoplasty: The difficult nose*, Philadelphia, 1988, Grune & Stratton.
2. Meyer R; Kesselring U: Sculpturing and reconstructive procedures in aesthetic and functional rhinoplasty, *Clin Plast Surg* 4:15, 1977.
3. Peck GC (ed): Rhinoplasty, in *Clinics in plastic surgery*, Philadelphia, 1988, WB Sanders.
4. Peck GC: Aesthetic rhinoplasty of the nasal tip, in Regnault P, Daniel RK (eds): *Aesthetic plastic surgery*, Boston, 1984, Little Brown.
5. Peck GC: Aesthetic rhinoplasty, in Grabb WC, Smith JW(eds): *Plastic surgery*, ed 3, Boston, 1979, Little Brown.

**A**

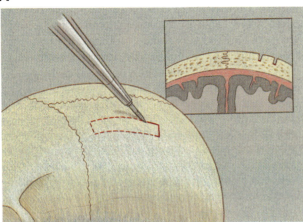

**B**

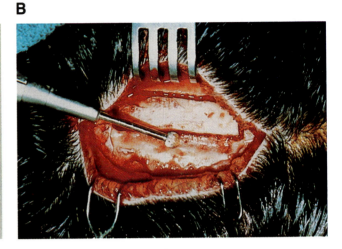

**C**

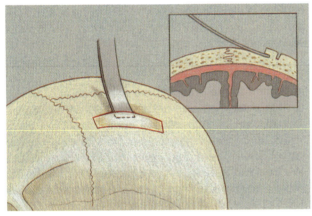

**FIG 10–3.**
Harvesting of split calvarial grafts. **A,** a side-cutting fissure burr is used to outline the bone graft and gauge the depth of the diploic space. **B,** a trough is cut with a pear-shaped burr to permit tangential introduction of the osteotome into the diploic space. **C,** removal of bone graft with a thin sharp osteotome directed tangential to the surface of the cranium.

loë. Continuous irrigation is essential to prevent burning the bone through friction from the burr. Once the proper level is encountered on all sides of the graft, an osteotome or large pear-shaped burr is used to cut a trough along the entire length of one side of the graft (see Fig 10–3). This trough allows the surgeon to introduce an osteotome in the correct manner for graft harvesting, that is, the osteotome is always introduced in a direction tangential to the calvarium. The osteotome is gradually worked into the diploic space, between the inner and outer table, by using a series of short, controlled taps. A sharp, thin osteotome is a prerequisite for successful graft harvesting. *It is of paramount importance to always keep the osteotome directed tangential to the skull at all times to prevent "plunging through the inner table"* (see Fig 10–3). If a second strip of bone is required, it is usually easier to harvest the second graft because the diploic space is well defined following harvesting of the first bone graft strip. Bone wax is used for hemo-

stasis along the donor site, and the wound is closed in layers. The use of a drain is optional.

The key to successful cranial bone graft harvesting is accurate delineation of the level of the diploic space. When first learning to harvest cranial bone grafts, the tendency is to be so concerned about violating the inner table that the graft is harvested superficial to the diploic space. This usually leads to splintering of the bone graft and harvesting an unsuitable piece of bone that cannot be used for dorsal augmentation. Careful delineation of the level of the diploic space with the use of a side-cutting burr along the entire periphery of the graft is essential. Following this, constructing a trough along one edge of the graft will clearly demonstrate the level of the diploic space and help ensure that the graft is harvested at the proper level between the inner and outer tables.

Another technical point to keep in mind when harvesting cranial bone is to be very patient and let the osteotome do the work of harvesting. Attempts at hurrying graft harvesting or levering up on the osteotome will usually lead to graft splintering and the need to harvest a second piece of bone. Also, great force is not required to harvest cranial bone grafts. If one is using a sharp osteotome, the amount of force required to gradually introduce the osteotome between the inner and outer tables is comparable to the force required to perform nasal osteotomy.

## Shaping the Graft

In most cases, the piece harvested will be fairly straight, unmalleable, and rectangular. The graft must be shaped to produce the desired contour. In general, we prefer a graft of fairly uniform and moderate width that gradually tapers as it descends toward the nasal tip. A hand-held burr is used to shape the graft, and continuous irrigation is necessary to protect the bone. After obtaining the proper shape along the dorsal surface of the implant, the undersurface is smoothed to allow the graft to sit within the recipient site in a stable fashion and prevent any rocking. The length and width of the graft will obviously vary from patient to patient, although most commonly measures approximately 1 cm in width and 3.5 to 4.0 cm in length (Fig 10–4).

If the nasal bone base is severely deficient, a multiple-tier graft may be required to provide adequate projection. Either this layered bone can be inserted individually, or preferably, the grafts are

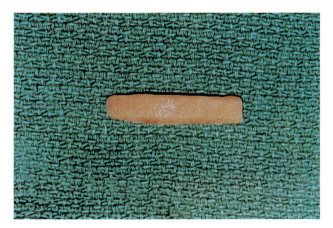

**FIG 10–4.**
A hand-held burr is used to shape the bone graft. In general, we prefer a graft of fairly uniform and moderate width that gradually tapers as it descends toward the nasal tip. The perimeter of the bone graft is beveled to prevent any sharp noticeable edges following graft insertion.

wired together and inserted as a single implant. If the graft is to be used as a cantilever, a fulcrum of bone must be fixated along the undersurface of the principal dorsal graft. This fulcrum should extend from the radix to the caudal border of the remaining nasal bone.

## Recipient Site Preparation

The recipient site is prepared by dissecting a precise pocket. The plane of dissection remains close to the nasal cartilages and subperiosteally along the nasal bones. Soft tissue is a surgeon's friend. As much of it as possible should be preserved to protect the graft.

Since bone-to-bone contact is a prerequisite for successful bone grafting, the periosteum of the remaining nasal bones must be reflected prior to graft insertion. The dissection is continued cephalad past the frontonasal angle so that the implant can clear the insertion site and then be manipulated retrogradely toward the nasal tip. It is helpful to smooth any irregularities present along the nasal dorsum with a rasp prior to graft insertion.

The bone graft can be inserted via many routes. We commonly use an intercartilaginous incision for graft insertion. Bilateral incisions are helpful in obtaining symmetrical mobilization of soft tissues and better access for manipulating the graft during placement. Bone grafts are most easily inserted via a transcolumellar open rhinoplasty technique, and this is our preferred approach when cranial bone grafting is performed in conjunction with cartilaginous grafting of the nasal tip.[3]

## Graft Immobilization

The prerequisite for successful bone grafting anywhere in the body is bone-to-bone contact followed by immobilization. Immobilization of the graft is essential to achieve rapid consolidation, attain bone graft revascularization, and minimize the tendencies to postoperative malposition or graft resorption. Graft immobilization is also essential when attempting to lengthen the nose or provide a cantilever support to the nasal tip. Many methods of immobilization are available, including interosseous wires or the use of miniscrew fixation. While each method has its advantages, our preference for immobilizing most of our cranial bone grafts is through the use of two 0.035-in. K-wires. The K-wires are placed percutaneously through the graft into the underlying na-

**A**

**B**

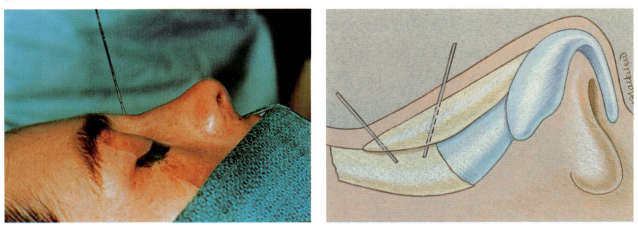

**FIG 10–5.**
The bone graft is immobilized through the use of K-wires percutaneously placed through the bone graft into the underlying nasal bones. Two wires are necessary. The first K-wire is placed to ensure that the graft is immobilized along the midline of the nasal dorsum. The second K-wire is necessary to prevent the graft from rotating either to the right or the left in the postoperative period.

sal bones. The first K-wire is placed to ensure that the graft is immobilized along the midline of the nasal dorsum. The second K-wire is necessary to prevent the bone graft from rotating either to the right or the left in the postoperative period (Fig 10–5). Following proper K-wire placement, the K-wires are cut short directly beneath the skin of the nose and remain in place for 3 to 4 weeks. These wires are then easily removed as an office procedure with local anesthesia[7] (Fig 10–6).

## Columellar Strut

A columellar strut is useful in the patient with a deficiency of caudal septum, a retracted columella, and a poorly projecting tip. The shape of the columella graft is that of an elongated rectangle, although it is thinner and shorter in length from what is used for the dorsal graft. These grafts commonly measure approximately 6 mm in width and between 18 and 25 mm in length. When a cranial bone graft is used to

**A**

**B**

**FIG 10–6.**
**A,** patient with iatrogenic collapse of cartilagenous septal support secondary to a previous septoplasty. Note the loss of cartilagenous support in the region of the dorsal part of the septum, as well as loss of caudal support with resulting columellar retraction and a plunging nasal tip. **B,** postoperative result following dorsal reconstruction with the use of a single strip of cranial bone. The retracted columella and support for the nasal tip were reconstructed with the use of a columellar strut of cranial bone placed through an intraoral incision.

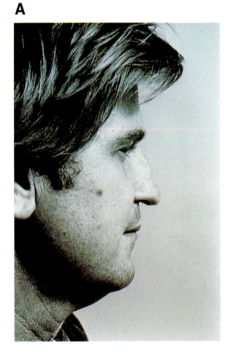

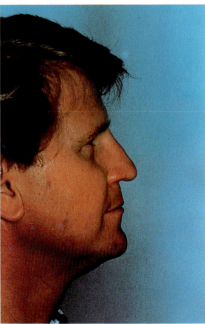

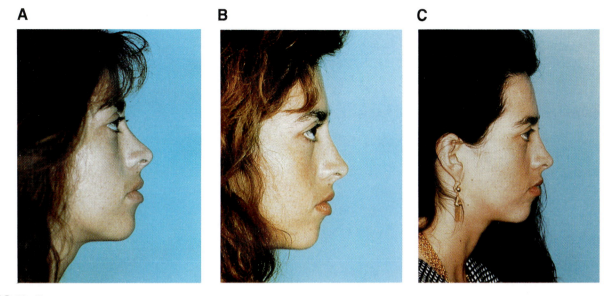

**FIG 10–7.**
**A,** preoperative appearance of iatrogenic saddle nose deformity. **B,** 6-month postoperative result following dorsal reconstruction with a single strip of cranial bone. **C,** 2-year postoperative result. Note essentially no resorption seen in the intervening period following dorsal reconstruction using cranial bone grafting.

augment the caudal port of the septum, our preference is to insert the graft through an intraoral incision. The anterior nasal spine is identified, and a pocket is made within the membranous septum. The graft is then placed into the nasal tip and can support the dorsal graft if required. We then prefer to secure the columellar strut securely to the maxilla in the region of the anterior nasal spine. If the anterior nasal spine is present, a "V"-shaped wedge of bone is removed from the base of the strut to allow a secure fit between the nasal spine and graft. If the spine is not present, the base of the graft is burred so that it is flush with the maxilla and will not rock or shift. The graft is then immobilized with either interosseous wires or miniscrews. Augmentation of the premaxilla with chips of cranial bone can then be performed if contouring in this region is required (see Fig 10–6).

### Postoperative Management

A dressing similar to that used in rhinoplasty is applied. Perioperative antibiotic administration is recommended. Light nasal packing is usually left in place for 24 hours.

In most of our patients the cast is removed at 1 week, and the area where the K-wires have been inserted along the nasal dorsum is managed with the use of topical antibiotic ointment and a small plastic strip bandage. These patients usually return some-where between 3 and 4 weeks following the procedure for removal of the percutaneously placed Kirschner wires.

### CONCLUSION

One of the great advantages of the use of cranial bone is that it is a membranous bone and theoretically exhibits less tendency to postoperative resorption when grafted within the craniofacial skeleton.[10] In our opinion, much of the problem seen with the use of cranial bone grafting has been when the cranial bones are not properly immobilized. In the serial follow-up of our patients who have undergone cranial bone grafting of the nasal dorsum, we have seen very little graft resorption when the principles discussed in this chapter have been applied (Fig 10–7). The key to the successful use of cranial bone grafting in these patients is a proper analysis of the deformity such that the reconstructive effort is precisely planned and executed. In our experience, these patients have been uniformly satisfied with the dorsal reconstruction, and there has been little need for later revisions following cranial bone grafting for the treatment of saddle nose deformity in secondary rhinoplasty patients (Fig 10–8).

**A**

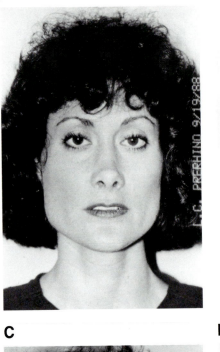

**B**

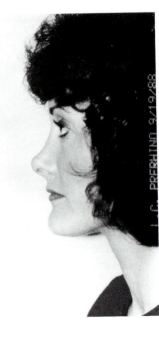

**C**

**D**

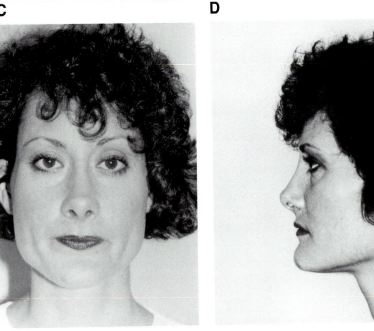

**FIG 10–8.**
**A** and **B,** preoperative appearance of a patient with iatrogenic saddle nose deformity. **C** and **D,** postoperative appearance following dorsal reconstruction with a single strip of cranial bone.

## REFERENCES

1. Converse J: Saddle noses, noses with a depressed dorsum, and flat noses. In Converse J, editor: *Reconstructive plastic surgery,* Philadelphia, 1977, Saunders, p 1135.
2. Craft PD, Sargent LA: Membranous bone healing and techniques in calvarial bone grafting, *Clin Plast Surg* 16:11, 1989.
3. Gruber RP: Open rhinoplasty, *Clin Plast Surg* 15:95, 1988.
4. Jackson LT, Smith J, Mixter RC: Nasal bone grafting using split skull grafts, *Ann Plast Surg* 11:533, 1983.
5. Posnick JC, Seagle MB, Armstrong D: Nasal reconstruction with full-thickness cranial bone grafts and rigid internal fixation through a coronal incision, *Plast Reconstr Surg* 86:894, 1990.

6. Sheen J: Cranial bone graft. In *Aesthetic rhinoplasty*, vol 1, ed 2, St Louis, 1987, Mosby–Year Book. p 383.

7. Stuzin JM, Kawamoto HK: Saddle nasal deformity, *Clin Plast Surg* 15:83, 1988.

8. Tessier P: Aesthetic aspects of bone grafting to the face, *Clin Plast Surg* 8:279, 1981.

9. Tessier P: Autogenous bone grafts taken from the calvarium for facial and cranial application, *Clin Plast Surg* 9:531, 1982.

10. Zins LE, Whitaker LA: Membranous versus endochondral bone: Implications for craniofacial reconstruction, *Plast Reconstr Surg* 72:778, 1983.

crosscutting and weakening the alar domes, the angle between the medial and lateral crura is narrowed.

## Clinical Case 1

This patient is a 19-year-old woman who presented to our office with a broad nasal tip and a long nose (Fig 11–2,A–C). The patient underwent sculpturing of the lower lateral cartilages and crosscutting of the alar domes to narrow the nasal tip. Elevation of the posterior two thirds of the columella and rotation of the tip were performed. The nasal bones were infractured, and a slight dorsal hump was appropriately reduced. Postoperatively, the patient has a defined nasal tip in balance with her nasal bridge (Fig 11–2,D–F).

## EXTREMELY BROAD TIP

Sculpturing the lower lateral cartilages and crosscutting the alar domes may not achieve the desired im-

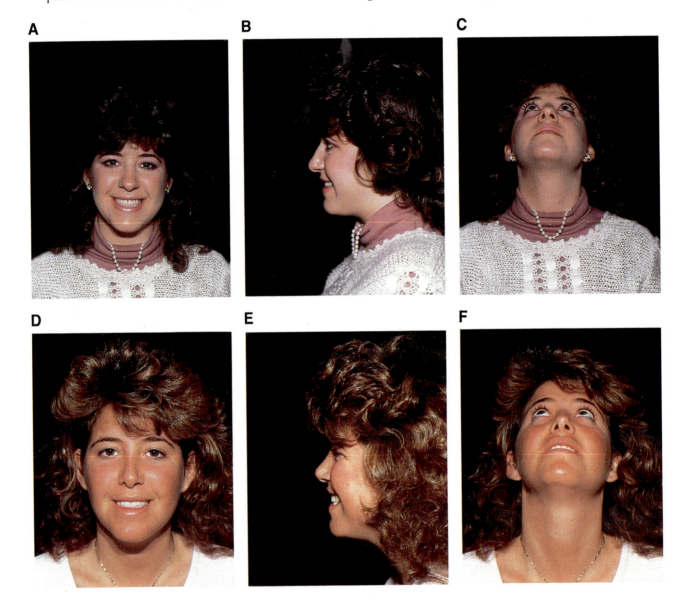

**FIG 11–2.**
**A,** a smiling preoperative frontal view shows a minimally broad nasal tip. **B,** a smiling preoperative left lateral view shows a long nose, a slight dorsal hump, and an inappropriate nasolabial angle. **C,** a preoperative worm's eye view reveals a broad nasal tip. **D,** a smiling postoperative frontal view shows a narrow bridge with a defined nasal tip. **E,** a smiling postoperative left lateral view shows an appropriate dorsal line and nasolabial angle. **F,** a postoperative worm's eye view reveals a more defined nasal tip pyramid.

provement in the patient with an extremely broad tip. For such a patient we use the lateral rotation technique. In all patients, we always begin by sculpting the lower lateral cartilages; then we evaluate our results. If additional narrowing is necessary, we proceed with the crosscutting technique and again reevaluate the results. If further improvement is necessary, we use the lateral rotation technique.

### Lateral Rotation Technique

Through the intracartilaginous incision the surgeon delivers the lower lateral cartilage. The crosscutting technique is performed at the level of the alar dome. A section of lower lateral cartilage is then excised from the lateral-most portion of the lateral crura (Fig 11–3). The lower lateral cartilage is rotated laterally and placed back in its bed (Fig 11–4). The nasal tip is tape-splinted to maintain and secure this position. The lateral rotation technique narrows the width of the nasal tip (Fig 11–5).

### Clinical Case 2

This patient is a 28-year-old female who has an extremely broad nasal tip as well as a wide bridge, long nose, slight dorsal hump, and an inappropriate nasolabial angle (Fig 11–6,A–C). A primary rhinoplasty was performed, including sculpturing of the lower lateral cartilages, shortening and elevating the nasal tip, rasping the dorsum, and lowering the supratip cartilage. The nasal bones were infractured, and two onlays from the lower lateral cartilage were placed over the alar domes. An alar base reduction was performed by using the modified Weir technique. At this point, the nasal tip was reevaluated. The crosscutting and lateral rotation technique were used to narrow the na-

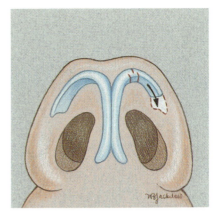

**FIG 11–4.**
Excision of the lateral-most portion of the lower lateral cartilage and lateral rotation of the cartilage.

sal tip. A small chin implant was also inserted. Postoperatively, the patient has appropriate facial lines with a more defined nasal tip (Fig 11–6,D–F).

## THE THICK-SKINNED NOSE

The patient with thick, heavy, sebaceous skin is a difficult problem since this type of skin will not contract around modified cartilage structures on the nasal tip pyramid. A reduction rhinoplasty will not substantially reduce the nasal tip. These patients should be well informed about the realistic expectations of surgery.

Many patients with a thick-skinned nasal tip also have inadequate tip projection. In these patients we perform a routine rhinoplasty and assess tip projection. Inadequate tip projection is treated with an umbrella graft. The horizontal onlay graft should be shorter (less than 9 mm) because of the thick skin.

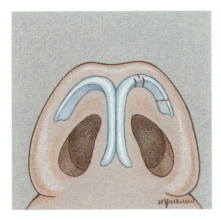

**FIG 11–3.**
Crosscutting technique and area of lower lateral cartilage to be excised.

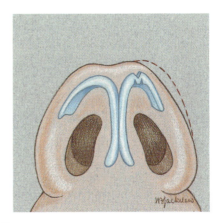

**FIG 11–5.**
The expected result of the lateral rotation technique.

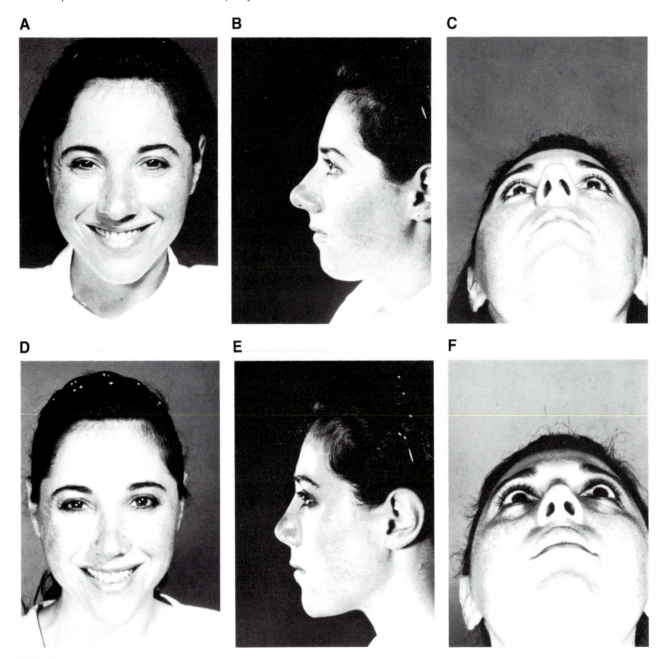

**FIG 11–6.**
**A,** a smiling preoperative frontal view shows an extremely broad nasal tip with a wide bridge. **B,** a preoperative left lateral view in repose displays a long nose, a slight dorsal hump, and microgenia. **C,** a preoperative worm's eye view shows an extremely broad nasal tip. **D,** a smiling postoperative frontal view shows a narrower bridge with nasal tip definition. **E,** a postoperative left lateral view in repose reveals an appropriate nasal length and facial balance. **F,** a narrower nasal tip pyramid can be seen in this postoperative worm's eye view.

The umbrella graft produces tip projection and enhances nasal tip definition.

When the skin is still too thick, we externally shave the skin, the same technique used to treat a rhinophyma. This technique can produce appropriate nasal tip definition. Complications of external shaving include changes in skin color and texture.

The skin may become hypopigmented, and the sebaceous pores may be more noticeable. These problems can be camouflaged with cosmetics.

It should be strenuously emphasized that only those patients whose skin thickness approaches that of rhinophyma are good candidates. Otherwise, scarring will be a severe problem.

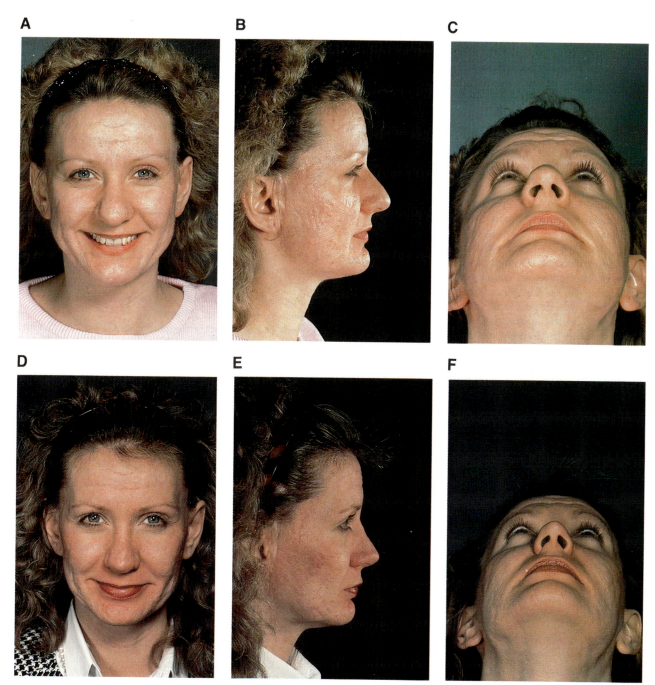

**FIG 11–7.**
**A,** a smiling preoperative frontal view shows an extremely broad nasal tip with thick sebaceous skin. **B,** a preoperative right lateral view in repose displays a long nose and drooping nasal tip. **C,** in the preoperative worm's eye view an extremely broad nasal tip with alar flaring can be seen. **D,** a smiling postoperative frontal view shows better nasal tip definition as a result of external shaving. **E,** a postoperative right lateral view shows an appropriate nasal length and nasolabial angle as well as adequate nasal tip projection. **F,** in the postoperative worm's eye view a more defined nasal tip pyramid is apparent.

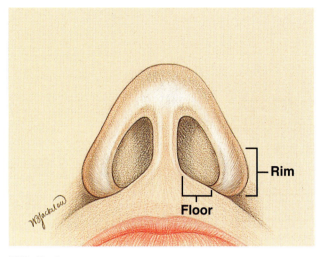

**FIG 12–9.**
Artist's drawing demonstrating the distinction between the alar rim and the alar floor.

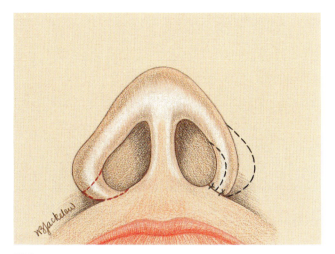

**FIG 12–11.**
Artist's drawing showing the reduction in alar flare eventuating from medial movement of the rim.

the alar-facial groove[10, 11] (see Fig 12–10). Inasmuch as Langer's lines, nasolabial folds, and glabellar wrinkles are anatomic creases that have historically served as the logical locations for surgical scars, so too are the natural junctions of the alae with the face. Incisions intentionally located above or outside of these landmarks are ill-advised. Also, staggered incisions render scars more visible, when so obvious means for camouflage are available.

Shaping of the alar base is achieved by bringing the ala closer to the columella.[2] This may be accomplished via a relatively short incision. Old literature describing incisions laterally skirting the nasal side wall are obsolete (see Fig 12–5). Both flare and width may be reduced by a short incision medially in the ala. Incisions laterally at the cheek have no ef-

fect on reducing flare of the rim or width of the floor.

Modified Weir excisions are indicated to reduce flare of the rims or width of the floor. They have no effect on tip height. Nasal tip height must be appropriate prior to alar surgery (see Figs 12–4 and 12–8). Likewise, variation in shape[1] of the resected alar segment has little effect on reducing flare or width.

### Summary of Surgical Principles

1. Modified Weir excisions reduce flare of the rims, width of the floor, or both.
2. Modified Weir excisions should only be done after all other nasal surgery is complete.
3. Scars should fall in natural creases.

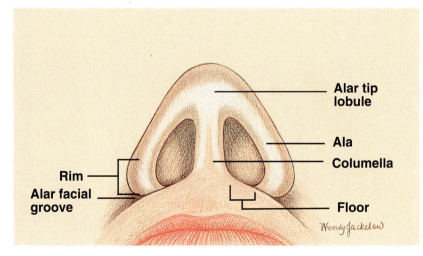

**FIG 12–10.**
Anatomy of the alae and adjoining structures.

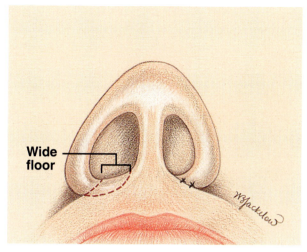

**FIG 12–12.**
Artist's drawing showing the reduction in floor width eventuating from excising a wedge from the floor.

4. Preservation of vestibular skin prevents notching.
5. Incisions should not traverse the lateral nasal wall.
6. Modified Weir excisions do not affect nasal tip height.
7. Altering the shape of the resection does little to reduce flare or width.

### Technique

**Reduction of Flaring Rims.**—An incision is made in the natural alar crease (Fig 12–13). The incision begins laterally and follows the crease to end at the vestibular (nostril) floor where the rim meets the floor. The incision follows the curve of the crease lat-

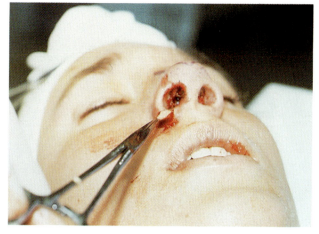

**FIG 12–14.**
Elevation of a wedge up to the rim margin.

erally and is generally 1.5 cm or less in greatest length. The incision is through the skin and subcutaneous fatty tissue but never traverses the intranasal vestibular skin.

The second incision is made superior to the first. It is based on judging the amount of rim flare and is never more than 0.4 cm above the first incision at the rim margin. It joins the first incision as a triangle laterally. Again, it incises the rim medially but does not cut the intranasal vestibular floor.

A triangular wedge of skin and subcutaneous tissue is elevated (Fig 12–14) and excised flush with the rim to preserve vestibular lining (Fig 12–15). Bleeding is controlled with cautery. The first suture is placed intranasally, the second exactly at the rim edge, and the third externally. The redundancy of vestibular skin or a dog-ear obvious after placement

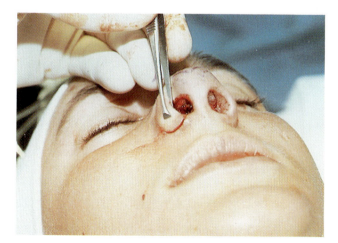

**FIG 12–13.**
Incision in a natural alar crease.

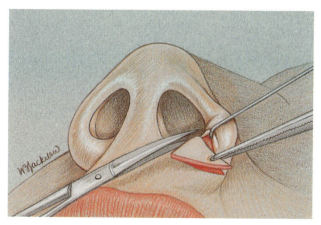

**FIG 12–15.**
Vestibular lining is always preserved as the wedge is excised flush with the rim.

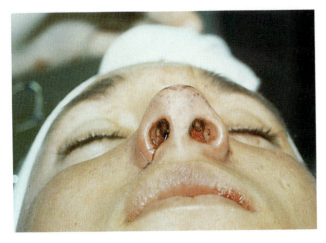

**FIG 12–16.**
After suturing of a modified Weir excision on the patient's right, the dog-ear has disappeared. Note the smooth contour at the suture line and the absence of any notching.

of the first suture disappears with healing. This redundancy prevents notching at the incision[6, 8] (Fig 12–16). If a fourth suture is necessary, it may indicate that the incision has been carried too far laterally on the nasal wall.

**Reduction of a Wide Floor With or Without Flaring Rims.**—As before, the incision follows the curve of the natural crease laterally but now ends in the floor 2 to 3 mm medial to the rim insertion (Fig 12–17; see also Fig 12–16). The incision again is 1.5 to 1.6 cm in greatest length. The superior (judgment) incision depends upon two factors: the width of the floor and flare of the rim. If there is just excess width and no flare, the second incision encompasses the floor

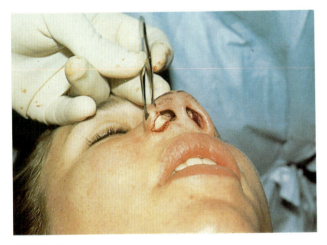

**FIG 12–17.**
The first incision for reducing a wide floor ends in the floor medial to rim insertion.

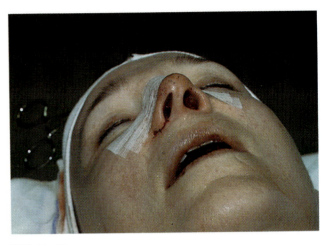

**FIG 12–18.**
Note reduction of the wide floor after a modified Weir excision on the patient's right.

only. If there is flare of the rim as well as excess width of the floor, then several millimeters of rim are included in the triangular wedge (Fig 12–18).

In the event that the nostril opening is small and it is feared that any further reduction in size might compromise the airway (Fig 12–19), then the procedure for flaring rims may be modified. In this case, the skin and subcutaneous tissue are excised as an ellipse instead of as a triangular wedge (Figs 12–20 and 12–21). Vestibular skin is again not excised (Fig 12–22). When sutured, this should produce little change in nostril size while it reduces rim flare bulk (Fig 12–23).

*Summary of Steps in a Modified Weir Excision*

A. Rim flare:
   1. The first incision follows the curve of the rim

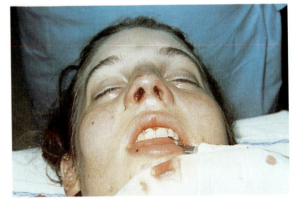

**FIG 12–19.**
Patient with small nostrils in whom reduction of nostril size might compromise the airway. Reduction of only the cutaneous portion of the alae is indicated.

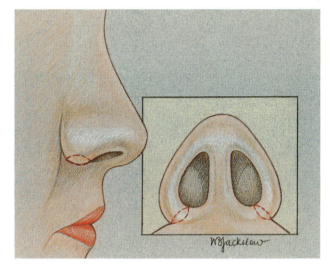

**FIG 12–20.**
Artist's drawing of an elliptical excision used for reduction of "bulky" alae in the presence of small nostrils.

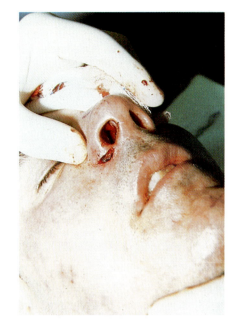

**FIG 12–22.**
Vestibular skin is always preserved, even with an elliptical excision.

to lie precisely in the crease. It ends where the alar rim meets the nostril floor.

2. The second incision depends upon the amount of flare. It begins at the rim edge superior to the first incision. It curves in a wedge or pie-slice shape to meet the lower incision laterally.

3. Both incisions are carried through the skin and the rim margin, but not into the vestibular intranasal floor.

4. Vestibular skin is never excised.

5. The vestibular skin is transected directly across the rim edge on the intranasal side.

6. The vestibular skin dog-ear should not be excised and prevents notching at the incision.

B. Wide floor:

1. The first incision begins laterally in the natural alar crease. It ends in the nostril floor, 2 to 3 mm medial to where the rim meets the floor.

2. The second incision depends upon the width of the floor as well as the flare of the rim.

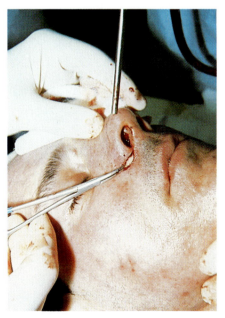

**FIG 12–21.**
Elliptical excision shown intraoperatively.

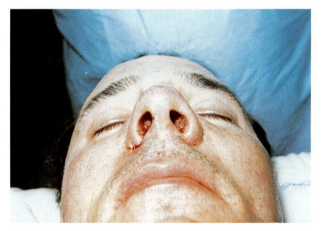

**FIG 12–23.**
While the elliptical excision reduces alar rim flare, it does little to decrease the size of the nostril opening.

3–6. Same as for A, "rim flare."
C. Small nostrils:
   1. The first incision is as for flaring rims or a wide floor.
   2. The second incision begins at the first incision laterally. It curves in an ellipse to meet the lower incision at the rim edge.
   3. Neither incision enters the vestibular intranasal floor.
   4. There is no vestibular skin redundancy because the two incisions form an ellipse, not a triangular wedge.
   5. The sutured ellipse should yield little change in nostril size.

### Postoperative Results

The patients shown have had modified Weir excisions (Figs 12–24 to 12–26). The surgical goals of decreasing rim flare, a wide floor, or both are achieved. Notching is not apparent. Scars are inconsequential in the worm's eye view (see Fig 12–24). After modified Weir excisions, scars should not be noticeable on the lateral nasal wall either in three-quarter (see Fig 12–25) or lateral views (see Fig 12–26).

### Complications and Untoward Sequelae

#### *Scarring*
Rarely, scarring at the site of sutures may be a problem. If a slight flare or excess width of the floor still remains a very conservative (1- or 2-mm) modified Weir excision encompassing the scar may be helpful.

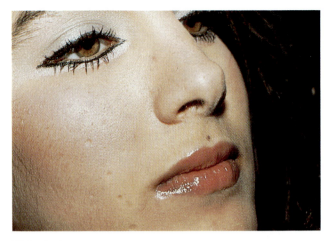

**FIG 12–25.**
Three-quarter view of a patient following modified Weir excisions. The scar is imperceptible at the alar-facial groove.

Excision and meticulous closure of the scar only may also be of benefit. Dermabrasion may be used alone or in conjunction with excision.

We see no absolute contraindication to performing modified Weir excisions in dark-skinned individuals, except if there is a known keloid diathesis after previous surgery. Even in these cases, a keloid on the nose or face is so rare that clinical judgment may permit judicious excision.

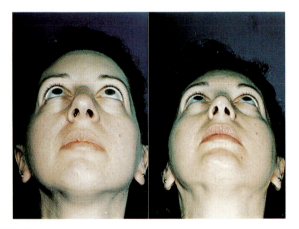

**FIG 12–24.**
Basal view before and after modified Weir excisions. Note the asymmetry of nostril openings that is present both before and after surgery. Cutaneous bases are, however, more symmetrical.

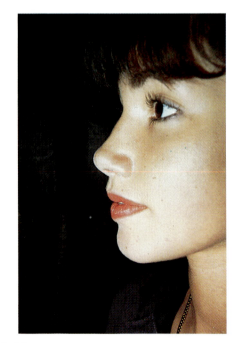

**FIG 12–26.**
Lateral view of a patient following modified Weir excisions. No scar is present on the lateral nasal wall.

### Notching

A notch at the incision in the nostril base is telltale evidence of alar resection. This appears unnatural because the smooth contour of the nasal sill has been interrupted.[10, 11]

If notching is evident, a conservative modified Weir excision with preservation of a vestibular skin bridge may eradicate the problem. The resection must incorporate the old scar and is always planned so as to lie in the alar crease. If the nostrils are already small, the excision is planned so that minimal change in size occurs (see above).

### Asymmetry

Slight asymmetry of the nostril openings and the alar bases is the rule in nature. An obvious asymmetry should be pointed out to the patient preoperatively.

Asymmetry that becomes pronounced after modified Weir excisions (Figs 12–27 and 12–28) may be due to several causes. One of the sutures may have come untied or may have been removed prematurely and allowed a minute dehiscence in the wound. The sizes of the excised segments may have differed on the two sides, or the advancement of the alar flap on the cheek may have differed on the two sides.

A small excision under local anesthesia may suffice to correct a minor discrepancy. However, many patients are not greatly concerned about this phenomenon provided that the remainder of the nose is to their satisfaction. If it is the nostril openings that are asymmetrical and not the alar bases, the problem may be of less import (see Fig 12–24).

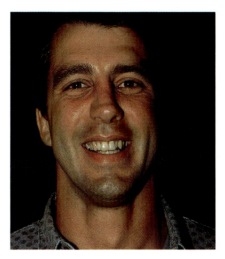

**FIG 12–28.**
Asymmetry of the cutaneous alar rims is visible as well (same patient as in Fig 12–28).

### Airway Compromise

This is the most feared sequela of too aggressive an alar excision. The thrust of the modified Weir excision should be to narrow the alae. The nostril will change as the rim and/or floor are moved medially toward the columella. This should not appreciably reduce the airway.

The alae are more important aesthetically than the nostril openings. The problem is not so much flaring *nostrils,* as described by Dr. Aufricht, but rather one of flaring *soft tissues.* As the soft tissues are realigned, then the nostrils follow proportionately.

Roughly, if the diameter of the nostril is less than the height of the tip lobule, then the excision must be elliptical, as in the above section "Small Nostrils." Nostrils of normal size should not be physiologically impaired if the greatest width of the triangular wedge is less than 0.4 cm at the rim margin. A wedge greater than 0.5 cm might indeed reduce the nostril opening to unphysiologic proportion.

### Conclusion

Modified Weir excisions may enhance the majority of rhinoplasties. The alar floor may be wide, the rims may flare, or both. Surgery of the alae aims at moving the floor and/or rims more medially. The procedure never changes tip height and should not compromise the airway. Scars should be inconsequential, and notching should not be observed. Modified Weir excisions may be performed in dark-

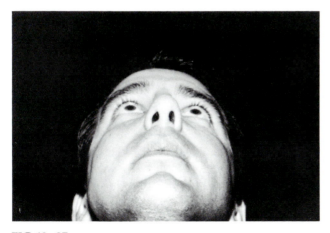

**FIG 12–27.**
Asymmetry of nostril openings following modified Weir excisions.

skinned patients. Asymmetry of the nostril openings is less a problem than is asymmetry of the rims. Asymmetry of the rims is often easily correctable.

## ALAR MARGIN SURGERY: MARGINAL (MILLARD) EXCISION

### History

In 1960, Dr. Ralph Millard addressed the problem of the bulky alar margin and elucidated a technique for its treatment.[4] Prior to that, external excisions, other than at the alar bases, were little used in aesthetic rhinoplasty.

### Indications

An alar rim that hides the columella in the profile view makes the nasal tip appear bulky and the nose overlong[7] (Fig 12–29). In the nose with "rather thick skin, broad alar wings, and long sidewalls, the columella will disappear as the sidewalls overhang the midcolumn. This relationship is unsatisfactory since the classic profile of the nose must show the delicate strength of its columella as the alae curve back and away."[3]

The overhanging sidewall can be corrected by the direct external excision of a strip along each alar margin. This approach is of value in the following conditions[3]:

1. A long and thick nose that when shortened develops overhanging sidewalls
2. A nose whose sidewalls overhang a columella that is already in the proper position

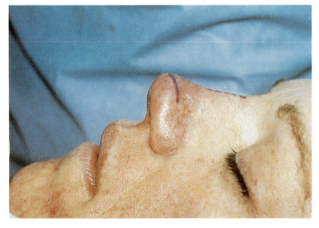

**FIG 12–29.**
Columella obscured by a veiling alar rim.

3. A nose with thick (bulky) alar rims
4. A nose in which the alar wings veil the columella in its posterior two thirds only

The above indications assume a proper columella position, a nasolabial angle of 90 to 95 degrees, an obtuse columella-lobule angle,[8] and a nontethered labial frenulum. As with other alar surgery, marginal excisions may be undertaken only after other nasal work is complete.

### Anatomy

The external nasal opening is formed by the alar rim laterally and the columella medially. Good profile aesthetics will have an arching alar rim with the columella showing below the rim in the profile view.[7] The alar rims should not obscure any portion of the columella in profile.

### Surgical Principles

As with other alar surgery, marginal excisions may be considered only after all other nasal work is complete. This is particularly important if the columellar septum is to be shortened, if the columellar-lobular angle is to be increased, or if the nose is to be lengthened with onlay grafts to the columella or lobule. Marginal excisions should, however, be done prior to modified Weir excisions. Judgment regarding width or flare of the rim may be altered by too bulky a rim. The two procedures may be performed on the same patient and often are.

### Technique

Estimate the amount of sidewall that needs trimming, and mark the excision. The excised strip should not exceed 3 to 4 mm in its greatest width. Starting at the height of the alar arch and continuing along the entire free border, excise the estimated strip (Figs 12–30 and 12–31). The alar margin should be kept under tension, with a hook at the height of the arch and gentle countertraction on the lip below the alar base. On cross section, the excised strip will be V shaped. This not only enables narrowing the thickness of the free edge but also facilitates closure of the defect.[3]

Interrupted 5–0 nylon sutures approximate the wound. The scar along the alar margin soon becomes unnoticeable. The procedure may be performed in non-Caucasian noses and is particularly useful in these cases. After completion of the mar-

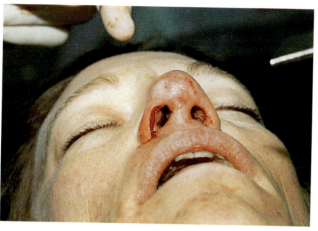

**FIG 12–30.**
Marginal (Millard) excision.

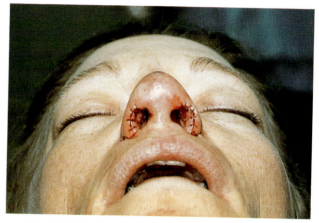

**FIG 12–32.**
Incision closed with interrupted 5–0 nylon sutures.

ginal excision, the modified Weir technique may be performed if needed (Figs 12–32 and 12–33).

### Summary of Steps in Marginal Excision

1. Mark the amount of sidewall that needs trimming.
2. Excise a strip that is elliptical en face and V shaped in cross section.
3. The excised strip should not exceed 3 to 4 mm in its greatest width.
4. The entire lateral rim (just short of the tip lobule) or only a portion (inferior) may be excised.

### Postoperative Results

The patients shown in Figures 12–34 and 12–35 have had marginal excisions. Veiling of the col-

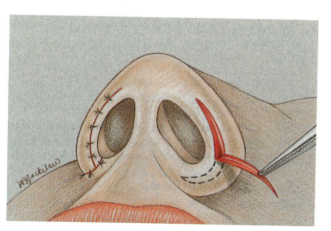

**FIG 12–31.**
The excised strip is V shaped in cross section.

umella by the alar wings has been eliminated. The columella "show" (2 to 3 mm) is proper (see Figs 12–34 and 12–35). Scarring is imperceptible.

### Complications and Untoward Sequelae

#### Scarring
The closure should lie at the alar margin proper, where confluence of light and shadow render an incision easy to conceal. Scar revision, dermabrasion, or a combination of the two may be used to treat visible scar deformities should they occur. We have observed no keloids or hypertrophic scars. Many patients have been dark skinned or non-Caucasian inasmuch as this group frequently has thick alar rims.

#### Excess Columella Exposure
This is a possibility since with healing and scar contraction, the rims tend to contract upward. Prevent-

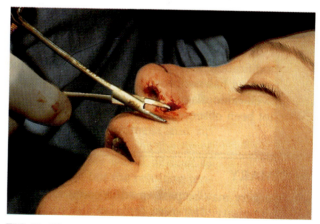

**FIG 12–33.**
Marginal excisions may be performed in conjunction with modified Weir excisions.

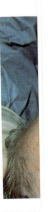

FIG 12·
Patient
colume

ing thi
or less
colume
rim au
treatm

*Asymi*

Asymi
notice
thesia
tively
perfor
excisic
ferred
ment

**Conclu**

Margil
menta
They :
fied V
margil
end o
this n
sian. S
to the
have i

**SUM**

Alar s
any rl
a mo
also b
modif

upper lateral cartilage from the lower lateral cartilage may be handled in one of two ways: (1) if the gap is small, it may be left as is to epithelialize from the vestibular skin, or (2) if the gap is large enough, a conchal composite graft (skin side down) should be applied. The conchal composite graft is sutured directly in place to fill the defect. Interrupted absorbable sutures are sufficient to hold it in position.

The mucoperichondrial flaps are secured to one another by using absorbable mattress sutures. In some cases thin sheets of silicone are placed on either side of the septum and held in place with 4–0 nylon mattress sutures.

### Additional Maneuvers

Additional maneuvers at the time of lengthening the short nose include all the other procedures that would ordinarily be done at the time of rhinoplasty. This includes tip grafting where necessary. It also includes dorsal grafting because many of these short noses are short in part because of inadequate length between the nasion and the tip-defining point. In some cases, the removal of dorsal septal scar tissue to perform the septoplasty has left a significant dorsal depression. By inserting a graft in this region, it not only improves the length of the nose but can also help keep the tip cartilages in a forward position. A single-thickness dorsal cartilage graft is usually adequate. The sides should be sanded or beveled so as to minimize sharp edges along the dorsum. To minimize mobility of the dorsal cartilage graft, two to three small holes are made with a no. 11 blade. This will permit the ingrowth of scar tissue

and stabilize the dorsal cartilage graft (Fig 13–18). A small-diameter hair punch can also be used to make these small holes.

One potential technical problem involves closure of the columellar incision after lengthening the nose. In spite of what appeared to be an adequate soft-tissue release of skin initially, the columellar flap may now not close without tension. At this time it is advisable to go back and look at the skin flap and try to find those areas where it is tethered. Further undermining may be necessary, not only laterally but also up high near the nasion, in order to allow the skin to advance over the newly lengthened cartilaginous framework. A small amount of tension is, however, permitted at the distal end of the flap where it is sutured to the columella.

Some of the short noses require straightening of the septum. They are either associated with a crooked nose and/or breathing difficulties. To do so, the usual techniques described elsewhere for septoplasty are employed. These include the hinge-door technique in which the septum is completely exposed following bilateral mucoperichondrial elevation. A single vertical incision is made near the junction of the cartilaginous septum with the bony septum (Fig 13–19). By releasing the floor of the septum from its vomerine groove it can be set to one side or the other. The caudal edge of that septum can be held in place by passing an absorbable suture through the buccal sulcus at the frenulum. This suture will secure the caudal edge of the septum in the most desirable position.

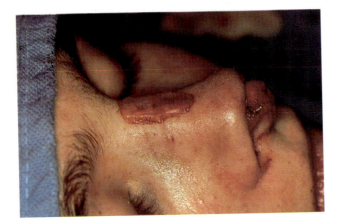

**FIG 13–18.**
The dorsal graft (if size permits) should receive two or more small holes. This will allow the ingrowth of scar to stabilize the graft.

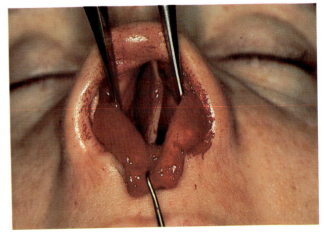

**FIG 13–19.**
Excellent exposure is achieved by the open technique. The septum can be scored on one side if needed, moved to a midline position, and held there with an absorbable suture that goes from the frenulum of the buccal sulcus to the cartilage.

## Technique for Correction of Apparent Shortness

The technique for the apparently short nose is considerably different from the absolutely short nose but deserves mention. The technique usually involves one or more of five steps:

1. A straight dorsal graft is often required to improve the distance between the nasion and the tip-defining point. This is because a straight nasal dorsum appears longer than a convex or concave dorsum. Moreover, by putting in a graft, the nasion can be raised to a more superior level to allow for an overall greater length between the nasion and the tip-defining point. In some patients, however, the nasion cannot be raised any higher without looking unnatural, and consequently absolute lengthening of the nose may be required.

2. Correction of the obtuse columella-labial angle itself may be very helpful in correcting the apparently short nose. It is often helpful to resect the posterior portion of the caudal septum as well as portions of the anterior nasal spine in order to improve the columella-labial angle.

3. If the tip is overprojecting, it should be lowered. Lowering of the tip is done by a transfixion incision that is taken deep toward the maxillary crest. Release of these soft tissues often in and of itself allows the tip to drop. Occasionally it will be necessary to incise the medial crura in the midportion and allow the cartilages of the medial crura to overlap one another (accordionate) and thereby shorten the height of the tip cartilages. Care should be taken in the process of improving the columella-labial angle that the lip is not unduly lengthened. If

the lip is long, absolute lengthening will be required.

4. The lower lateral cartilages should also be released by an intercartilaginous incision. This in conjunction with the transfixion incision will allow the tip cartilages to rotate inferiorly and allow the downward movement of the tip-defining point (Fig 13–20).

5. Finally, the dorsal slope of some apparently short noses is much too shallow and contributes to the overly projecting tip. By making a steeper dorsal slope, the apparent length of the nose can be increased. The normal slope of the female dorsum is 34 degrees. For a male it is 36 degrees.

## CASE EXAMPLES

### Absolutely Short Noses

*Classic Short Nose*

The first patient (Fig 13–21) is a 55-year-old woman who some 30 years previously underwent a primary closed rhinoplasty. Shortly after the first surgery she was quite satisfied with the result. It provided her with a short, "cute" nose that she appreciated for some years. However, as the patient advanced in years, the short turned-up nose did not fit her facial features. This is often the case for middle-aged patients. Examination of this patient reveals the fact that the distance between the nasion and the tip-defining point is in fact absolutely short in comparison to the height of the nose. The columella-labial angle is somewhat obtuse, and her nostrils show too much on frontal view. Since the lip is already at its maximum length, it would not be advantageous to resect tissue to improve the columella-labial angle. Rather, it would be advantageous to advance the tip of the nose and lengthen the distance between the nasion and the tip-defining point. Drawing on the preoperative photographs gives a good preview of what is desired postoperatively. Not only is length desired but also a correction of the dorsal concavity.

At surgery a stair-step incision was made just posterior to the waist of the columella. A great deal of scar tissue was seen, along with twisted and misshaped cartilages. Of interest is the fact that the external appearance of the tip was better than would be indicated by the internal appearance of the tip cartilages. The dorsum was shaved until cartilaginous tissue was seen. A fair amount of scar tissue made up the vertical height of this nose. The mucoperichondrium was elevated bilaterally and carried

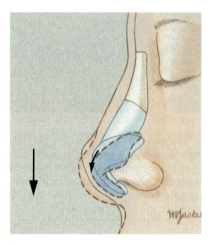

**FIG 13–20.**
The tip-defining point can be relocated by releasing the upper from the lower lateral cartilage.

or whether an absolute lengthening would be needed, i.e., the use of a baton graft. Drawing on the preoperative photographs helped make the decision. The patient clearly needed additional length along the entire columella because of the long lip. In fact, a lip-shortening procedure (excision of the skin of the upper lip under the nose) was considered as an ancillary procedure but was refused by the patient.

At surgery, through an external approach, the scar tissue was cleared off the dorsum until dorsal cartilage could be seen. Because an easy entry into the mucoperichondrial plane could not be made, the upper lateral cartilage (with its lining) was separated from the septum. This made it easier to dissect the mucoperichondrium off the cartilage bilaterally. Staggered releasing incisions were made bilaterally, as well as separation of the upper from the lower lateral cartilages. Care was taken not to separate the tip cartilages, so that the baton graft would not fall between them. A full centimeter of lengthening was thus obtained. A baton graft made of concha was fastened to the septum and pointed toward the middle of the columella in an attempt to lengthen the lip rather than push the anterior caudal septum forward and just rotate the tip forward. A thin, one-layer dorsal graft was added to the dorsum to remove some of the dorsal concavity.

At 16 months following surgery, one can see improvement. The vertical height of the nose is now what it should be, the nose is longer, and the lip actually shows some shortening. The scar (as is usually the case) is inconspicuous.

## COMPLICATIONS AND UNDESIRABLE RESULTS

### Insufficient Lengthening

This patient (Fig 13–24) sustained a midfacial fracture, including fracture of the nasal bones and ethmoid region, which went untreated for over 1 year. The patient was seen subsequently when he presented with a very shortened nose. Upon examination, one can see that the distance from the nasion to the tip-defining point is quite short and is aggravated by the fact that the nasion is quite low and deeply recessed. There is also an obtuse columella-labial angle, and the nostrils show considerably. This patient's problem also consisted of a severe airway obstruction due to accordionation of the septal and cartilaginous elements upon one another.

Surgery consisted of an open approach. From the dorsum the mucoperichondrium was elevated bilaterally. The patient exhibited a large amount of bony and cartilaginous material that created a thickening of the septum. This material was removed and used for grafting material, and an L-shaped septum was left. The mucoperichondrium was released in the standard fashion to allow advancement of the columella. A baton graft was made from the cartilage removed from the septum and was applied to the dorsal L-shaped septum. It held the tip of the nose in a more caudal position. In addition, the upper lateral cartilage had to be separated from the lower lateral cartilage. Fortunately, the soft tissues between the upper and lower lateral cartilages permitted this to happen without having to transect the vestibular skin, thus precluding a composite graft.

A cranial bone graft was taken from the parietal region by using standard techniques. With rongeurs it was trimmed to the appropriate length. A double graft was necessary. The existing nasal bones were rasped so that the bone grafts could have a flush contact with the existing nasal bones. A small percutaneous pin held the bone grafts to the nasal bone. One of the dorsal bone grafts extended all the way to the tip cartilages and helped hold them in their newly advanced position. The domes of the tip cartilages were sutured together and a tip graft applied. Although even more lengthening was desired, the skin simply would not stretch much further and yet allow closure of the columellar incision.

Postoperatively at 13 months one can see that there is considerable improvement in the absolute length of the nose. However, in comparison to the patient's pretrauma condition, one sees that complete restoration of the length was not achieved. Further lengthening of the nose in the future can be considered.

### Donor Site Complications

Prior to the advent of leaving behind a portion of the ellipse removed from the concha, flattening of the ear was more likely to occur following extensive conchal removal (Fig 13–25). Also, an occasional patient will exhibit an unaesthetic scar along the anterior aspect of the concha (Fig 13–26) when that approach is used. Fortunately, the frequency of ear flattening and a noticeable anterior scar is such that the advantages of the technique far outweigh the disadvantages.

**A**

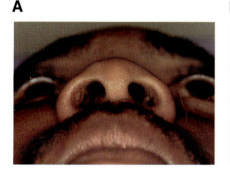

**B**

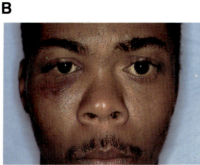

**C**

**D**

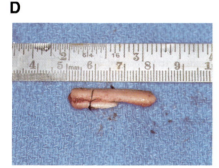

**E**

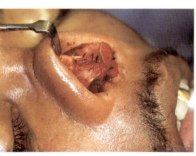

**F**

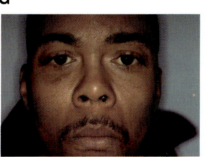

**G**

**H**

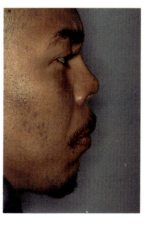

**FIG 13–24.**
This patient's nasoethmoid fracture went untreated. He exhibits absolute shortness including a deeply recessed nasion, nostril show, and an obtuse columella-labial angle **(A–C).** At surgery a cranial bone graft (double layer) was used along the dorsum **(D).** The mucoperichondrium was released, and a cartilage baton graft attached to the septum held the tip cartilages in a more normal anatomic position. A tip graft was also added **(E).** Early results looked quite good **(F).** After several months, however, some bone absorption was seen that may have been due to inadequate securing of the bone graft to the nasal bones. After 1 year, however, considerable improvement does remain **(F-H)** in comparison to his pretrauma condition.

## Miscellaneous Potential Complications (Undesirable Results)

The columella scar is not a common or significant complication (undesirable result). In fact, the potential problem with the scar is no different for the short nose (despite potential problems in skin closure) than for any other type of open rhinoplasty.

The incidence of severe columella scarring (including retraction) that requires surgical correction is estimated at 1 in 100 cases. If, however, the patient with a short nose has had a prior open approach, a local flap rotation may be needed. Otherwise scar contracture and a receding columella may result. Although septal perforation would appear to be a significant problem when bilateral mucoperichondrial crushed with a Tessier forceps and modeled to the desired shape. The cartilaginous portion is carved by following the biomechanical principles described by Gibson and Davis[1] and is always fairly short to avoid the danger of postoperative distortion. It can be located at the caudal or the distal end of the graft depending on where more augmentation is desired (Fig 14–6).

To increase tip projection a septal cartilage graft is carved to the shape and size required by the individual case by following the design described by Sheen.[8] It is introduced through a small rim incision into a pocket dissected between the skin of the tip and the caudal extension of the fascia of the superficial musculoaponeurotic system (SMAS). It is maintained in position by a nonabsorbable suture that enters the skin above the graft, passes through the cartilage, and emerges again through the skin; the two ends are fixed to the skin with tape (Fig 14–7). The tip graft increases the anterior projection of the tip, as well as produces angularity and camouflages the thickness of the skin. It is always complemented by a second strut of cartilage introduced into the columella between the medial cruces to increase the structural support.[2] When the columella is receding, a larger graft is used. It is shaped as a triangle 15 to 20 mm in height and 5 to 8 mm in width. It is introduced into the columella in a pocket different from the tip graft and placed in a sagittal position between the medial cruces. The base of the triangle is located at the level of the nasal spine. In this manner the base of the columella is projected caudally, and the vertex of the acute columellar-labial angle is obliterated to produce an obtuse angle without undesirable exposure of the nares (Fig 14–8).

The ear concha is an alternative donor area for the cartilage. Excellent material can be harvested for the tip and columellar grafts, but in my opinion, it is not adequate for the dorsum. In spite of careful carving and limited crushing (which is not well tolerated by ear cartilage), I find it difficult to achieve the precision required for an aesthetic procedure, and visible irregularities may appear 6 to 12 months later. It is, however, an excellent complement when the septal graft is small or when most of the septum is used for dorsal augmentation. When rib grafts are used, a large supply of cartilage is available.

It is easy to carve into any shape to fill the requirements for the columella and the tip. It has the extra advantage of rigidity, which is important to provide a stronger structural support in very small noses or when the skin coverage is very thick. The use of alloplastic implants is not indicated for this

**A**

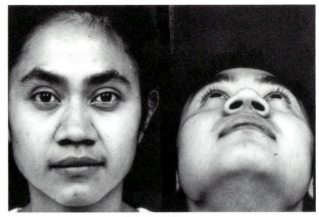

**B**

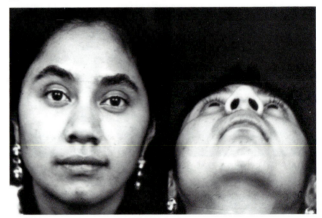

**FIG 14–9.**
**A,** preoperative photographs of a 45-year-old female with a small thick-skinned nose, small alar cartilages, short columella, and wide alar bases. **B,** postoperative photographs after a chondrocostal bone graft to the dorsum, a rib cartilage graft to the columella and the tip, alar base resection, and sliding genioplasty.

type of surgery. My personal experience with this material is very limited except for numerous cases of previously operated noses arriving at our clinic with exposed implants perforating the skin. It may produce acceptable results when small pieces are used to augment the dorsum in Oriental noses, but no consistent long-term results can be obtained when tip projection and angularity are the goals. The correction of the wide alar base is the last step of the operation because the amount of resection can only be assessed after the tip projection has been increased. Weir excision of the alar base is done to achieve an adequate width-to-height ratio of the triangle formed by the base of the nose (Fig 14–9).

As previously stated, the angle of convexity of the Amerindian face is larger than that of the Cauca-

**A**

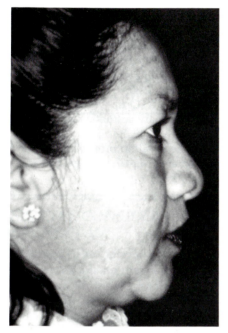

**B**

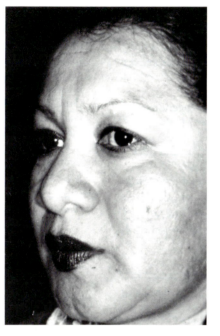

**C**

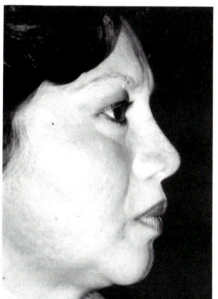

**D**

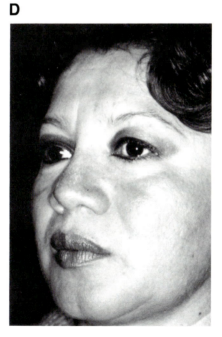

**FIG 14–10.**
A and B, preoperative photographs of a patient with a hypoplastic nasal pyramid, thick skin on the caudal half of the nose, very wide nasal bone, and receding columella. C and D, postoperative views after an osteocartilaginous rib graft to the nasal dorsum, a rib cartilage graft to the columella, and a wedge excision of alar bases. The procedure was complemented by remodeling of mandibular angles and partial resection of the masseter muscle performed through the intraoral route.

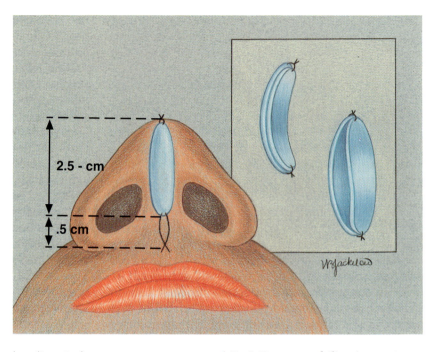

**FIG 15–12.**
If more anterior projection is desired, then the concave side can be sutured to the convex side by bending (scoring) it anteriorly. It is then placed concave side forward.

be sutured to the convex side by scoring it anteriorly. It is then placed with the concave side forward. Mastoid soft tissue can be added to the tip to soften the area in the case of thin tip skin (Fig 15–13). Apical and base markings are made on the skin, and the

temporary external 5–0 Dexon stabilization sutures are used for closure (Fig 15–14).

The base of the graft is placed first and then the apex. Slight but acceptable pressure against the tip apex is often necessary for proper projection. Cau-

**A**

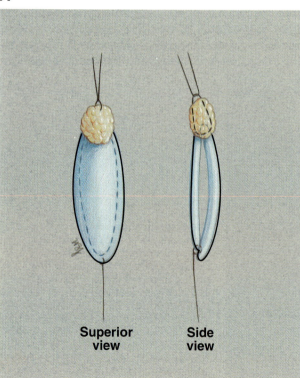

Superior view    Side view

**B**

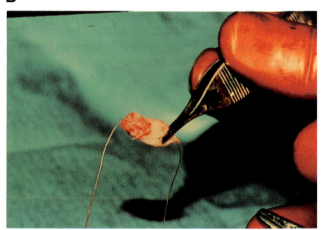

**FIG 15–13.**
**A,** in cases where additional soft-tissue covering over cartilage is needed, mastoid soft tissue can be incorporated with the graft. This is particularly important in thin-skinned tips to avoid cartilage "pointing." **B,** intraoperative view.

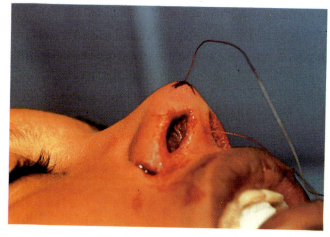

**FIG 15–14.**
The superior tip of the pea-pod graft is positioned by using a 5–0 Dexon pullout suture. This is pulled anteriorly and superiorly under reasonable tension until the graft is in the correct location.

tion should be exercised to ensure that tip vascularity remains intact. After irrigation, complete soft-tissue closure is mandatory. Supportive tape should be used for 5 days. The pullout stabilization suture can be held secure by the tape to ensure good graft positioning.

The graft stabilization sutures are normally pulled up and trimmed 5 days after surgery. If any graft movement or distortion has occurred, adjustments can be made by applying tension to the su-

ture and then waiting another 2 to 3 days before trimming it. These stabilization sutures can also be incorporated with additional deeper sutures from the graft to the surrounding soft tissue and alar cartilage. This will help to avoid lateral or posterior drift of the tip graft.

Nighttime nasal tip taping should be carried out for 6 to 12 weeks postoperatively in order to decrease swelling.[3]

Figure 15–15 exhibits what tip grafting can do. This preoperative view shows a male patient with a depressed, unsupported tip. Postoperatively, good projection has been achieved with the placement of a 2.5 × 0.75-cm pea-pod graft. Minimal dorsal reduction, caudal septal shortening, and minimal alar cartilage reduction were also performed on this patient.

Figure 15–16 also illustrates the benefits of pea-pod tip grafting. The preoperative view shows a female patient after two previous rhinoplasties. A previously placed small tip graft failed to provide adequate projection. Postoperatively, the nose has greater projection due to the placement of a 3.5 × 1-cm pea-pod tip graft. No tip defatting was possible due to scarring, but the amount of projection gives the illusion of a thinner tip.

The male patient in Figure 15–17 had a very thick, bulbous nasal tip. To correct this, a very stiff, double-layered 3 × 1-cm conchal cartilage graft was used, and minimal tip thinning was performed.

**A** 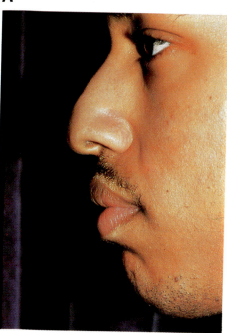 **B**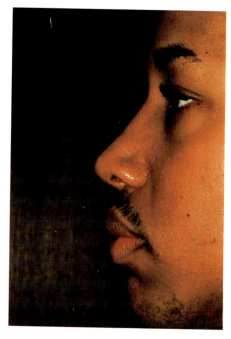

**FIG 15–15.**
**A,** this preoperative view shows a male patient with a depressed, unsupported tip.
**B,** postoperatively, good projection has been achieved with placement of a 2.5 × 7.5-cm pea-pod graft. Minimal dorsal reduction, caudal septal shortening, and minimal alar cartilage reduction were also performed.

**A**

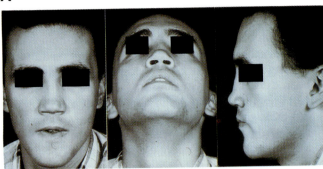

**B**

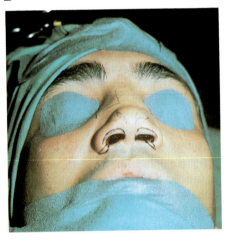

**C**

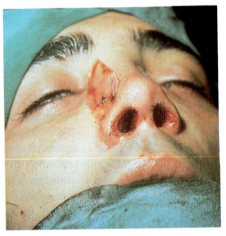

**D**

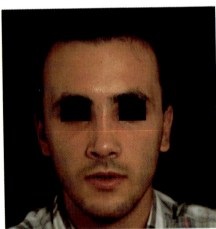

**E**

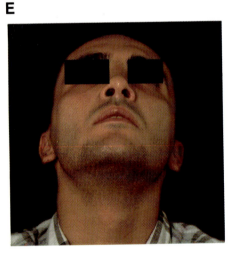

**FIG 16–16.**
A 24-year-old man with thick distorted nasal bones, deviated septum, and loss of support of the tip-columellar complex. Correction was achieved by straightening of the nasal pyramid and septum and insertion of a cartilage graft from the quadrangular plate into the columella, membraneous septum, and dorsum. **A,** preoperative view. **B** and **C,** intraoperative view. **D–E,** postoperative view.

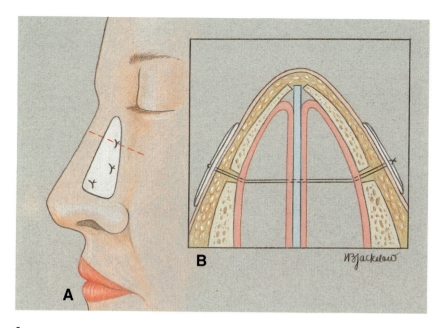

**FIB 16–17.**
Transnasal mattress suture for fixation of the narrowed bony pyramid. The thread is passing through the lateral osteotomy and through the septum. **A,** lateral view. **B,** sagittal view.

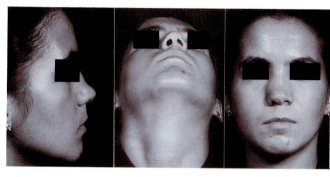

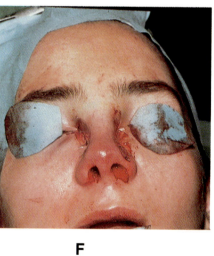

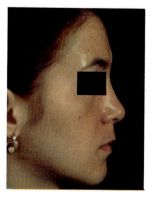 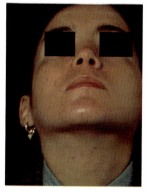 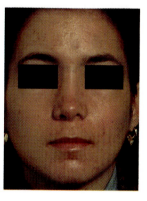

**FIG 16–18.**
Broad and crooked nose in a 23-year-old female. For stabilization of the narrowed bony pyramid, the transnasal mattress sutures were left in place for 10 days.
**A,** preoperative view. **B** and **C,** intraoperative view.
**D–F,** postoperative view.

**A**

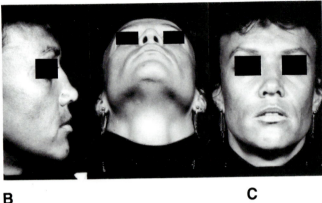

**FIG 16–19.**
Use of a Doyle nasals splint for keeping the mobilized septum in a straight position after correction of a crooked nose with secere septal deviation. Preoperative (**A**), intraoperative (**B** and **C**) and postoperative views (**D–F**) are shown.

**B**

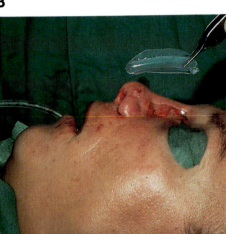

**C**

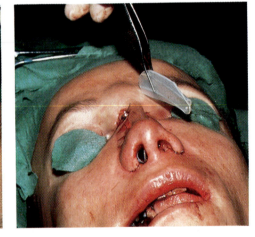

**D**

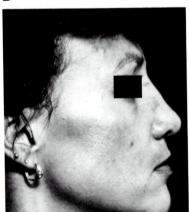

**E**

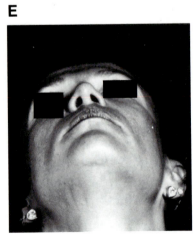

**F**

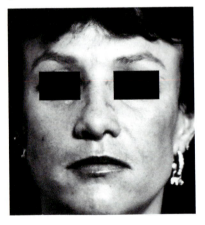

vault of the nose. More particularly, the paramedian osteotomy and the paramedian section of the upper lateral cartilages from the septum must be controlled because failure to correct the dorsal cartilaginous and bony arch would again be the cause of a late-recurring deviation and crookedness of the dorsum months after the procedure, even if the result on the operating table showed a symmetrical positioning of the bones.

For the same reason, the bony as well as the cartilaginous median transposition should be overcorrected, i.e., at the end of the operation the nasal dorsum has to deviate slightly to the opposite side because of the memory of the corrected structures. This dogma is more important in revision cases than in primary rhinoplasty.

In many cases the packing is applied firmly only in the inferior part of the nasal cavities and loosely upward to avoid moving the realigned bones apart. Before packing I insert plastic tubes bilaterally along the nasal floor in order to permit nasal breathing if the packing has to be left more than 2 days, which is necessary in difficult cases of septoplasty. The tube may be a custom-made Doyle airway Silicone splint (Fig 16–19).

In cases of severe preoperative deviation, I use a plastic sheet or small plates of x-ray film as a splint that can be placed on either side of the septum (Fig 16–20).[22]

The overcorrecting plaster dressing should be left in place at least 10 days or even better 2 to 3 weeks. Due to swelling of the skin, the plaster might have to be changed after 1 week or 10 days.

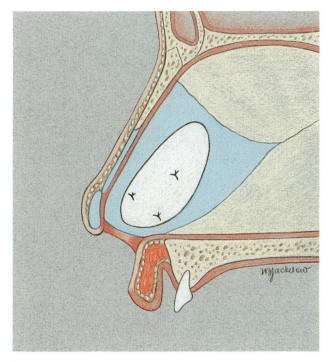

**FIG 16–20.**
For stabilization of the repositioned septal plate I occasionally use a plastic sheet in apposition unilaterally or bilaterally.

## REFERENCES

1. Barsky AJ: *Principles and practice of plastic surgery*, Baltimore, 1950, Williams & Wilkins.
2. Cottle MH: Surgical corrections of the septal deformities, *Ann Rhinol Soc* 7:14, 1960.
3. Denecke HJ, Meyer R: *Plastische Operationen an Kopf und Hals. Korrigierende und Rekonstruktive Nasenplastik.* Berlin, 1964, Springer-Verlag.
4. Dupont C, Cloutier GE, Prevost Y: Autogenous vomer bone graft for permanent correction of the cartilaginous septal deviations, *Plast Reconstr Surg* 38:243, 1966.
5. Eitner E: *Kosmetische Operationen.* Vienna, Austria, 1932, Springer-Verlag.
6. Feuerstein SS: Personal communication, 1985.
7. Fomon S: *Corrective surgery: principles and practice,* Philadelphia, 1960, Lippincott.
8. Goodman WS: Recent advances in external rhinoplasty, *J Otolaryngol* 10:433, 1981.
9. Gorney M: Correction of the deviated nose, *Ann Plast Surg* 8:201, 1984.
10. Gorney M: The septum in rhinoplasty form and function. In Millard D Jr, editor: *Symposium on Corrective Rhinoplasty,* vol 13, St Louis, 1976, Mosby–Year Book.
11. Ivy RH: *Nelson's loose leaf surgery.* New York, 1932, Thomas Nelson & Sons.
12. Jost G, Meresse B: Etude de la fonction entre les cartilage lateraux du nez, *Ann Chir Plast* 18:175, 1973.
13. Killian G: The submucous window resection of the nasal septum, *Ann Otol Rhinol Laryngol* 14:363, 1905.
14. Koechlin H: New instruments in rhinoplasty, *Plast Reconstr Surg* 8:132, 1951.
15. Lautenschlager A: Die Eingriffe am Ohr und an der Nase. In *Kirschners Operationslehre,* Berlin, Springer-Verlag, 1934.
16. Maliniac JW: *Rhinoplasty and restoration of facial contour,* Philadelphia, 1947, FA Davis.
17. Meyer R: In Denecke HJ, Meyer R, editors: *Plastische Operationen an Kopf und Hals I, Korrigierende Nasenplastik,* Berlin, 1964, Springer-Verlag.
18. Meyer R: Nasenplastik mit dem zahnärztlichen Bohrer, *Kosmetikerinnen Fachzeitung* 26, 1954, p 99.
19. Meyer R: *Secondary and functional rhinoplasty—the difficult nose,* Orlando, Fla, 1988, Grune & Stratton.
20. Meyer R: Secondary rhinoplasty in secondary nose,

Transactions of the Seventh International Congress of Plastic and Reconstructive Surgery, Rio de Janeiro, 1979.

21. Meyer R, Kesselring UK: Fibrinogen tissue adhesive glue in aesthetic plastic surgery, Abstracts of the 6th Congress of the International Society of the Aesthetic Plastic Surgery, Tokyo, 1981.

22. Meyer R, Kesselring UK: Secondary rhinoplasty. In Regnault P, Daniel RK, editors: *Aesthetic plastic surgery*, Boston, 1984, Little Brown.

23. Mir Y, Mir L: El periostio y la reconstrucción estética nasal, *Cir Plast Ibero-Latinoam* 9:4, 1983.

24. Ortiz-Monasterio F, Olmedo A: Rhinoplasty on the mestizo nose, *Clin Plast Surg* 4:89, 1977.

25. Planas J: The tile graft: a method of building the roof of the nose using preserved homograft septal cartilage, *Eur J Plast Surg* 9:140, 1987.

26. Planas J: The twisted nose, *Clin Plast Surg* 4:55, 1977.

27. Planas J: Total extirpation of the septum. In *Transactions of the Third International Congress of Plastic Surgeons*, Washington 1963, Amsterdam, 1964, Excerpta Medica.

28. Pollet J, Baudelot S: La rhinoplastie extra-muqueuse. Ses indications, *Ann Chir Plast* 15:61, 1970.

29. Robin JL: Considération techniques sur la chirurgie réductrice des arêtes nasales, *Acta Otorhinolaryngol Belg* 22:704, 1968.

30. Sarnoff J: Pitfalls and safeguards in plastic surgery, *Plast Reconstr Surg* 5:168, 1950.

31. Schrudde J: La osteotomia subperiostica total en el estrechamiento de la nariz, *Rev Esp Cir Plast* 3:41, 1970.

32. Schuffenegger J, Gubisch W: La reconstruction fonctionnelle et esthétique de la pyramide nasale antérieure par implants cartilagineux septocolumellaires, Abstracts of the Tenth Congress of the Society of European Rhinology, Nancy, 1984.

33. Seltzer AP: *Plastic surgery of the nose*, Philadelphia, 1949, Lippincott.

34. Tamerin JA: Five most important points in reduction rhinoplasty, *Plast Reconstr Surg* 48:214, 1971.

35. Tardy M E: Rhinoplasty tip ptosis: etiology and prevention, *Laryngoscope* 83:983, 1973.

36. Tardy ME: Practical suggestions on facial plastic surgery—how I do it. Sublabial mucosal flap: repair of septal perforations, *Laryngoscope* 87:275, 1977.

37. Webster RC, Davidson TM, Rubin FF: Practical suggestions on facial plastic surgery. How I do it. Recording projection of nasal landmarks in rhinoplasty, *Laryngoscope* 87:1207, 1977.

# The Aging Nose

Bernard L. Kaye, M.D.

## RHINOPLASTY IN THE OLDER PATIENT

The older patient can benefit from rhinoplasty as much as the younger patient. The operation can be an independent procedure, or more often, it can be a useful ancillary procedure with rhytidectomy. Some older patients may notice that their noses are undergoing changes associated with age, including increased drooping and increased bulbousness of the tip, overgrowth of the dorsum, retrusion and increased sharpness of the labial-columellar angle, and widening of the nostrils. Other older patients may have long-standing nasal deformities that they always wanted to have improved but were not able to do so for one reason or another, such as a lack of time or financial wherewithal. Some older patients who always wanted rhinoplasty may have hesitated to have it done for fear of criticism or derision by colleagues at work or by family members, particularly if the deformity was a family trait.

Rhinoplasty in an older patient may be complete or partial. In either case, conservatism and artistic judgment are key to obtaining patient satisfaction. The goal of surgery should be to obtain a nasal appearance that the patient may have had (or should have had) during youth. Most older patients do not want a new nose. They particularly do not want a "nose-bobbed" appearance. Most such patients want a relatively straight nose without excess dorsal concavity. Also, many are terrified at the thought of a piglike look, with elevated, flaring nostrils.

In contrast to younger individuals, older patients may have more systemic health problems such as hypertension, arteriosclerosis, and cardiopulmo-nary disease. These patients require more thorough preoperative medical evaluation than most young people do. I have such patients evaluated by an internist preoperatively. The presence of the conditions cited above is not in itself a contraindication to rhinoplasty, provided that the patient is judged to be able to safely tolerate the surgery and anesthesia.

When performing rhinoplasties in older patients, one can notice significant tissue differences from younger patients. Cartilage tends to be more brittle. It is more difficult to shave down the cartilaginous dorsum. Alar cartilages are more likely to fracture during excision. Bone is more brittle and may be more likely to comminute during osteotomy. There is little likelihood of obtaining greenstick fractures. Septal mucosa tends to restretch more, and when raising the tip by septal mucosal excision, one should remove a little more than would be removed in a younger patient. Nasal skin, particularly near the tip, is more coarse. If the patient also has rhinophyma, it may be necessary to excise some excess skin.

## NASAL CHANGES WITH AGE

There are a number of changes that take place in the nose with age (Fig 17–1):

1. The tip becomes more bulky due to overgrowth of the alar cartilages.

2. The tip tends to droop lower than 90 degrees due to overgrowth of the alar cartilages as well as laxity of the covering soft tissues.

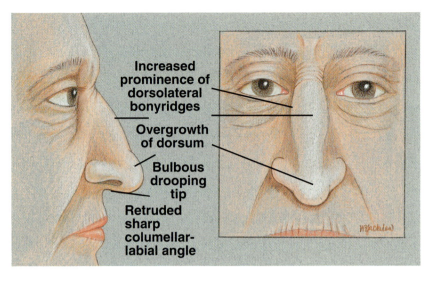

**FIG 17–1.**
Nasal changes with age. (Adapted from Kaye BL: *Facial rejuvenative surgery,* Philadelphia, 1987, Lippincott.)

3. The labial-columellar angle becomes more acute and retrudes, thus losing its gentle, obtuse fillet-like shape of youth (Fig 17–2).

4. The bony dorsum overgrows and produces humps and lateral bony ridging that were not present in youth.

5. The nostrils may widen.

To correct these changes, with or without rhytidectomy, two types of rhinoplasty may be performed, partial or complete rhinoplasty.

## PARTIAL RHINOPLASTY

Many older patients can benefit from a partial rhinoplasty, a procedure that modifies the nasal tip and may or may not involve conservative reduction of the nasal bony dorsum or lateral bony ridges, without infractures (Fig 17–3). This operation is particularly useful as an ancillary procedure with rhytidectomy because it takes little time and does not add to the healing time of a rhytidectomy. It omits the two steps that many believe cause the most morbidity in

**A** **B**

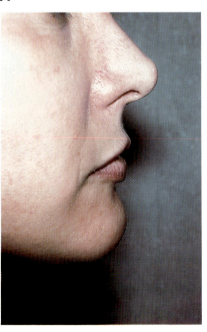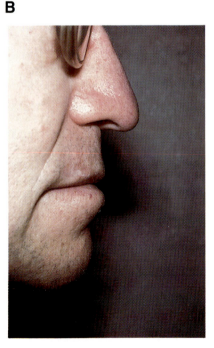

**FIG 17–2.**
**A,** youthful, obtuse columellar-labial angle. **B,** sharp, retruded columellar-labial angle that can appear with age.

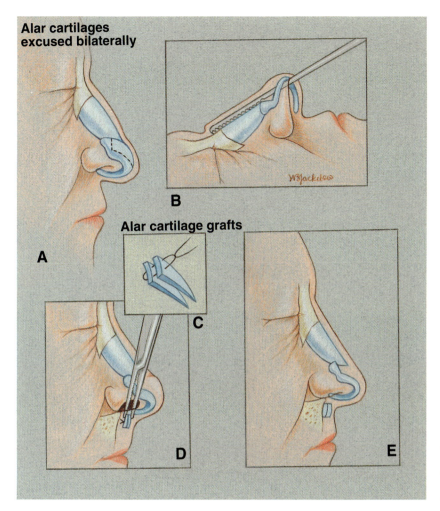

Alar cartilages
excused bilaterally

B

Alar cartilage grafts

A

C

D

E

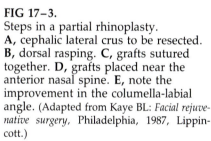

FIG 17–3.
Steps in a partial rhinoplasty.
**A,** cephalic lateral crus to be resected.
**B,** dorsal rasping. **C,** grafts sutured
together. **D,** grafts placed near the
anterior nasal spine. **E,** note the
improvement in the columella-labial
angle. (Adapted from Kaye BL: *Facial rejuvenative surgery,* Philadelphia, 1987, Lippincott.)

rhinoplasty: total hump reduction and infractures. Partial rhinoplasty may involve any or all of the following steps (Fig 17–3):

1. Reduction of tip bulk by removal of predetermined cephalic portions of the alar cartilages. This maneuver, in itself, will serve to raise the tip to some extent.

2. Conservative reduction of a bony hump by rasping (not enough to open the "roof" to require infractures). Lateral bony ridges can also be reduced by rasping.

3. A sharp, retruded labial-columellar angle can be improved by insertion of a retrolabial cartilage graft just behind the angle. The graft can be made up of the two segments of alar cartilage that were removed; the segments are sandwiched and sutured together and inserted, convex surfaces anteriorly, through a transfixion incision or an incision in the nostril floor. This maneuver also helps to increase tip projection and raise the tip somewhat (Fig 17–4).

4. If a drooping tip is not elevated enough by tip reduction or insertion of a retrolabial graft, one may shorten the tip by conservative excision of an antero-inferior triangle of septal mucosa or septal cartilage and mucosa. Whereas the membranous septum has more tendency to stretch in older patients, it is wise to take 0.5 to 1 mm more lining than cartilage. Some older patients are reluctant to have their nostrils showing. It is best to tell them preoperatively that they may benefit from secondary tip elevation later. Tip elevation may be of benefit physiologically as well as aesthetically. A number of older patients have told me that they breathe better after tip elevation.

5. Nostrils often widen with age, and raising the tip makes them more apparent. Alaplasties are useful to narrow them.

6. Some older patients present with rhinophyma as well as the other changes mentioned

**A**

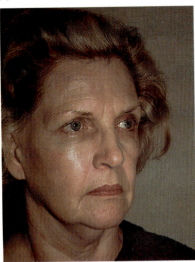

**B**

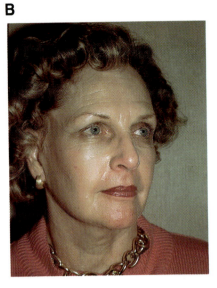

**C**

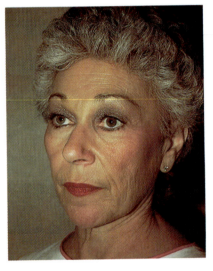

**D**

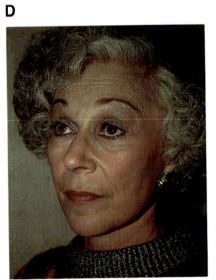

**FIG 17–4.**
**A** and **B,** partial rhinoplasty in a patient who also had cervicofacial rhytidectomy and dermabrasion of the upper and lower lips. **C** and **D,** partial rhinoplasty. The patient also had a forehead lift, rhytidectomy, and a perioral chemical peel.

**A**

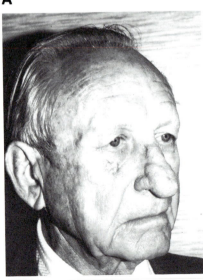

**B**

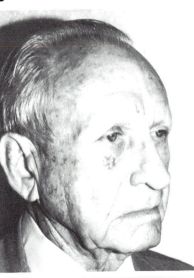

**FIG 17–5.**
**A** and **B,** bulbous drooping tip and rhinophyma in an older patient treated by a combination of shaving, lower rhinoplasty, and external transverse skin excision. Upper-lid blepharoplasty was also done. (From Kaye BL: *Aesthetic Plast Surg* 3:57–63, 1979. (Redrawn with permission.)

above. Skin shaving as well as skin excision can be useful for such patients (Fig 17–5).

## COMPLETE RHINOPLASTY

Some older patients can benefit from a complete rhinoplasty (Fig 17–6). The additional steps consist of removal of the entire osteocartilaginous hump and infracture of the nasal bones. A complete rhinoplasty can be done as an individual operation or along with a rhytidectomy, depending on the preference and operating rate of the individual surgeon. I believe that a complete rhinoplasty may be done with a face-lift. In my opinion, the tapes and splint for the rhinoplasty do not interfere with the results of a rhytidectomy.

Combining rhinoplasty, partial or complete, with rhytidectomy helps to produce a more complete facial rejuvenation without adding to the patient's recovery time from the rhytidectomy.

**A**

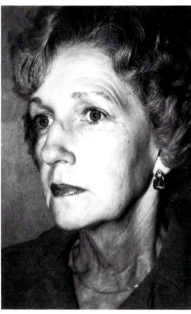

**B**

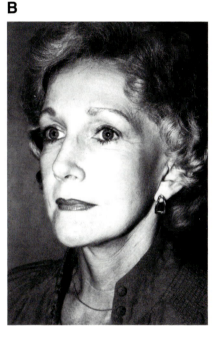

**C**

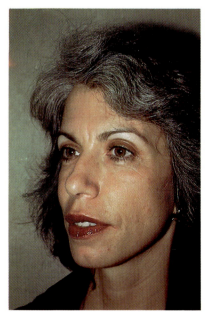

**D**

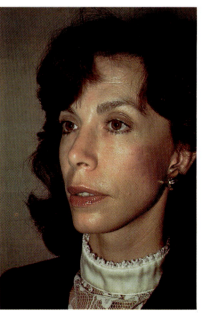

**FIG 17–6.**
**A** and **B**, complete rhinoplasty. The patient also had rhytidectomy, a forehead lift, blepharoplasty, and perioral peel-abrasion. **C** and **D**, complete rhinoplasty in a patient who also had rhytidectomy, a forehead lift, and chin augmentation.

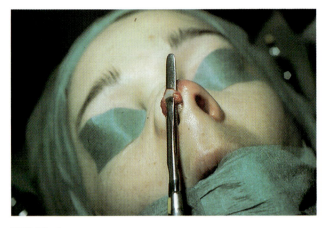

**FIG 18–4.**
Luxation technique. The cephalic two thirds of the lateral crus are from the vestibular skin resected.

## PINCHED NOSE

A pinched nose is a permanent sinking of the vestibular wall that obstructs the nostril and creates an unaesthetic alar groove on one or both sides. Excessive resection of the lateral crus of the alar cartilage and the intranasal lining leads to scar retractions in the vestibules and compensatory scar hypertrophy in the soft tissue found between the upper and the lower lateral cartilage. Correction is done by careful removal of the scar tissue but in extreme cases the vestibular lining may need restoring with small composite skin grafts taken from the inner aspect of the crus helicis of the ear after removal of scar tissue. When the vestibular lining is intact, one just has to reconstruct the alar cartilage framework. For that, I meticulously insert a discoid cartilage graft from the septum. This graft is carved in a slightly convex shape and fixed, like a bridge, over the remaining parts of the lateral crus with transalar mattress sutures (Fig 18–6).

## VALVE COLLAPSE

Reduction of the angle at the luminal valve may externally be a deformity similar to a pinched nose, which has the same etiology and often the same secondary treatment. When the ala collapse is due to inherent weakness or flaccidity, it is sufficient to perform an extramucosal dissection with section of the upper lateral cartilage at its insertion to the sep-

**A**

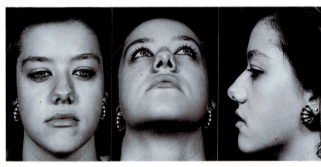

**B**

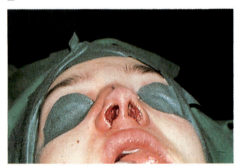

**C**    **D**    **E**

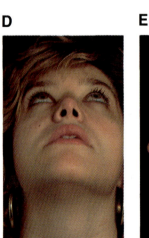

**FIG 18–5.**
A bulbous tip in a 26-year-old girl is corrected with resection of nearly the whole dome bilaterally during the revision surgery. The depression of the upper border of the alar cartilage (alar-nasal crease), which is usually a secondary cartilage deficiency problem, is corrected with small sliced cartilage inlays fixed with mattress sutures. **A,** preoperative views. **B,** markings made at surgery. **C–E,** final result.

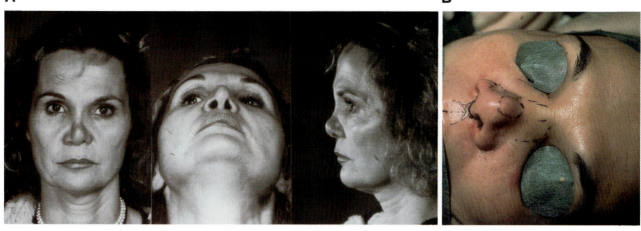

**FIG 18–6.**
Middle-aged woman with severe alar pinching, obstruction in the valve area, and a mass of fibrous tissue in the tip and at the level of the upper and lower lateral cartilages. In addition to correcting the external and internal walls with interposition of sliced cartilage grafts, a septal perforation of more than 4 cm in diameter could be reduced considerably in a one-stage procedure (see the later section on septal perforations), at least in the anterior two thirds of the defect. A complete closure with a three-stage method was not necessary in this case. **A,** preoperative views. **B,** correction areas outlined. **C–E,** result after 1 year.

tum and fixation of this mobilized upper lateral cartilage by transalar mattress sutures. Eventually one can remodel the lower lateral cartilages and hold the lateral crus in a more convex position with the same mattress sutures.

## DEPRESSIONS AT THE UPPER BORDER OF THE ALA (ALAR-NASAL CREASE)

These depressions are also a problem of secondary cartilage deficiency. They have to be corrected by means of small cartilage inlays fixed with mattress sutures.

## HANGING (HOODING) ALA

The alar rim must have a harmonious line, not too low, not too high, not too straight, and not asymmetrical. When the aesthetic relationship between the columella and the alar rim does not exist or when the nose is significantly shortened by raising the columella, it may be necessary to raise the alar rim in addition to the columellar correction. I employ the following technique for accomplishing a rim elevation: (1) marginal resection and (2) trimming the caudal rim of the lateral crus of the alar cartilage. Actually I perform marginal resections in about 10%

of all rhinoplasties. As I proposed in 1977[17] I mostly cut the edge of the nostril along its whole length when the entire lower lateral rim is too low (Fig 18–7).

On request I correct other anomalies and resect the border only posteriorly or anteriorly or at either end. The outline of the wedge resection is carefully marked with a scalpel, and the resection is carried out with fine, curved scissors. After cautious cauterization with a no. 15 blade, the cut edges are meticulously approximated by over-and-over sutures of 6–0 nonabsorbable material. These lower lateral rim resections are often combined with alar base resections. In some patients the chief secondary deformity is not the thickness of the entire nasal tip, but merely the thickness of the nostril margins. Reduction of such marginal thickness can be performed at the same time as the marginal resection by removing

celluloadipose or fibrous tissue between the two skin layers of the nostril (Fig 18–8).

## RETRACTION OF THE ALAR BORDER

A slightly pronounced height of the alar ridge may have an attractive sensual look, but excessive retraction of the alar border becomes quite unattractive. In most cases, I use a technique that I advocated in 1977,[17] which consists of adequate dissection of the nostril and insertion of a cartilage spacer.

If at the beginning of the operation such a correction is planned, I perform an intracartilaginous instead of an infracartilaginous incision. With this incision or the intracartilaginous one, the upper part of the lateral crus should, if possible, not be resected. With the intracartilaginous incision a pocket

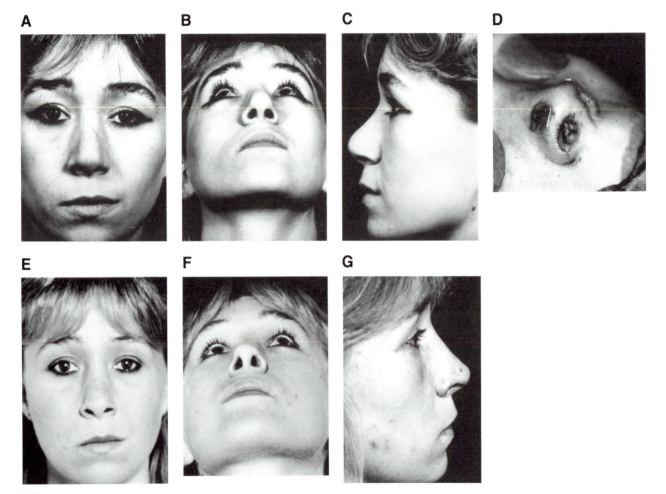

**FIG 18–7.**
A 25-year-old female wtih a deep and straight alar rim corrected with marginal resection and meticulous 6–0 over-and-over suturing. **A–C,** preoperative views. **D,** end of the operation with marginal over-and-over sutures. **E–G,** late results show improvement.

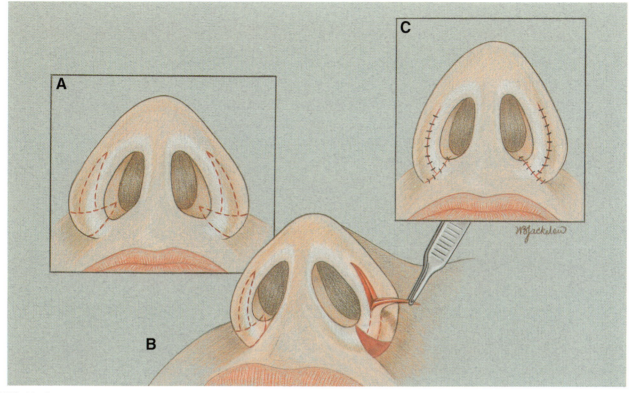

**FIG 18–8.**
Thinning the thick ala combined with alar base wedge resection. **A,** outline of the excisions. **B,** after the marginal resection a beveled incision at the alar border permits a keel resection of celluloadipose tissue between the external and the internal skin layer of the ala. **C,** "over-and-over" suture at the alar rim and separate sutures at the base.

between the external skin and vestibular skin can be created by approaching the margin with fine blunt scissors in the region of the alar retraction. The pocket is enlarged with the curved Trelat elevator and pushed down with the marginal skin in order to make room for the rectangular or oval piece of cartilage harvested from the upper part of the lateral alar crus or from the septum. Two or three transalar mattress sutures tied over a plastic sheet with 5–0 nonabsorbable thread will keep the cartilage transplant in situ and the alar rim in the new position. A slight overcorrection at the end of the operation is of benefit to achieve a good permanent result (Fig 18–9).

## SHORT NOSE, PIG SNOUT NOSE

For lengthening the whole nose, the external skin can usually be stretched downward and forward much more easily than the mucosa of the nasal cavity and the skin of the vestibule. Thus it is rather difficult to lengthen a nose that has been previously overshortened. A cartilage graft can correct the ob-tuse nasolabial angle. An inner degloving maneuver has to be added to the external one. This procedure can be combined with correction of a tethered upper lip by removal or reduction of a too prominent nasal spine; section or reduction of the depressor septi nasi muscle; freeing the upper lip and the gingiva from the anterior surface of the maxilla between the spine and the teeth; and inserting a cartilaginous, bony, or alloplastic spacer. Depending on the degree of shortness of the nose, one can apply different techniques. Once the mucoperichondrial vault is brought downward and forward by using the extramucosal technique, a cartilage spacer must be provided to adequately lengthen the septum and with it, the whole nose (Fig 18–10). Then the two mucosal flaps cover the graft and are joined to the columella with interrupted and mattress sutures. The cartilage can be obtained from the posterior part of the septum as a straight or L-shaped graft and sutured to the anterior border of the septal cartilage by mattress sutures. Extreme cases of short nose have to be treated by using augmentation with an L-shaped rib cartilage.

**A**

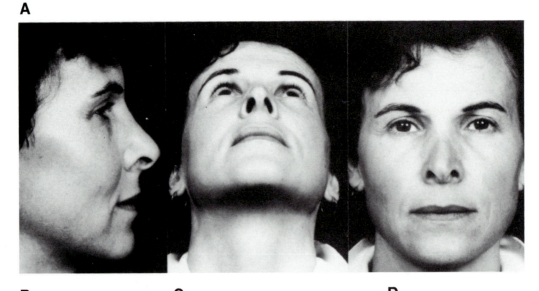

**B**          **C**          **D**

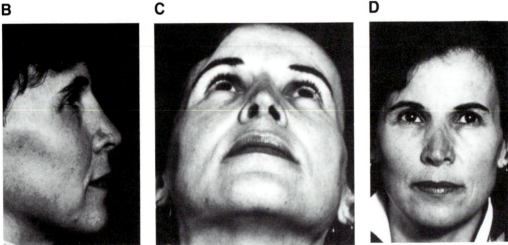

**FIG 18–9.**
Alar retraction in a young lady after two previous rhinoplasties. Lowering of the alar rim is combined with tip-plasty.
**A,** preoperative views showing the retracted alae. **B–D,** final results show improvement.

## INADEQUATE OSTEOTOMIES AND SECONDARY BONE DEFORMITIES

Many secondary deformities result from inadequate or irregular osteotomies and particularly from insufficient mobilization of the nasal bones and approximation of their median borders, i.e., the cut edge after hump removal. Any hump removal calls for an exact and symmetrical narrowing of the nasal bones in the same way that a large flat nose needs narrowing without hump removal in order to reconstruct the nasal arch and build a triangular pyramid in cross section.

Incomplete lateral and transverse osteotomies and incomplete infracturing are among the more common postrhinoplasty problems. Refracture with eventual comminution of that bone complex helps to correct these problems. After the lateral osteotomies are performed, I check to ensure that the osteotomies have been made at the appropriate level. If the testing finger finds a step at the lateral edge of the lateral osteotomy, the cut has not been placed laterally enough. A parallel osteotomy must be added immediately and the resulting bone strip left in place. This can be done with a 2-mm osteotome.

After precise approximation of the dorsal edges of the nasal bones, it becomes obvious whether the transverse osteotomy is truly horizontal or is angulated with medial spur formation. This defect occurs most often in noses with thick bones. If such a spur

**A**

**B**

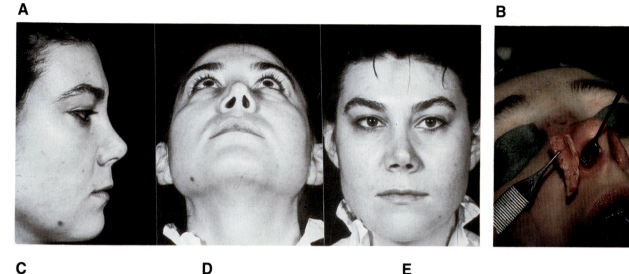

**C**

**D**

**E**

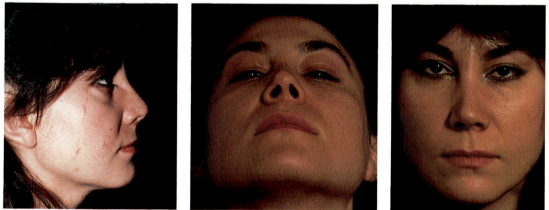

**FIG 18–10.**
The nose of this 25-year-old girl was overshortened during the primary surgery **(A).** For lengthening a conchal cartilage graft **(B)** was placed into the membraneous septum and the columella. In addition, the tip had to be corrected by symmetrically remodeling the lower lateral cartilages. Skin and lining of the lengthened nose have been fixed by transnasal mattress sutures for 1 week. **C–E,** the results show improvement.

is present, it must be mobilized with a curved chisel and removed with the Luer or Levignac biting forceps as when correcting a flat nasal pyramid. Occasionally, when the base of the bony pyramid is very broad in flat noses, a transnasal suture is necessary for holding the bony and cartilaginous structures in their new position for 7 to 10 days. The suture material is 4–0 nylon on a straight needle going through the nasal cavity, the septum, and the other nasal cavity with the osteotomy bone gap used for passage.

## CROOKED NOSE

In cases of deviation of the bony pyramid, I proceed by performing all the usual osteotomies and by resecting a strip of bone from the dorsal edge of the overly large side. Many authors correct such deviations by resecting bone at the lateral osteotomy site on the flatter side, which permits one to pivot the whole nasal pyramid toward that side. I prefer to manage the mobilization and displacement of the bony and cartilaginous elements of the pyramid by detaching them from each other and placing them in a new straight and equilibrated position.

In all cases, but especially in S-shaped dorsal deviation, it is important to section the upper lateral cartilages at their insertion into the septum by using extramucosal technique. These cartilages must be trimmed paramedially and placed into a symmetrical position.

In many cases a crooked nose is due to a *deviation of the septal cartilage* beginning at its junction with the vomer and contracting toward the roof with

**A**

**B**

**C**

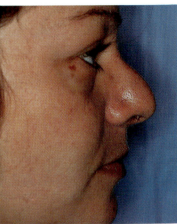

**D**

**E**

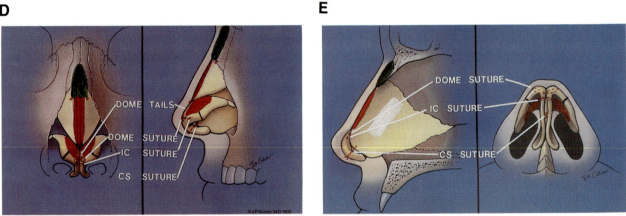

**F**

**G**

**H**

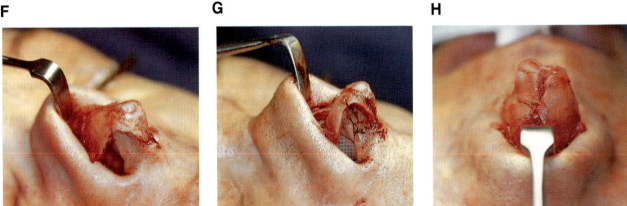

**FIG 19–8.**
Dorsal deformity. **A–C,** preoperative views show that the patient has a dorsal deficiency in the upper portion of the nose but a residual dorsal hump in the lower aspect of the dorsum. The tip is broad also. **D** and **E,** Gunter diagrams indicate that the plan included sutures for the domes, intracrural sutures, a crural-septal suture, and the formation of dome tails. In addition, a graft for the upper half of the dorsal aspect of the nose was planned along with a resection of the dorsum in the lower half. A transection of the lateral crus was planned to reduce the convexity in the tip of the nose. **F–I,** intraoperative views show the ill-defined tip cartilages and excess convexity in the area of the lateral crus. After scoring the domes and lateral crus, dome tails were preserved. These were sutured to the dorsal edge of the septum so as to prevent the tip from dropping postoperatively. **J** and **K,** postoperatively there is an improvement in the profile because the dorsal deficiency was recognized. Resecting the lower half of the dorsum alone would not have sufficed. The nose is narrower in the tip as well. The basal view shows improvement in the triangulation and also exhibits the fact that a columellar scar in this region is usually inconsequential.              *Continued.*

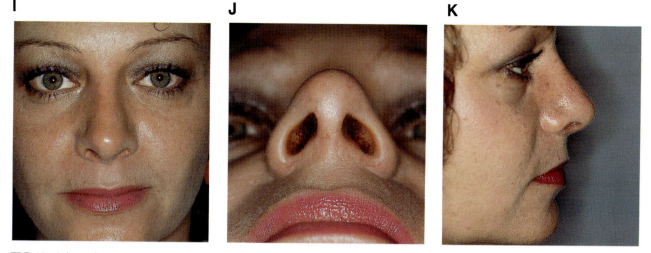

**FIG 19–8 (cont.).**

sion in the area of the left upper lateral cartilage. The nose itself was also slightly long, and there was a hanging columella.

Drawing on photographs of the patient preoperatively helped ascertain what needed to be performed (i.e., tip reduction). In drawing on these pictures it also appeared that a slight shortening of the nose would be helpful. The Gunter diagram indicates the exact operative steps that were taken. This included transection of both the middle and lateral crura. Sutures were required to control the shape of the existing tip cartilages. These included the intercrural suture as well as dome sutures and a crural-septal suture. The convexity of the lateral crus had to be corrected by transecting the lateral crus in its most convex portion. A graft had to be added to the region of the left upper lateral cartilage, and some shortening of the caudal edge of the septum was done. Finally, some additional intracrural sutures were necessary to maintain the narrowness of the middle crura region.

At surgery the cartilages could be seen after reflecting the skin by making an external columellar incision (stair-step). The abnormal cartilages showed eversion of the middle crura. The domes themselves were not narrow enough, but the width of the lateral crus seemed to be appropriate. The surgical maneuvers described in the Gunter diagram were performed. In the intraoperative view one can see that the clamp is pointing to the area of the transection of the middle (medial) crura. This simple transection results in overlap of the elements. In order to control the amount of height reduction, some undermining of the cartilage on one side was performed. Usually it is not necessary to suture the elements of the middle crura after the transection is made (as was the

case here). However, if undermining is significant and there is a drop of 2 to 3 mm the elements of the crura then begin to separate. Sutures are then required to prevent the elements from becoming displaced in the anteroposterior direction.

The dome was scored and dome sutures placed. Intercrural sutures were required not only at the usual location, at the cephalic part of the middle crura, but also in this case at the region of the caudal aspect of the middle crura in order to correct the eversion that was seen intraoperatively. The final result can be seen intraoperatively where there is now narrowing of the domes. Although not visible on these particular intraoperative views, a transection of the lateral crura was performed that resulted in a slight overlap of the elements and an improvement in the convexity of the lateral crura. A graft was added as an onlay to the region of the left upper lateral cartilage to correct a slight depression noted here. This graft was sutured directly in place. Finally, a crural-septal suture of 4–0 nylon was used by passing between the middle crura, which then picked up the cartilage of the septum (after it was shortened). The suture was then brought back out between the middle crura and tied. This maintained the tip cartilages in the desired location. It also corrected the hanging columella.

Postoperative results at greater than 1 year indicate an improvement in the profile view with a slightly shorter nose that no longer has as much columellar hang as it had previously. There is not as much tip projection either. The frontal view shows an improvement in the depression that caused the patient's complaints of asymmetry and also an improvement in the width of the tip of the nose due to

**A**

**B**

**C**

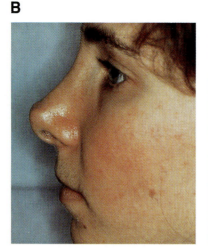

**D**

**E**

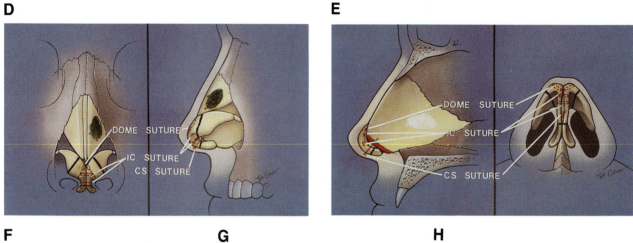

**F**

**G**

**H**

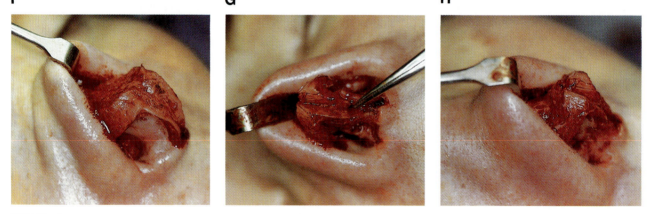

**FIG 19–9.**
The overprojecting tip. **A–C,** the preoperative views exhibit depression on the left lateral side and a boxiness to the tip, especially on the basal view. There is a slightly hanging columella. **D** and **E,** Gunter diagrams indicate that the plan included several sutures to hold the cartilages of the tip together, as well as some shortening of the caudal edge of the septum, a graft to the left upper lateral cartilage, a transection of the midportion of the lateral crus, and a transection of the midportion of the medial or middle crus. **F,** an intraoperative view after the exposure shows that the middle crura are everted and there is a lack of dome narrowness. **G** and **H,** after sutures are applied to hold the cartilages in the proper position, the middle crus is transected to correct the overly projecting tip. The clamp points to the area of the middle crus transection.

*Continued.*

**I**     **J**     **K**

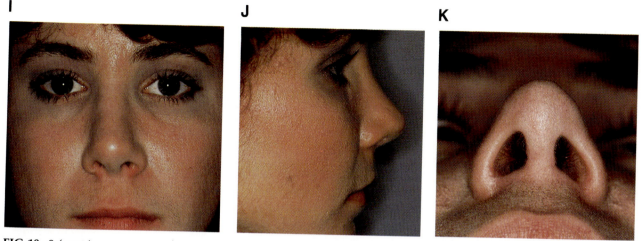

**FIG 19–9 (cont.).**

**I–K,** postoperatively one can see an improvement in the overly projecting tip as well as an improvement in the boxy nature. The depression on the left side is no longer seen, nor is the columella hanging. The basal view exhibits a very satisfactory scar.

the prominent and convex lateral crura. The domes themselves are not as sharp and prominent or as separated. This is due in part to the bringing together and stabilization of the middle crura. A basal view shows that the boxy, squared-off tip is now much more triangulated, as is desirable. Although this view is important to plastic surgeons, it is only occasionally important to the patients themselves. In this case, however, the view indicates not only an improvement as a result of relocating the tip cartilages but also the fact that the stair-step columellar incision was well worth the price of having the ability to execute maneuvers with a great deal more precision.

### Short Nose

See Chapter 13 in this book.

### Alloplastic Problems

Alloplastic complications are well known. When silicone or some other type of form material is used to augment the nose, one of the potential complications is implant exposure. When this becomes the case, it is usually necessary to replace the alloplastic material with autogenous material. The open approach allows for ease of replacement and execution of the reconstructive process. The patient in Figure 19–10 is a case in point. This is a middle-aged Vietnamese woman who had a previous augmentation rhinoplasty using silicone. She was seen to have partial implant exposure upon physical examination.

It was decided to remove the existing alloplastic material and replace it with autogenous material from the septum if possible but, if not, from the concha.

At surgery a stair-step, external columellar incision was made and the skin retracted. A large silicone implant was seen to traverse the dorsum. It went between the tip cartilages and not only gave the patient some dorsal prominence but provided a good deal of tip projection as well. Upon removal of the alloplastic material at surgery it was apparent that the patient required a good deal of dorsal fill as well as tip projection. A double-layered cartilaginous graft was fashioned to a size that was similar to the alloplastic graft that was removed. By elevating the mucoperichondrium bilaterally the graft could be harvested from the septum. The double-layered graft was then fashioned, and sutures were used to hold the components to one another. The graft was laid along the dorsum and held there with nylon sutures. This dorsal graft also maintained nasal length.

Sutures were used to secure the existing cartilages to one another. For example, in order to prevent splaying of the tip cartilages, an intercrural suture was required. In order to maximize narrowing of the tip, dome sutures were utilized. Because a transfixion suture was not required here, a crural-septal suture was not used. Despite the dorsal graft there was a need for further tip projection, and therefore a small tip graft was fashioned and sutured to the existing, somewhat deficient tip cartilages by using a 5–0 nylon suture. The final result of grafting the tip and dorsal aspects of the septum can be seen in the intraoperative view. Finally, the pa-

## The Underlying Facial Skeleton

This supportive structure may present specific abnormalities reflected in nasal changes. The nasal sill and floor may be more or less deficient of maxillary bone and cause depression or notching externally. The premaxillary procumbency (forward projection) markedly disturbs the nasal-columellar-lip relationship, especially in bilateral complete cleft lip cases. It is compounded with a relative or real lack of anterior projection of the lateral maxillary segment or segments to create an abnormal differential placement of the columellar base and alar bases in the anterior-to-posterior direction. These bony relationships are widely variable from case to case, and they may also vary in any individual situation with time, growth changes, and the effects of surgical treatment and dental orthopedic maneuvers. As time passes, the reverse of procumbency (retroplacement or retrusion of the premaxilla) may develop, and generalized hypomaxillarism and midface depression may result in a class III malocclusion (see Figs 20–14 and 20–16). These problems can well affect the nose directly and/or relatively. The basic deformities of the CLTND complex are a result of not only the skeletal abnormalities intrinsic to the nose itself but also its underlying facial bony support.

## Accessory Deformities

Many accessory anatomic aberrations of the nasal features can accompany the basic characteristic cleft deformity complex,[4, 9] and these are in large part iatrogenic and result from failings in lip "repair" or nasal "reconstruction." As a result of lip repair, accessory nasal problems may include nostril enlargement or constriction and asymmetry; misplacement of the alar base in any direction; distortion of the alar base, nasal floor, or sill; and scar contractures influencing the nose. As a result of attempts at nasal reconstruction, accessory deformities may include destruction of the normal nasal columellar-lip junction and angle; every variety of distortion of the columella; abnormal lengthening of the columella; enlargement, constriction, and asymmetry of the nostrils; unnecessary external or internal scarring; subdermal scarring with destruction of the elastic capabilities of the skin drape; damage or destruction of essential cartilaginous framework parts; abnormal islands of bone, cartilage, or synthetic graft material; obstruction from several sources, including abnormal added mass or scarring internally, neglected septal deviation or turbinate hypertrophy, or a lack

of alar wing positional corrections; and a myriad of inadequate or inappropriate "corrections." These may be due to either a lack of understanding of the basic problem complex, a lack of ability to effect a desired change, or both. These iatrogenic problems greatly encumber or prevent the successful efforts of any other surgeon coming later with a desire to improve the situation. The surgeon can no longer concentrate on the actual virgin CLTND, which may have been relatively straightforward, but he must deal with many other problems that may be far more unyielding to the best efforts or even irreversible. In the bilateral cleft lip repair, irreverence for the normal columellar-lip junction and transposition of flaps into the nasal columellar area to "lengthen the skin" or any other method of "lengthening" the columellar skin directly will likely create everlasting and gradually worsening problems of abnormal-looking distortion with growth and the passage of time.[7] A method of bilateral cleft lip repair that "puts it all together" has previously been set forth; it avoids injury in this area and presents a rational, contemporary approach.[2] Noniatrogenic accessory problems also occur and are the same as those special problems presenting in non–cleft-related nasal reconstruction candidates. The worst of these is abnormally thick skin. While this virtually is not seen in very young children, it is an occasional later seriously limiting factor. The surgeon will be wise to identify this problem before surgery and greatly reduce expectations of improvement. There may also be a relatively smaller alar soft-tissue mass on the side of the cleft. This is reflected by slightly diminished vertical height of the lateral external alar prominence and a somewhat less pronounced convexity. Also, persons with CLTND may have any other set of inherent features that may be considered less than ideal in non–cleft-affected persons. Included would be abnormally large nasal tip cartilages, a dorsal hump, the effects of trauma, etc. These features may be dealt with simultaneously while the specific cleft deformity changes are made, especially in late cases.

## THE TREATMENT GOAL

The goal of treatment is to translate a solid understanding of the CLTND problem complex into a rational and appropriate program to modify form and function toward normalcy without causing harm. (Normalizing the anatomy means making modifications of existing structural distortions to more nearly resemble normal. It does not mean a complete change of structure from one thing to another.) The physical aspects of the developing nose and face and the psychological aspects of the person as a whole must be carefully considered together.

## TIMING THE RECONSTRUCTION

There are three categories of timing CLTND reconstruction (CLTNDR). When the surgical approach is made on an infant either immediately with or in concert with (staged) primary cleft lip repair, it is referred to as *"primary CLTNDR."* When the nasal surgery is deferred until early childhood, it is called *"early CLTNDR."* When the surgical effort is begun later, usually in teenage years or adulthood, it is referred to as *"late CLTNDR."*

### Primary Cleft Lip–Type Nose Deformity Repair

It is natural and proper for surgeons to want to promptly "fix" any structural abnormality. And so it has been with the CLTND. [3, 5–9] But there ought to be a distinct physical or psychological requirement why a specific structural abnormality should be "fixed" at a given time. And this ought to take into account risks and disadvantages as well as supposed advantages of the treatment.

**Arguments in Favor of Primary CLTNDR.**—The purported indications include the "prevention of a later deformity" and the "avoidance of psychological problems."

**Arguments Against Primary CLTNDR.**—"Prevention of later deformities" is certainly not ensured by primary reconstructive attempts. If there is lessening of the deformity, it may be only a matter of degree, and these cases are likely to need further corrections that may be made much more difficult by previous surgery. Controlled studies do not exist and are virtually impossible since cases vary.

The "avoidance of psychological problems" is unacceptable as an indication for primary repair. Children do not develop complexes or psychological problems related to facial features ordinarily until 6 or 7 years of age or later.

There are remarkable spontaneous changes in the physical relationships of the nose, the premaxilla, and lateral maxillary segments as well as intrinsic nasal growth changes in the first few years and later. So there are significant difficulties in making lasting definitive primary CLTND correction judgements.

In the unilateral condition, some uncontrolled evidence suggests that primary CLTNDR may be helpful to some extent in certain cases in certain surgical hands. [3, 6, 9] But follow-ups until 17 to 18 years would be necessary for absolute conclusions, along with proper controls. All surgeons dealing with unilateral cleft lips have been amazed from time to time at how good the nose may look after lip repair and only adjustment of the nasal floor and alar base position (Fig 20–5,A and B). And at other times the surgeon may be equally dismayed at the poor appearance of the nose in cases that seemed similar (Fig 20–5,C and D). So it is not possible to make a clear prediction as to which patients might benefit most from CLTNDR primarily. Furthermore, the likelihood of unnecessary scarring or of irreversible damage to the tiny fragile lower cartilaginous framework in an infant's nose is considerable—especially in the hands of the occasional surgeon. Experienced surgeons will have a healthy respect for this risk as well as for the multitude of iatrogenic problems that so often compound the issue after previous CLTND surgery. It is still questionable whether primary unilateral CLTNDR is generally advisable, what the proper candidate selection process should be, and whether the potential advantages outweigh the potential disadvantages. [1, 4] In bilateral cleft cases, there is clear evidence that columellar skin flap elongations result in abnormal distortions with growth and time—to say nothing of the additional scarring and atypical "operated-on" look. [7] In severe bilateral CLTNDR cases, probably no conservative primary reconstruction attempt is likely to have significant success, and in mild conditions such attempts may be of little usefulness. Generally speaking, bilateral primary CLTNDR methods raise all the same questions as in unilateral cases. In addition, they carry magnified risks of unnecessary scarring and tissue harm, incompletely "correct" the problem, are uncontrolled and mostly inadequately followed for solid conclusions, and may make later reconstructive attempts more difficult or impossible.

Compare the congenital CLTND for a moment with congenital microtia. There is no significant pressure in favor of immediate primary "reconstruction" of this anomaly, which is subject to change with growth. Why, then, "repair" the nose primarily (perhaps an even more complex structure subject to remarkable change)?

No surgeon will be at fault for not doing primary CLTNDR, but grievous error may be committed by

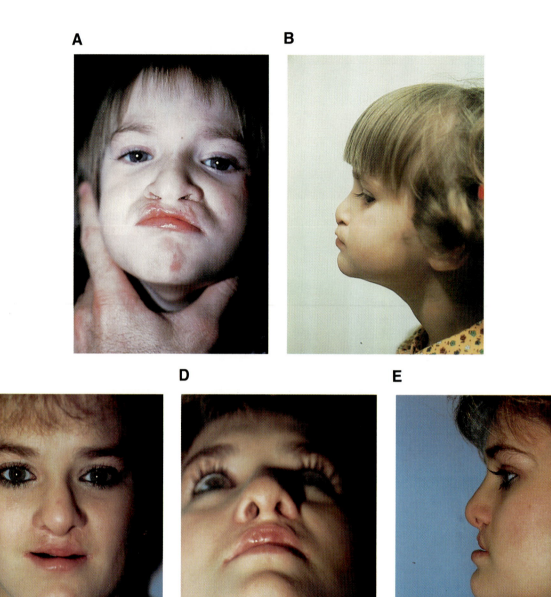

**FIG 20–16.**
Bilateral case example. **A,** frontal-infranasal view with an "absent" columella. **B,** lateral view. **C,** frontal view at 17 years of age (12 years after reconstruction of the lower cartilages). **D,** infranasal view, 17 years of age. **E,** side view at 17 years of age with midface retrusion. (From Black PW, Hartrampf CR, Beegle P: *Ann Plast Surg* 12:128, 1984. Used by permission.)

normal anatomy and comparative anatomy of the deformity condition. If one side of the lip cleft is complete and the other incomplete, an asymmetrical nasal deformity will be present while both sides are abnormal, and it adds interest to the challenge of bilateral CLTNDR. Of course, no direct columellar skin surgical alterations are made. Bilateral cases are presented in Figures 20–15 to 20–17.

### The Internal Components of the Nose

The factors of importance pertinent to the internal structure of the nose have to do with obstruction and projection.

**Obstruction.**—The technique of correction of the inner nasal components relates to the septum and the turbinates. With unilateral cleft lips the nasal septum is usually convexly deviated on the side of the cleft. The other side is likely to have lower turbinate hypertrophy. In the bilateral condition the septum may be central or deviated depending on the asymmetries of clefting, and the turbinate situation is likely variable. Although not usual, when severe obstruction is present in early childhood, the surgeon may wish to relieve it while doing early CLTNDR. It has been stated that septal resection does not interfere with growth of the nose. There are still reservations, however, and it is rarely if ever required to

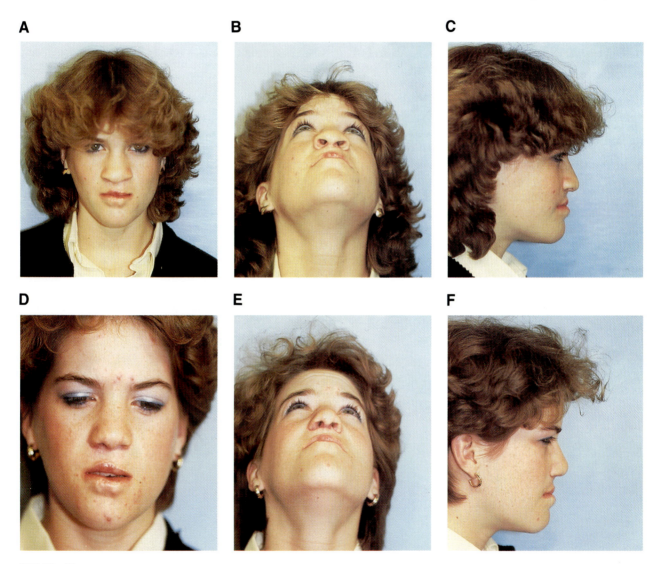

**FIG 20–17.**
Bilateral case example. **A,** frontal view—wide nose. **B,** infranasal view—wide and large nostrils. **C,** lateral view. **D,** frontal view showing postoperative lower cartilage reconstruction and narrowing of bone and alar bases (wedge resections). **E,** infranasal view. **F,** lateral view.

carry out extensive nasal septal surgical resection in young children. It is virtually always possible to establish adequate airways by a manipulative re-alignment of the septum; more definitive septal resection-reconstruction can be done later if needed. If septal resection is done in late CLTNDR cases, it may be done prior to elevating the MFF (or LNF) by using whatever approach is familiar to the surgeon. Or with the flap elevated, the septum can be approached directly from its caudal margin by going between the medial crura. This will probably seem more unfamiliar and difficult for most surgeons accustomed to other approaches. Some very conservative turbinate reduction in children may be helpful, but it is very uncommonly necessary.

**Septal Projection.**—In perhaps 10% of bilateral CLTND conditions septal development is profoundly inadequate, and this is associated with a *profound flattening* of the tip of the nose (the septum is short from maxilla to tip and from nasion to tip). The condition of profound septal inadequacy permits nasal collapse (flattening, loss of tip projection) toward the facial plane. This CLTND profound flattening is a separate problem from that of the lower nasal cartilage framework derangement and its unnatural tip depression and caudal rotation. Recognizing the problem may be impossible until later growth simply does not keep up with expectations. And it probably should not be dealt with surgically at early CLTNDR, but instead as a separate later procedure some years after the early cartilaginous correction has been made and when the surgeon is convinced that this diagnosis is correct (although no

exact knowledge about appropriate timing exists). Previous knowledge of what the normal septum *ought* to look like from experience is essential. The straightforward technique of reconstruction is, once again, to directly reverse the septal deformity, i.e., to elongate the septum in both dimensions by a cartilage graft extension (Fig 20–18). This graft can be harvested from the septum itself and applied directly to the septal "tip" margin as a boomerang-like right triangular graft. It is fixed by interrupted sutures of 6–0 clear nylon along the attached fitted margin and stabilized forward to prevent lateral bending by two sandwich splint grafts (one on each side) of full-thickness septal cartilage material placed several millimeters below the dorsum (parallel to it) so as not to interfere with the normal A-frame upper lateral cartilage relationship to the septum. These sandwich splint grafts overlap the junction between the septum and the tip boomerang graft and are secured by several through-and-through mattress sutures of 6–0 clear nylon. Of course, the long-established principles of balanced cartilage grafting must be respected, i.e., all opposing graft sides must be the same with respect to perichondral coverage (either intact or denuded) to maintain straightness and avoid warping. If lower cartilage work is done at the same time, it should be done as always, and it may or may not be attached along the caudal septal margin as appropriate. The occasional surgeon may think that *most* bilateral CLTND cases have septal inadequacy and "profound flattening"— this is *not* so (see Fig 20–16). And caution is recommended so as not to overreact and perform unnecessary septal tip surgery. The patient in Figure 20–20 received a boomerang graft.

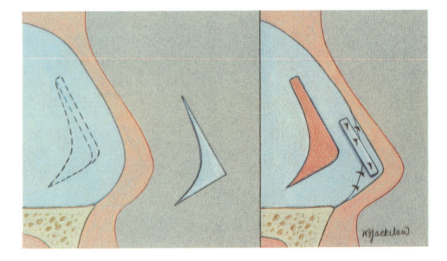

**FIG 20–18.**
Diagram of septal boomerang graft enhancement.

## Technique of Correction of Bony Skeletal Deformities

Bony problems may relate to the nasal bone structure or the non-nasal facial bones.

### Nasal Bone Problems

In some cases the nasal bony structure is unusually wide while the dorsal profile is satisfactory (see Fig 20–17). A straightforward method of correction is to remove a segment of tissue directly alongside the septal dorsum from tip to glabella. The upper lateral cartilages are separated from the dorsum, and a strip of cartilage along this margin some several millimeters wide is resected. Then continuing directly cephalad in the bony nose, the same width of bone is removed up to the nasion with a small straight bone-biting instrument. The same is done on each side. Lateral osteotomies are performed, and infracturing narrows the entire nasal pyramid without changing the profile (see Fig 20–17).

### Non-Nasal Bone Problems

Problems affecting the nose at the maxillary level are commonly relative to bone insufficiency in the nasal floor ("notching"), inadequate forward projection of the maxilla on the cleft side in unilateral cleft cases, and bilateral hypomaxillarism and premaxillary retrusion (midface retrusion) in bilateral cleft cases (see Figs 20–14 and 20–16). Panhypomaxillarism can present with other clefts as well— even with solitary secondary palate clefts.

The exposure provided by the MFF presents a perfect simultaneous opportunity for certain grafting procedures. The insufficiency in the bony nasal floor can be corrected by grafting, and forward movement of the alar base away from a "depressed" maxilla also may be accomplished by bolster onlay graft support. These grafts may come from excess nasal septal cartilage or bone. They may be done simultaneously with grafting the bony maxillary arch cleft— so-called alveolar bone grafting. Iliac or cranial bone can be used; there is no practical difference in the results. Iliac bone is preferred, and most patients agree. Bone grafts to maxillary clefts are usually done between the ages of 9 to 11 (8 to 12) years, depending upon dental and bony development (and with orthodontic-orthopedic arch compatibility preparation) prior to eruption of the incoming permanent canine lateral to the cleft. There seems to be no significant adverse consequence on growth at these ages.

Some cases of severe maxillary retrusion will be inadequately responsive to orthodontic orthopedics and will require maxillary advancement surgery. This may involve LeForte II or LeForte I surgery and may favorably or unfavorably affect the nasal-facial profile relationships. Occasionally mandibular surgical adjustments also may be required.

## Technique of Correction of Accessory Deformities

While there are a multitude of variations and combinations, certain of these accessory problems are seen with considerable regularity. The treatment of some of these can therefore be addressed. In every case the surgeon needs to rely on judgement, aesthetic sense, and experience in planning and executing the specific changes in individual situations to reverse the deformities.

### Abnormal Nostril Enlargement

This is usually associated with a widened nasal floor and misplaced alar base and can usually be corrected simultaneously with the lower cartilages. It is most directly improved by a properly planned wedge resection as appropriate or a Y-V–plasty at the alar base (see Fig 20–17).

### Abnormal Nostril Constriction

This is one of the most difficult problems to correct nicely.[9] It may be amenable to a V-Y–plasty at the alar base if this is where the problem is. The next most likely consideration is a moon-shaped takeout around the anterior rim of the nostril (Fig 20–19). This is also likely to elevate the nostril rim (cephalad) in the frontal view. The surgeon must be cautious in this judgement to avoid an overcorrection. At other times a wedge transfer of full-thickness tissue on a subcutaneous casual pedicle may be slid into the nasal floor–alar base area. If the lip is too long on the side of the cleft and the alar base too high, the wedge can be taken caudal to the alar base to help both problems. Alternatively, it can be taken lateral to the alar base in other cases. Often nostril constriction is best dealt with as a second stage in the CLTNDR. Complete correction of severe nostril constriction may be virtually impossible surgically. Perhaps a properly designed "tissue expander" will answer this problem (a "nostril expander").

### The Hanging Anterior Nostril Rim Skin

Even if the cartilage framework is nicely corrected, there may tend to be excessive skin on the side of

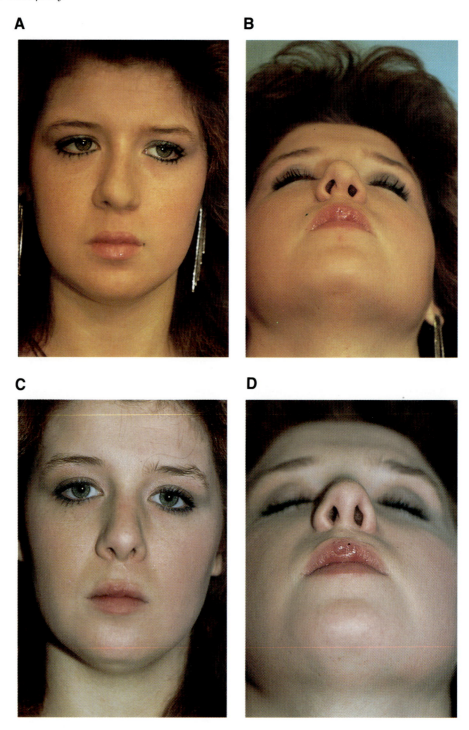

**FIG 20–19.**
**A** and **B**, preoperative views of unilateral deformity with nostril constriction. **C** and **D**, postoperative cartilage reconstruction, septoplastic and anterior rim reaction on constricted side.

the deformity relative to the elongation of the skin on that side of the nose due to the original caudal malpositioning of the lower cartilage. If this skin is not successfully adjusted cephalad at the original surgery, the anterior rim may still droop caudally due to skin alone. A very carefully positioned anterior nostril rim excisional ellipse (as mentioned in the previous paragraph) may ameliorate this problem at a second stage.

*Alar Base Misplacement*
This has been mentioned in conjunction with nostril size adjustment. Frequently the alar base needs to be moved in more than one direction (such as medi-

ally *and* superiorly or inferiorly). A slanted Y-V–plasty can do this nicely, or a slanted V-Y–plasty may be proper (for lateral *and* superior or inferior movements). A floor or alar wedge takeout or tissue transfer may also be appropriate in some cases. Obviously these maneuvers must be "custom planned" and can usually be done at the original surgery.

### Unusually Large Alar Mass

Generous alar base lateral takeouts may be needed in some noses when the alar formations are unusually large (see Fig 20–17). These takeouts may be designed and positioned to or not to significantly affect the nostril size by either taking a full-thickness wedge (externally and through the nostril side) or only an external wedge (without entering the nostril).

### Residual and New Postoperative Defects and Asymmetries

In all second-stage CLTNDR cases, planning is on an individual basis. If the evaluation suggests that the basic cartilage maneuvers required for success have not been accomplished, then the open approach by an MFF or LNF is likely to give the best opportunity for definitive improvement (tissues permitting). But if the basics have been handled well and only a slight local depression or asymmetry is present, then perhaps some limited camouflage subcuticular cartilage graft work may help. Alternatively, in cases where previously very extensive surgery has been done and the proper skeletal support may not be retrievable, supportive and/or contour grafts may be helpful together with whatever external modifications still may be reasonable within the residual ability of the tissues to respond. Occasionally, in cases where the lower lateral cartilage framework support has been destroyed or where the external alar prominence is relatively too slight, a properly chosen arched graft (like a rib) from the concha to the alar area is very helpful (oriented anteriorly to posteriorly from tip to alar base).

In some cases the elasticity and conforming capabilities of the nasal skin drape has been destroyed by external scarring and/or extensive postsurgical subdermal scarring. This may lead to flattening and may possibly restrict forward nose growth because of its unyielding external force. (The Flathead Indians and the Chinese understood this principle and molded foreheads and tiny feet. This is also the basis of the Fränkel orthodontic appliance in reverse.)

In India, nasal septal destruction and flattening secondary to leprosy has been reversed for more than 25 years by graduated acrylic fitted blocks inserted through incisions in the upper labial sulcus to expand the nasal lining and skin in preparation for cantilever bone grafts. It seems quite feasible that a subcutaneously placed inflatable expander on an unyielding platform anchored to bone by a tripod (at the nasion and the two lateral inferior nasal-maxillary wall margins) may provide a solution to the very occasional inadequate nasal skin problem so that proper skeletal reconstruction can be accomplished.

What may be a satisfactory result at a given age may become newly unsatisfactory either intrinsically or in relationship to other facial proportions with growth and development.[7] These changes can be anticipated to some extent but may come as a surprise as well (see Figs 20–14 and 20–16). The surgeon should avoid overoperating at every whim and should follow through with an overall plan coordinated with dental and other team members.

It is always amazing and somewhat disconcerting how many patients are satisfied with a basic good improvement and fail to see a need to continue with relatively smaller changes that would take the result from third base to home plate (Fig 20–20). For instance, they are often unconcerned with nostril size discrepancies since they do not see this as a problem in the mirror.

### Combinations of Nose and Other Problems

It may be expedient to consider CLTNDR and nonnasal reconstructive needs at the same time surgically. A frequently coexisting problem is an upper labial or alveolar fistula. With the MFF these areas are directly amenable to treatment, and if the timing is right, an alveolar bone graft is an easy simultaneous procedure. Certain lip revisions may be convenient at the same time also. If the MFF is used, lip changes are marked and "red-lined" with the knife first—then the actual surgical changes are made last (after the MFF is replaced).

### Ordinary Non–cleft-related Unflattering Nasal Features

The same individuals with cleft problems may also have any other undesirable nasal features genetically related or on the basis of trauma. It may be appropriate to make corrections for such features as dorsal humps, bulbous tips, receding chins, lower lip protrusions, or post-traumatic external or internal prob-

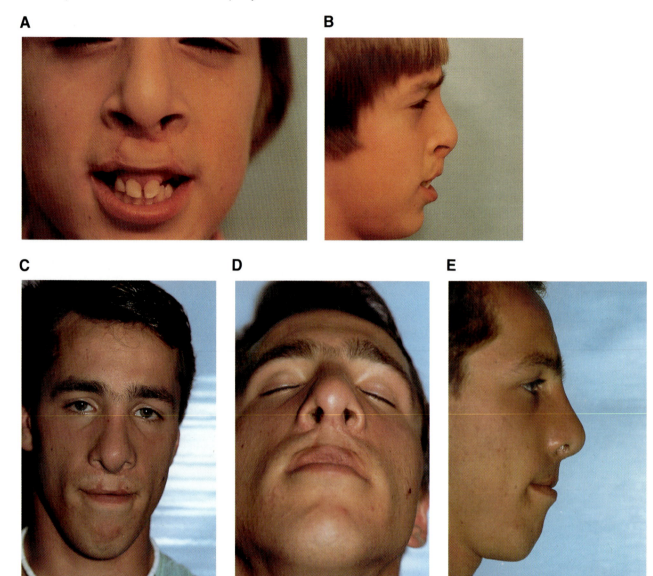

**FIG 20–20.**
**A** and **B,** this patient has had previous attempts nasal columellar "lengthening" elsewhere by prolabial flaps but has a residually flat nose. **C–E,** after lower cartilage reconstruction and a septal boomerang graft, the patient still needs further lip scar work and chin augmentation, but further help was declined.

lems at the same time that CLTND features are being corrected, especially in late CLTNDR or second-stage cases.

*Residual Overall Facial Considerations*
Even with the very best efforts to normalize the CLTND complex, the nose and other facial features may not be as flattering as hoped. Good dental rehabilitation together with the skilled addition of cosmetics and appropriate hair styling may enhance the overall presentation (Fig 20–21). Good advice in these areas should be made available when appro-

priate. In some cases psychological assistance may be indicated, and this important aspect of care should not be overlooked.

## CONCLUSIONS

CLTNDR, according to the methods outlined, provides good lower nasal symmetry and satisfactory tip projection and columellar length without changing the nose in abnormal ways. Results improve dramatically with experience. Good lower nasal form

A B

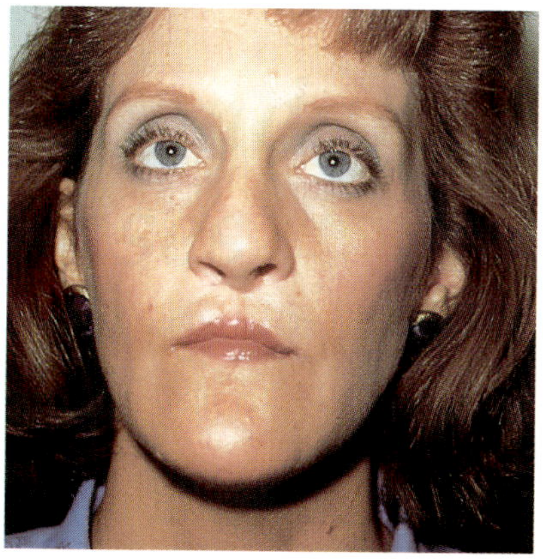

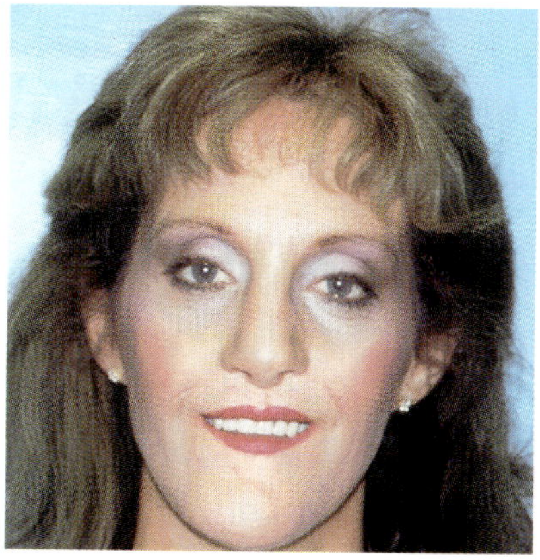

**FIG 20–21.**
**A,** bilateral cleft adult with a wide nose and unflattering presentation. **B,** after nasal surgery and dental, hair, and makeup enhancements.

and symmetry is predictable. When results are short of expectations, the reasons fall into certain categories: inadequate exposure, inadequate mobilization of the lateral alar wing, inadequate or timid execution of the treatment plan, lack of attention to "accesory" problems, and handicaps presented due to previous lip or nasal surgery. It is perfectly reasonable to anticipate some secondary additions to the basic CLTNDR, especially relative to nostril constriction (an error in the lip repair) or the "hanging," caudally elongated nasal skin on the side of the cleft. It is much easier to provide nostril narrowing than enlargement at the same time as basic CLTNDR. It appears that corrections made "early" are retained with growth (longest follow-ups for early unilateral and bilateral reconstructions are to 17 years of age). There is no added morbidity with these procedures when compared with any other rhinoplastic procedures.

## SUMMARY

Reconstruction of the CLTND presents a remarkable challenge. The conditions have basic commonalities, variations on the theme, many accessory problems and constant change until maturity. The aim of surgical treatment is to normalize anatomic derangements while avoiding harm due to direct injury or unnatural changes. Often surgery may be hampered by previous efforts and may need to be devoted as much or more to problems created by unsuccessful previous lip or nose surgery as to cleft-type problems. A plea is made for careful understanding of the CLTND complex and a rational conservative approach to its management aimed at reducing the

physical, psychological, and social stigmata associated with uncorrected deformities of this type that tend to mark individuals as "different" and as cleft-afflicted persons.

## REFERENCES

1. Black PW, Hartrampf CR, Beegle P: Cleft lip type nasal deformity: definitive repair, *Ann Plast Surg* 12:128, 1984, *and Cleft Lip Type Nasal Deformity: Definitive Repair.* The Educational Foundation of the American Society of Plastic Surgery, Teaching Film Library.
2. Black PW, Scheflin M: Bilateral cleft lip repair: "putting it all together," *Ann Plast Surg* 12:118, 1984.
3. Broadbent TR, Woolf RM: Cleft lip nasal deformity, *Ann Plast Surg* 12:216, 1984.
4. Cronin TD, Denkler KA: Correction of the unilateral cleft lip nose, *Plast Reconstr Surg* 82:419, 1988.
5. Matsuo K, Hirose T, Otagiri T, et al: Repair of cleft lip with nonsurgical correction of nasal deformity in the early neonatal period, *Plast Reconstr Surg* 83:25, 1989.
6. McComb H: Primary correction of unilateral cleft lip nasal deformity: a 10-year review, *Plast Reconstr Surg* 75:791, 1985.
7. McComb H: Primary repair of the bilateral cleft lip nose: a 15-year review and a new treatment plan, *Plast Reconstr Surg* 86:882, 1990.
8. Nakajima T, Yoshimura Y, Sakakibara A: Augmentation of the nostril splint for retaining the corrected contour of the cleft lip nose, *Plast Reconstr Surg* 85:182, 1990.
9. Salyer KE: Primary correction of the unilateral cleft lip nose: a 15-year experience, *Plast Reconstr Surg* 77:558, 1986.
10. Salyer KE: Primary repair of the bilateral cleft lip nose: a 15-year review and a new treatment plan, (discussion), *Plast Reconstr Surg* 86:890, 1990.

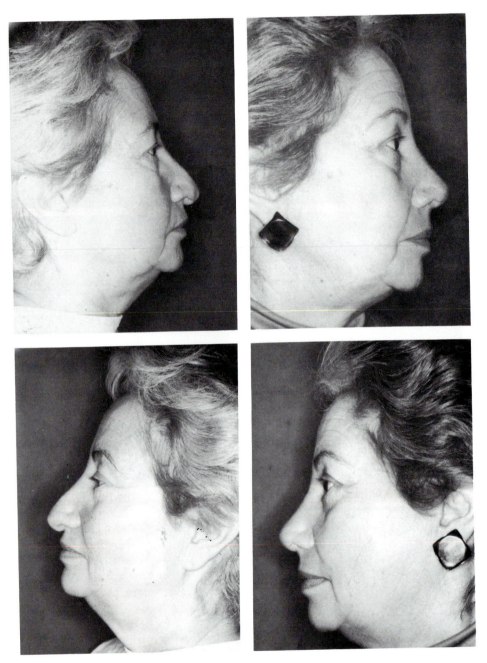

**FIG 21–4.**
Patient with a drooping tip treated by a septal graft to the columella and an auricular graft to the dorsum. *Left*, preoperative views; *right*, postoperative views.

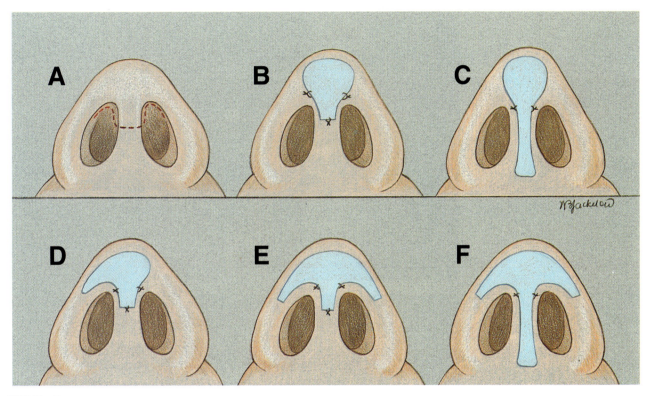

**FIG 21–5.**
Schematic representations. **A,** marking of Rethi's incision (for the open approach). **B,** placing of the shield graft.
**C,** shaping the graft into the form of a champagne cup to be used in cases of collapsed columella. **D,** half an anchor graft to correct an asymmetrical nasal tip and unilateral alar collapse. **E,** anchor graft to correct an asymmetrical nasal tip and bilateral alar collapse. **F,** anchor graft used for the same purposes previously described, as well as when there is columellar collapse.

# Airway Obstruction and Inferior Turbinates

Lorelle N. Michelson, M.D.

George C. Peck, M.D.

The most common cause of nasal airway obstruction in plastic surgical practice is enlargement of the inferior turbinates.[1, 6, 7, 12, 18, 19, 25] This may be observed preoperatively and may occur postoperatively, often resulting merely from the stimulation of surgery. The inferior turbinates should be addressed routinely, their size and potential for enlargement taken into consideration with every rhinoplasty.

## OBSTRUCTION

In the past, surgeons treated *all* airway obstruction, regardless of cause, by septal surgery.[8] The attitude all too often was "when in doubt, do a submucous resection."[2] While this may improve breathing in some cases, persistent nasal obstruction from inferior turbinate hypertrophy is not necessarily improved by septal surgery (Fig 22–1). Failure to achieve a satisfactory airway has thus occurred frequently.[6]

Nasal obstruction is subjective. It is a *symptom* of which the patient is aware. However, not every patient who is aware of this symptom will have physiologic deformities. And conversely, not every patient with deformities will feel obstructed. It is common, for example, to observe a markedly deviated septum in the asymptomatic individual. Patients may likewise complain of breathing difficulties and

have "midline" septa, invisible inferior turbinates, and no other obvious structural etiology for the complaint.

The history, examination, and the surgeon's clinical judgment remain the most reliable means for diagnosing and treating nasal obstruction. It is not necessary to treat "obstruction" determined, for example, only on rhinomanometric evaluation if the patient is unaware of the problem. Prophylaxis against obstruction may, however, be prudent in some instances. This is particularly true in the case of enlarged inferior turbinates incidentally encountered in the "allergic" patient undergoing cosmetic nasal refinement.

Increased airway resistance produces symptoms of obstruction. Resistance is increased by pathology near the internal valve. Most pathology near the valve and hence many etiologies of obstruction, may be diagnosed at office examination. Problems at the valve include scar contractures (Fig 22–2), maxillary crest spurs (see Fig 22–7), septal deviations, collapsing upper lateral cartilages,[13] and hypertrophied inferior turbinates.[19] The etiology of obstructive symptoms can be determined prior to surgery in the vast majority of patients.

The plastic surgeon may occasionally see a patient complaining of obstruction where no etiology can be determined from the history or examination. Allergic, sinus, and emotional problems may be ex-

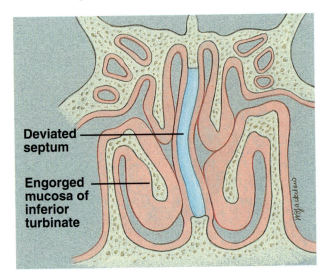

**FIG 22–1.**
Coronal section through the midnose showing both a deviated septum and enlargement of the inferior turbinates. One can appreciate why straightening the septum without simultaneously treating the turbinates may fail to adequately open the airway.

plored but represent diagnoses of exclusion. There will remain a small number of patients for whom no etiology can ever be documented.

Thus, patients concerned with the shape and size of their nose may also be concerned with the ability to breathe properly. The most common cause of complaints referable to breathing in plastic surgical practice is deformity near the valve. The most common deformity near the valve in the presence of obstructive symptoms is enlargement of the inferior turbinates.

Treatment of most nasal obstructions fall within

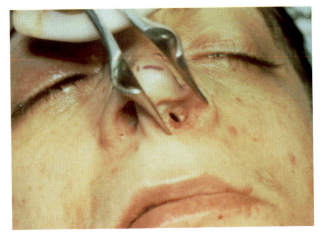

**FIG 22–2.**
Patient with marked scar contracture near the nasal valve.

the realm of the expertise of the plastic surgeon. Most patients can be treated for obstruction concurrent with cosmetic rhinoplasty.

Some obstructions have an iatrogenic basis. The surgeon undertaking rhinoplasty should be aware of ways to avoid iatrogenic breathing problems.

## RHINITIS

Many types of inflammatory states of the nasal mucous membranes are described. These include acute infectious rhinitis (coryza, "upper respiratory tract infection" [URI]), allergic rhinitis, vasomotor rhinitis, hyperplastic or hypertrophic rhinitis, rhinitis medicamentosa ("nose-dropitis"), and postrhinoplasty rhinitis.

Rhinitis, with the exception of the atrophic form, is characterized by inflammation of the nasal mucosa as well as the mucosa of the inferior turbinates. Since the inferior turbinates are located in the area of highest airway resistance, one can appreciate why their reduction produces so marked an increase in airway patency in the "rhinitis" patient of most any etiology.

## NASAL CYCLE

In the normal nose, there is a rhythmic variation between congestion and decongestion. One nasal airway is opening, and its turbinates are shrinking while the opposite nasal airway is closing. This has been termed the "nasal cycle." The cycle occurs over periods of 30 minutes to 4 hours.[2, 32]

## NASAL VALVE

Airflow through the nose is limited by the smallest diameter in its course, specifically, the internal valve.[1, 30] It is easy to understand why even minor deformities near the valve can create the feeling of obstruction.

The nasal valve was first described by Mink in 1903.[20] The nasal valve is the opening between the caudal end of the upper lateral cartilage and the nasal septum.[17]

The nasal valve is a portion of the nasal valve area (Fig 22–3). The nasal valve area includes the distal end of the upper lateral cartilage, the caudal edge of the septum, the head of the inferior turbinate, and the remaining tissues surrounding the pir-

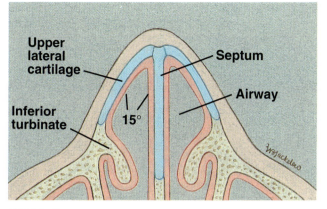

**FIG 22–3.**
Diagramatic representation of the nasal valve area showing the important angle between the upper lateral cartilage and the septum (sagittal section).

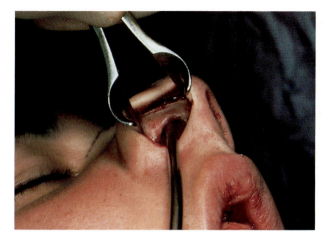

**FIG 22–4.**
Visualizing the nasal valve area. (Courtesy of Dr. George C. Peck.)

iform aperture. The tissues associated with the piriform aperture include the floor of the nose, fibrofatty tissue, and the frontal process of the maxilla.[17, 25]

The nasal valve area, the narrowest portion of the nasal passage, has many synonyms. These include the os internum, ostium internum, the valve area, and area 2.

The projecting anterior portion (head) of the inferior turbinate has congestive capabilities. It is the most important regulator of airflow in the nasal valve area. This has been reaffirmed scientifically.[14]

The nasal valve angle is measured in degrees and represents the angle between the upper lateral cartilage and the nasal septum (see Fig 22–3). The valve angle normally ranges between 10 and 15 degrees in the leptorrhine (Caucasian) nose.[17] The nasal valve area is the inflow regulator and accounts for most of the inspiratory resistance to airflow.[10, 14, 15, 31] The head of the inferior turbinate, which is within the valve area, plays a dominant role as an inflow regulator.[17]

As airflow increases during inspiration, the valve narrows, thereby increasing resistance. The valve opens again as the process is reversed with expiration. It is obvious that rigidity (scar) or flaccidity of the cartilage and soft tissues near the valve can affect valvular function and breathing.[13, 16, 17, 29]

The nasal valve area requires examination in every patient who has symptoms of obstruction (Fig 22–4). The nasal valve may be examined without a speculum,[27] which can distort the important relationship of the caudal end of the upper lateral cartilage to the septum (Fig 22–5). The tip of the nose may be gently elevated digitally. The caudal

end of the upper lateral cartilage should normally form an angle of 10 to 15 degrees with the nasal septum. A smaller angle is consistent with symptomatic narrowing of the valve. A larger angle is termed *ballooning* and is normal in the platyrrhine (black) nose, yet it may be associated with symptoms in the leptorrhine nose because of a decrease in resistance.[17]

Any disturbance of the nasal valve area may produce breathing problems. These disturbances include valve (1) narrowing, (2) widening (ballooning), (3) flaccidity,[13] (4) rigidity, or (5) any combination of the above. Space-occupying masses such as large

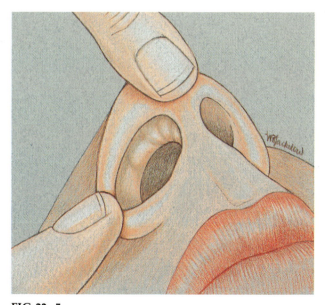

**FIG 22–5.**
The nasal valve area may be examined without the use of a speculum.

turbinates or ectopic cartilage or bone at the maxillary crest will also limit valve function.

Valve flaccidity occurs with loss of skeletal support,[13] such as loss of portions of the upper lateral cartilage from trauma or surgery. Valve rigidity is caused by scar contracture (see Fig 22–2). This may be produced by incisions located intentionally at the valve area. This is true of the intercartilaginous incision practiced in the classic Joseph rhinoplasty. Purposely connecting the sculpturing and transfixion incisions may also be conducive to this complication,[22, 23] but less so (see below).

## AVOIDING OBSTRUCTION

Although enlargement of the inferior turbinates is the most common cause of persistent breathing obstruction, it cannot be denied that sequelae from previous rhinologic surgery represent another cause. Many common surgical practices unwittingly set the stage for postoperative obstruction.

Nasal obstruction may occur following rhinoplasty either as a direct result of the surgery or as an exacerbation of some underlying factor. The most common reasons for postrhinoplasty obstruction include hypertrophied turbinates, persistent septal deviation, intranasal adhesions and webs,[1] and scarring at the valve.

Historically, an intercartilaginous incision was used to access the nasal dorsum as well as the lower lateral cartilages in some everting techniques (Fig 22–6, incision 1). This incision is unnecessary in

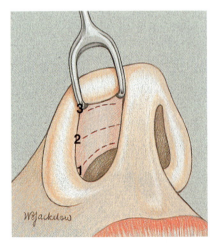

**FIG 22–6.**
The three commonly used incisions for access to the lower lateral cartilages. The transcartilaginous incision *(2)* is preferred. (Courtesy of Dr. George C. Peck.)

light of its potential for valve distortion. All surgery of the lower lateral cartilages and bridge, as well as of the upper lateral cartilages, where necessary, may be performed via a transcartilaginous incision.[11, 23] The intercartilaginous incision may be considered an obsolete technique and is almost never necessary (see Fig 22–6, incision 1).

Likewise, if a transfixion incision is to be employed for caudal septal access, it is possible to preserve a bridge of tissue between it and the transcartilaginous sculpturing incision. This avoids a circular scar contracture.[23] In those unusual cases where the two incisions are inadvertently connected, the resultant scar predisposes to less of a problem because it remains in a wider portion of the nasal passageway, several millimeters distal to the valve area proper.

One must also be careful to preserve the lateralmost portion or tail of the lower lateral cartilage when sculpturing this structure.[23] Removal of too much cartilage here may not only produce an unaesthetic pinched appearance but may also weaken the cartilages physiologically. With inspiration, this may allow the nares to collapse near the valve area, thus producing symptoms of obstruction.

Older rhinoplasty techniques that resected large portions of the upper lateral cartilages should also be relegated to history. Resection of upper lateral cartilage reduces support near the valve and can lead to inspirational collapse and obstructive symptoms.[1, 21, 23]

Routine transmucosal separation of the upper lateral cartilages from the septum will also produce scarring and narrowing of the valve angle. This maneuver may be employed in those cases where narrowing of the middle third of the nose can only be achieved in this fashion. Routine transmucosal separation is unnecessary.[23]

Excising mucosa and, particularly, excision of mucosa near the valve is conducive to scar contracture with obstructive sequelae.[21–23, 25, 27] Except when trimming the caudal edge of the septum, nasal mucosa should never be excised.

There are a myriad of causes of inferior turbinate hypertrophy, including allergy, dust, tobacco, pregnancy, trauma, and compensatory—often in response to deviation of the septum. We commonly observe *unilateral* enlargement of one turbinate when the septum deviates to the opposite side.

It is therefore reasonable that the mere instrumentation from nasal surgery with its concomitant "trauma," edema, and introduction of nasal packing and foreign materials may produce a temporary or prolonged enlargement of the inferior turbinates. In a review of 1,000 consecutive rhinoplasties, Beekhuis found that approximately 10% of patients developed a persistent enlargement of the inferior turbinates postoperatively that caused obstructive symptoms.[3]

We therefore advocate cauterization of inferior turbinates in those aesthetic rhinoplasties where the turbinates are even slightly enlarged. This is true even in those "purely aesthetic" cases where no symptomatic obstruction was present preoperatively. This is an exception to our belief that only symptomatic patients should be treated for obstruction. The practice of turbinate fulguration is a safe, rapid, and simple prophylaxis against future symptoms.

The septum and its treatment are amply covered elsewhere. As stated, most obstructive symptoms are referable to some abnormal structure around the valve, which may, of course, include the septum. One common error of omission in the operative treatment of patients with obstruction secondary to septal deviation is worthy of emphasis.

When the septum is deviated, it is common to find an abundance of ectopic cartilage, bone, and callus at the maxillary crest around the valve area. This is especially true following trauma to the septum. If this area is not meticulously debrided during submucous resection, obstruction is likely to persist or be accentuated postoperatively.

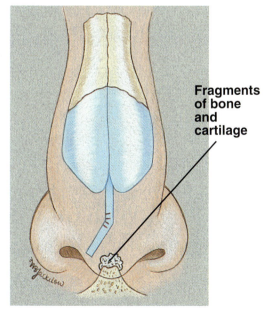

**FIG 22–7.**
The area at the maxillary crest may contain obstructing fragments of bone and cartilage. This area must always be examined and, if necessary, debrided during submucous resection of the septum.

When submucous resection of the septum is performed, it is important to check this key portion of the valve area located at the base of the septum near the maxillary crest (Fig 22–7). If the Frazer suction canula cannot easily pass into the posterior part of the pharynx, then further debridement may be necessary. This often requires sharp resection with rongeurs, osteotome, or chisel.[19, 24]

While not an etiology of obstruction, septal perforations nevertheless often represent an iatrogenic problem that relates to treating patients with obstruction. We feel that this entity may suffer from overemphasis. The majority of patients we have seen with septal perforations, whether iatrogenically or otherwise caused, report no adverse symptomatology. They in fact usually report *improvement* in their breathing if the surgery were performed for that purpose. Septal perforation may be one of the *bêtes noires* of our specialty and one that deserves a special perspective.

## INFERIOR TURBINATES

The turbinates are thin semicircular bones covered by a dense periosteum and a thick, highly vascular mucous membrane. They project from the lateral nasal wall and subdivide each nasal cavity into "meatuses."

There are three pairs of turbinates: superior, middle, and inferior. There is occasionally a fourth, the supreme.[27] Embryologic appendages of the maxilla, the inferior turbinates are responsible for the nasal obstruction commonly seen in plastic surgical practice.[1, 7, 18]

The main functions of the turbinates are filtration, humidification, and warming of inspired air. They also protect the respiratory passages against noxious agents by reflex swelling and obstruction of the nasal passages when stimulated.[1] The inferior turbinates are the most susceptible to enlargement.[18]

In their classic study of the nasal valve, Haight and Cole confirmed that the anterior ends of the inferior turbinates were responsible for the greater portion of nasal resistance. They found little additional resistance to airflow as one traveled posteriorly in the nose. They performed histamine stimulation of the inferior turbinates and found that the anterior tip of the turbinate increased in size by as much as 5 mm in some cases.[14]

An enlarging turbinate progresses from hypertrophy to hyperplasia to polypoid degeneration.[18, 27] The advanced stage, or polyps, is characterized by edematous areas of mucosa engorged with interstitial fluid.[26]

The degree and chronicity of turbinate obstruction range from the normal transient swelling of the turbinates, which occurs when passing from a cold to a hot environment, to the chronically enlarged turbinate, which develops on the contralateral side of a markedly deviated septum.[1] In most instances only the soft tissues of the turbinate hypertrophy. It is the soft tissue and not the bone that usually blocks the airway (see Fig 22–1).

According to Goode,[12] in the absence of prior nasal surgery or trauma, nasal obstructive symptoms occurring at ages 20 to 60 years are rarely due to abnormalities of the septum or external nose. Since the nose completes growth by the early teens,[23] symptoms secondary to congenital septal deflections or external narrowing should have appeared by that time. Thus in the 20- to 60-year-old age group, in the absence of surgery or trauma, the septum is not changing, but the turbinates probably are.[12] Obstructive symptoms in this age group are more frequently related to the turbinates than to the septum.

Most authors agree[2, 5, 6, 12, 18, 25] that the most common cause of nasal obstruction is a gradual, chronic enlargement of the turbinates. A history of hay fever or allergic disorders should forewarn the surgeon of a potential postoperative exacerbation of nasal obstruction.[1] Dust, tobacco, pregnancy, and emotional factors are commonly cited as etiologies for enlargement of the turbinates. However, certain drugs such as aspirin and some tranquilizers as well as certain diseases such as hypothyroidism have also been implicated.[4, 18, 28] Nasal surgery may also predispose to enlargement.

## TREATMENT OF ENLARGED INFERIOR TURBINATES

Since it is primarily the engorged mucosa that occludes the airway, electrocoagulation of the offending mucosa should ablate the occlusion. While surgical resection or partial resection[6, 9, 17, 25] may offer much improvement, we invariably elect to use fulguration rather than resection because we feel that this offers the following advantages:

1. Cauterization of the turbinates is rapid. Less than ten seconds per side is required to completely dissolve the offending mucosa.

2. Improvement is immediate. Patients operated under local anesthesia have on occasion reported immediate subjective relief after cauterization.

3. There is no bleeding.

4. No packing is necessary.

5. The procedure is simple.

6. There is no intraoperative or postoperative pain.

7. No "bridges are burned." After cauterization, resection of additional turbinate is certainly possible either at the same time or subsequently if symptoms persist. We have thus far not found this to be necessary.

8. There have been no recurrences of hypertrophy.

9. There has been no postoperative dry nose.

10. All patients remain asymptomatic at 1 year.

We have not had occasion to reoperate on a turbinate following electrofulguration or to surgically excise additional turbinate tissue. In the patient who remained symptomatic, however, we would not hesitate to do so.

We do not agree with the allegation in the otolaryngologic literature[26] that "surgery on the allergic nose is contraindicated during the hay fever season." In fact, many of our patients report vast improvement in allergic symptoms after cauterization.

The bipolar Elektrotom cautery produces a clean "circumferential" dissolution of the soft tissue overlying the bony turbinate (Fig 22–8). While the Valleylab (Bovie) cautery has been tried and a similar method was described in the literature in 1963,[18] the Bovie has proved less than satisfactory for this purpose. The Valley device requires several passes before one begins to see any effect. Two or three passes of the bipolar device are generally sufficient to produce dissolution.

Enlarged inferior turbinates encountered incidentally during aesthetic rhinoplasty in patients

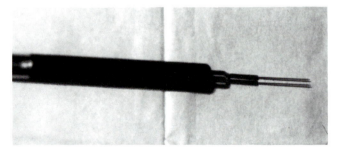

**FIG 22–8.**
Bipolar cautery is used for turbinate fulguration.

with no breathing problems are cauterized to ensure a patent airway postoperatively. We cauterize the inferior turbinates in approximately half of all rhinoplasties we perform.[19]

## SURGICAL TECHNIQUE

We inject local anesthesia with a 5-cc syringe and a long 25-gauge needle (Fig 22–9). Opening the speculum reveals the projecting soft tissue of the inferior turbinate into which 0.5 to 1 cc of a freshly prepared solution of 1% lidocaine with 1:200,000 epinephrine is injected as the needle is withdrawn. Cocaine packs are not used.

We use the Dennis Bipolar Turbinate Probe (Elmed, Inc., Addison, Ill) (see Fig 22–8). We grasp the turbinate on either side with the two tips of the bipolar forceps (Fig 22–10). We perforate the presenting edge of the turbinate longitudinally and cauterize it for 5 seconds. An immediate destruction of the blocking tissue occurs. A second pass of the probes is frequently necessary, again for 5 seconds. It is usually unnecessary to resect any additional soft tissue or bone.

No postoperative bleeding or "dry nose" has been observed. On reexamination after 3 months, a scarred 2 × 2-mm zone may be visible intranasally at the lateral wall. Crusting is also seen early postoperatively. This may be treated with bland or antibiotic ointment for comfort. At 6 to 12 months, scarring is barely evident along a clean, intact mucosa. Thus far, recurrence has not been observed.[19]

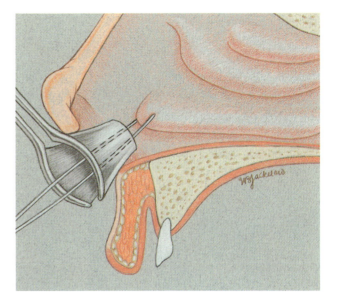

**FIG 22–10.**
The projecting edge of the inferior turbinate is perforated and cauterized with the bipolar instrument.

## SUMMARY

In the patient complaining of obstruction, the internal valve area is the likely offender. The inferior turbinates, key structures in the valve area, are the suspected cause of the obstruction until proved otherwise.

Prevention of obstruction necessitates prudent placement of intranasal incisions and avoiding resection of upper lateral cartilage and mucosa. When enlarged, prophylactic cauterization of the inferior turbinates should be considered.

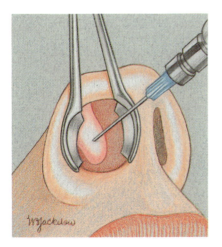

**FIG 22–9.**
Local anesthesia is injected prior to cauterization.

## REFERENCES

1. Baker DC: Physiology. In Rees TD, editor *Aesthetic plastic surgery*, Philadelphia, 1980, Saunders, p 66.
2. Baker DC, Strauss RB: The physiologic treatment of nasal obstruction, *Clin Plast Surg* 4:121–129, 1977.
3. Beekhuis GJ: Nasal obstruction after rhinoplasty: etiology and techniques for correction, *Laryngoscope* 86:540–548, 1976.
4. Blue JA: Rhinitis medicamentosa, *Ann Allergy* 26:425–429, 1968.
5. Courtiss EH: Diagnosis and treatment of nasal airway obstruction due to inferior turbinate hypertrophy, *Clin Plast Surg* 15:11, 1988.
6. Courtiss EH: Nasal physiology, patient evaluation, and effects of surgery, In Rees TD, Baker DC, Tabbal

N, editors: *Rhinoplasty problems and controversies,* St Louis, 1988, Mosby–Year Book.

7. Courtiss EH, Gargan TJ, Courtiss GB: Nasal physiology, *Ann Plast Surg* 13:214, 1984.

8. Courtiss EH, Goldwyn RM: The effects of nasal surgery on airflow, *Plast Reconstr Surg* 72:9, 1983.

9. Courtiss EH, Goldwyn RM, O'Brien JJ: Resection of obstructing inferior nasal turbinate, *Plast Reconstr Surg* 62:249, 1978.

10. De Wit G, Kapteyn TS, van Bochove W: Some remarks on the physiology, the anatomy and the radiology of the vestibulum and the isthmus nasi, *Int Rhinol* 3:37–42, 1965.

11. Elliott RA Jr: Personal communication, 1981.

12. Goode RL: *Diagnosis and treatment of turbinate dysfunction,* American Academy of Otolaryngology, 1977.

13. Goode RL: Surgery of the incompetent nasal valve, *Laryngoscope* 95:546–555, 1985.

14. Haight JSJ, Cole P: The site and function of the nasal valve, *Laryngoscope* 93:49–55, 1983.

15. Hinderer KH: *Fundamentals of anatomy and surgery of the nose,* Birmingham, Ala, 1971, Aesculapius.

16. Hinderer KH: Surgery of the valve, *Int Rhinol* 8:60–67, 1970.

17. Kern EB: Surgery of the nasal valve in Rees TD, Baker DC, Tabbal N, editors: *Rhinoplasty problems and controversies,* St Louis, 1988, Mosby–Year Book, pp 209–222.

18. Little SW: Management of enlarged turbinates, *Va Med Monthly* 90:484, 1963.

19. Michelson LN, Peck GC: Septal and turbinate surgery. In Peck GC, editor: *Techniques in aesthetic rhinoplasty,* ed 2, Philadelphia, 1990, Lippincott, pp 178–179.

20. Mink PJ: Le nez comme voie respiratorie, *Presse Otolaryngol Belg* 481–496, 1903.

21. Peck GC: Basic primary rhinoplasty, *Clin Plast Surg* 15:23–27, 1988.

22. Peck GC: Secondary rhinoplasty, *Clin Plast Surg* 15:34, 1988.

23. Peck GC: *Techniques in aesthetic rhinoplasty,* ed 2, Philadelphia, 1990, Lippincott, pp 22, 23, 26, 118, 187.

24. Rees TD, editor: *Aesthetic plastic surgery,* Philadelphia, 1980, WB Saunders, pp 300 ff.

25. Rees TD, Baker, DC, Tabbal N, editors: *Rhinoplasty problems and controversies,* St Louis, 1988, Mosby–Year Book, pp 189–239.

26. Sanders SH: Allergic rhinitis and sinusitis, *Otolaryngol Clin North Am* 4:565, 1971.

27. Sheen JH: *Aesthetic rhinoplasty,* St. Louis, 1978, Mosby–Year Book, pp 26, 40–43.

28. Stahl RH: Allergic disorders of the nose and paranasal sinuses, *Otol Clin North Am* 7:703–718, 1974.

29. van Dishoeck HAE: Inspiratory nasal resistance, *Acta Otolaryngol* 30:431–439, 1942.

30. van Dishoeck HAE: Some remarks on nasal physiology, Lectures read for the American rhinological society at Yale University, New Haven, Conn, June 1957, pp 23.

31. van Dishoeck HAE: The part of the valve and the turbinates in total nasal resistance, *Int Rhinol* 3:19–26, 1965.

32. Williams HL: Nasal physiology. In Paparella MM, Shumrich DA, editors: *Otolaryngology,* vol 1, Philadelphia, 1973, Saunders.

# CHAPTER 23

# Airway Obstruction: Turbinectomy

Eugene H. Courtiss, M.D.

Robert M. Goldwyn, M.D.

In 1973 an executive came into one of our offices (E.H.C.) complaining of difficulty in breathing through his nose. He stated that the condition existed for many years and that his only relief followed the use of oxymetazoline (Afrin) nose drops, which he used four times a day. He was truly a nasal spray addict. A submucous resection of his nasal septum 3 years previously had failed to improve his airway. At this time, a speculum was inserted into his nose, and large inferior turbinates that were blocking his airway were observed.

Although treatment of nasal airway obstruction due to turbinate hypertrophy by turbinate resection was alleged to cause adverse sequelae, we were unable to find documented evidence of such a sequence.[3] That fact plus the belief that bilateral inferior turbinate resection appeared to be a direct and permanent treatment of his problem was discussed with the patient. He opted for surgery, which was performed as described below. After his packs were removed and the edema subsided, the patient had a clear airway that was present when he was examined 16 years after his operation. Subjectively and objectively his airway obstruction has been successfully treated, and he has not used any nasal sprays or drops since his operation.

As the result of that and subsequent experiences, when patients complain of airway obstruction that is due to inferior turbinate hypertrophy, we offer them treatment by inferior turbinate resection. We believe that it produces predictable and permanent results [2, 4–6] and have not observed any adverse sequelae even when patients were followed as long as 10 years.[2, 3]

## PATIENT SELECTION

Careful and complete internal examination of the nose is crucial to treatment.[1] The nose should be examined before and after the lining has been contracted with an agent. This allows complete examination of the internal nose. If the constriction of the lining also improves the airway, treatment of the inferior turbinates can also be expected to improve the airway. Shrinking decreases the size of the turbinates; it does not straighten a deviated nasal septum nor treat obstruction due to pathology in the internal or external valves. However, if examination indicates that the obstruction is due to septal or valvular problems, then the latter should be treated.[1]

## TECHNIQUE OF TURBINATE RESECTION

The patient should be anesthetized with either a topical and local anesthetic or a general anesthetic. The inferior turbinate is fractured in a cephalad direction, and then one blade of the turbinate scissors is placed on top and the other blade below the turbinate (Fig 23–1) and the obstructing segment removed. Because of the thickness of the scissor blade, part of the turbinate remains. Removal of the most posterior segment is not necessary, although if this is done, no apparent harm results.

Because of the vascularity of the turbinates, the cut stump of a turbinate bone may bleed significantly. As a result, the nose should be packed. We prefer compressed Gelfoam[7] coated with bacitracin;

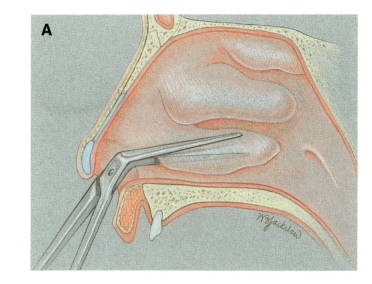

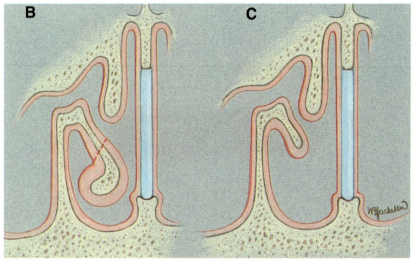

**FIG 23–1.**
Technique of turbinectomy. Note the application of scissors to the leading edge of the turbinate **(A)**. Note the level at which the turbinate is excised **(B)** and the final result **(C)**.

however, any pack may be used. The advantage of the Gelfoam pack is that it does not need to be removed. The patient blows it out at 7 to 10 days, at which time the stump of the turbinate has healed.

## LONG-TERM RESULTS

The long-term results of this surgery have proved to be excellent.[5]

## REFERENCES

1. Courtiss EH: Diagnosis and treatment of nasal airway obstruction due to inferior turbinate hypertrophy, *Clin Plast Surg* 15:11, 1988.
2. Courtiss EH, Gargan TJ, Courtiss G: Nasal physiology, *Ann Plast Surg* 13:214, 1984.
3. Courtiss EH, Goldwyn RM: Resection of inferior turbinates, *Plast Reconstr Surg* 62:249, 1978.
4. Courtiss EH, Goldwyn RM: Resection of inferior turbinates: A 6-year follow-up, *Plast Reconstr Surg* 72:913, 1983.
5. Courtiss EH, Goldwyn RM: Resection of inferior turbinates: A 10-year follow-up, *Plast Reconstr Surg* 86:152, 1990.
6. Courtiss EH, Goldwyn RM: The effects of nasal surgery on airflow, *Plast Reconstr Surg* 72:9, 1983.
7. Gorman JB, Courtiss EH: Another nasal pack, *Plast Reconstr Surg* 70:233, 1982.

# The Septum in Rhinoplasty: "Form Follows Function"

Mark Gorney, M.D.

In contrast to Mies Van Der Rohe's classic architectural dictum, quite the opposite applies in septorhinoplasty: function is almost wholly dependent on form.

No septum is really straight. Heredity, birth, and repetitive trauma all combine to give most of us some degree of septal irregularity. As long as the nasal vault is adequate, minor septal deviation is of little concern. However, it is self-evident that any narrowing or lowering of that vault without simultaneous correction of the septum will lead to some limitation of airflow. The externally deviated nose calls for aesthetic as well as functional correction. What we are concerned with is the essentially straight or slightly deviated nose, inside of which there is a potential for both functional and aesthetic failure. A crooked nose cannot be straightened without correcting the septum; a simple rhinoplasty can create a crooked nose if the septum is not corrected.

A structurally sound and straight septum is the foundation of a satisfactory rhinoplasty result. As obvious as this may seem, there is still substantial disagreement among plastic surgeons as to appropriate corrective techniques. There is also significant misunderstanding of nasal physiology, particularly of the valve area, and sometimes there is a cavalier disregard for the integrity of the nasal airway. It is a safe bet that the rate of obstructive complications is higher than rates officially reported in the literature. In other words, is it enough to make them beautiful if they cannot breathe?

Volumes have been written on the functional aspects of nasal surgery. Neither this material nor the internal anatomy or function of the nose will be belabored here. In a text directed at trained aesthetic surgeons it is appropriate to limit our attention to one facet of a broad field: an overview of the structural aspects of septoplasty as it relates to cosmetic rhinoplasty.

## INFORMED CONSENT

In a consultation with the patient who has potential nasal obstruction, you must offer sufficient explanation of the anticipated procedure to allow the patient to make an intelligent decision. In order to do this it is useful to draw the following metaphor: "Your nose is like an A-frame cottage. The front half of the cottage is made of canvas, and the back is made of wood. Down the middle, from front to back, there is a main bearing wall that supports the spine of the roof. If a giant tree were to fall on the house, the spine of the roof would cave in, and the central bearing wall would probably bend to a much greater degree on the weak front than on the hard rear. The bearing wall will buckle to varying degrees, thereby obstructing the rooms on either side. Imagine further that the bottom of this wall is set into a trough that also runs from the front to the back of the structure. Both sides of the central bearing wall and the sides of the trough are covered with thick, red velvet wallpaper. On the slanting side walls of the roof there are some broad shelves that protrude into the room. If the center wall is bulging into the space on either side, it will be difficult to pass from one end to the other. If the wall is crooked enough that the shelves on each side touch it, there is no passage at all. If the wall is only partly crooked and I wish to make the house narrower by moving the side walls in, I will achieve the same obstructive effect (no pas-

sage) unless I straighten out the main bearing wall first. To do this I must raise the wallpaper. Since I do not want the roof to collapse, I must leave at least an L-shaped support at the front and under the roof. If this portion is also crooked I must also try to straighten it out. The wallpaper on both sides is then rejoined, back to back, to leave a better passage on either side."

This may seem an oversimplified version, but in

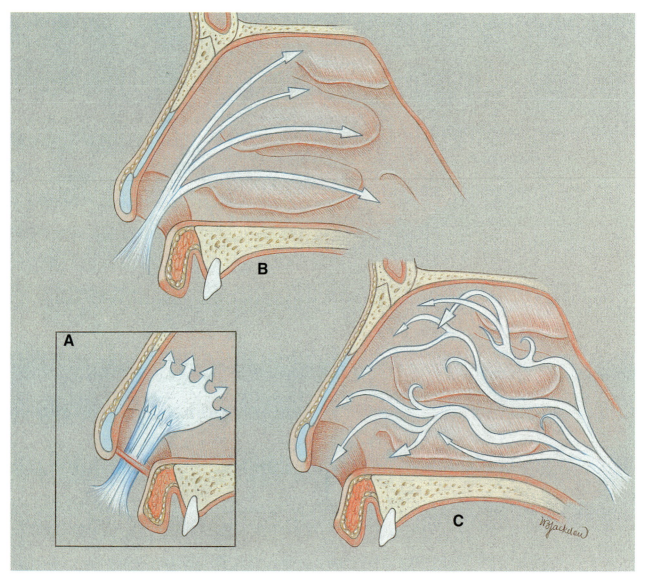

**FIG 24–1.**
**A,** the way in which air currents traverse the nasal conduits, their direction, their shape, and the speed of the stream are determined as much by nasal configuration as by the natural anatomic constriction found approximately 2 cm inside the nostrils. **B,** on normal inspiration in the intact nose, the air is directed upward and backward and arches up between the septum and turbinates to the face of the sphenoid and then down through the choana and into the pharynx. Relatively little air passes along the floor. The choana has essentially no effect on the stream. **C,** on expiration air passes through the lower portion of the choana and is thrown into the eddies by the baffle effect of the posterior aspect of the turbinate and the nozzle effect of the nostrils.

cases where results have been less than optimal, it will strongly refute any claim that the patient did not understand the technical aspects of the operation.

## NASAL PHYSIOLOGY

For the purposes of this chapter we will focus on several limited but important facets of internal nasal physiology of significance to the plastic surgeon.

The way in which air currents traverse the nasal conduits, their direction, their shape, and the speed of the stream are determined as much by nasal configuration as by the natural anatomic constriction found approximately 2 cm inside the nostrils (Fig 24–1,A). This area, commonly referred to as the internal valve, is the confluence of the caudal edge of the upper lateral cartilages and the septum (under the overlap of the upper border of the alar cartilages). This valve converts a round column of air into a flat stream. The length and capacity of hose mean nothing; the stream it throws and its direction are determined by the shape of the nozzle.

On normal inspiration in the intact nose, the air is directed upward and backward and arches up between the septum and turbinates to the face of the sphenoid, down through the choana and into the pharynx (Fig 24–1,B). Relatively little air passes along the floor. The choana has essentially no effect on the stream.

Over the turbinates air becomes humidified to approximately 90% relative humidity before reaching the larynx.

On expiration air passes through the lower portion of the choana and is thrown into the eddies by the baffle effect of the posterior aspect of the turbinates and the nozzle effect of the nostrils (Fig 24–1,C).

As the air currents are moved over the ciliated surfaces, particulate matter is deposited, probably by electrostatic effect. The mucosal glands deposit a lubricating blanket, which is moved by the cilia and carries off debris. Tear flow assists this mechanism.

The function of the nasal cilia is well known. Cilia line the inner surface of the nose except for the olfactory areas. Going back to the metaphor, one can visualize a house through the center of which run two corridors covered with thick, velvet-pile, self-cleaning wallpaper. The dust entering the house is passed along the wall, ceiling, and floor, down the corridor, through the back door, and into the ash can; it makes the complete trip in 20 minutes. This self-cleaning wallpaper works 24 hours a day unless something happens. Cilia are tough and have only one natural enemy: drying. This eliminates their ability to function and move mucous.

The principal iatrogenic enemy of cilia is scar tissue. It makes hurdles over which cilia cannot move the mucous blanket. Annular scars not only bar the flow but further narrow the nozzle, thus creating not only a mechanical but also a physiologic barrier (Fig 24–2,A and B).

The valves must be of sufficient size to allow free flow of air, and they should be nearly identical. If disproportionate amounts of air are allowed to enter one side only, that side will tend to dry and undergo metaplasia. This may be reported by the patient as a feeling of nasal obstruction. Underventila-

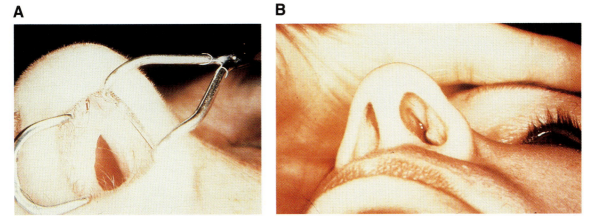

**A**      **B**

**FIG 24–2.**
**A,** annular scars not only bar the flow but further narrow the nozzle, thus creating not only a mechanical but also a physiologic barrier. **B,** sometimes the stenosis is severe.

tion, on the other hand, will lead to constant accumulation of mucous.

## ARCHITECTURAL SIGNIFICANCE OF THE SEPTUM

It is generally agreed that if one drops an imaginary line from the nasion to the nasal spine, anything posterior to that line can be resected from floor to ceiling without fear of collapse. Anything anterior to it must be resected with discretion and forethought to avoid insufficient support and subsequent functional (and aesthetic) distortion. Even if there seems to be an adequate dorsal cartilaginous support remaining, beware of the effect of contracture of the mucosal leaves and the plane of scar between them. (If there have been perforations, this contracture will be more significant.) Contracture of this plane of scar can exert sufficient pull to create a saddle nose if the remaining dorsal strut is too narrow or weak.

If one considers the upper lateral cartilages as the wings sprouting from the dorsal edge of the septum (an embryologically correct concept), then the upper edge of the deviated septum must be freed from the wings that tether it. If one fails to do this, their guidewire effect will eventually deviate the

dorsum again. This separation should be done at the submucoperichondrial level. If one keeps the mucoperichondrial flap attached to the underside of the upper lateral cartilages except where they join the septum, then the mucoperichondrial flaps will not sag. In this way, one can avoid cutting away the upper lateral cartilages through the mucosa. Cutting through cartilage and mucosal lining creates scar and synechiae, which later may restrict inspiratory airflow.

High septal deflection, often undetected, can frustrate a perfect rhinoplasty. The hump, which is in the normal midsagittal plane, may be covering a crooked septum just below it, a configuration easy to miss in a cursory preoperative examination. Operative edema may deceive the surgeon. After infracture is finished, the nasal bones and upper lateral cartilages are then brought together against an undiscovered deviation of the new upper border of the septum. Two weeks later when the edema recedes, the beautiful result at the end of the operation may appear distinctly off center.

The sequence of the septal correction at surgery is important. Figure 24–3 shows a typical subluxation and override of the septum-vomer junction at the anteroinferior corner of the quadrilateral cartilage. What happens here can have a profound effect

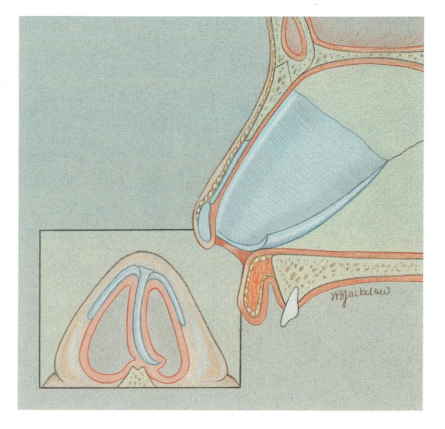

**FIG 24–3.**
Typical subluxation and override of the septum-vomer junction at the anteroinferior corner of the quadrilateral cartilage.

on the new profile line. If the dislocated lower edge of the cartilage is freed up and replaced within the vomer, this will tend to lift the lower end of the nose (Fig 24–4). On the other hand, if the extremely deviated lower edge of the septum must be cut off or the vomer groove must be chiseled out and removed to allow the septum back into the midline, the surgeon may end up lowering the end of the nose, whose support depends on the remaining vertical cartilaginous strut. Thus, the surgeon must know what he intends to do ahead of time. It is poor planning to make a beautiful profile and then correct the septum only to find the profile lowered in the tip area. It is wiser to do the septal correction first and leave more

than adequate dorsal buttress so that the profile line can still be corrected or the nose shortened at the end of the rhinoplasty without weakening the remaining support. This takes preoperative planning. If in doubt, the hump resection and dorsal correction must be done first, and then the septoplasty, so that enough cartilage is left behind to guarantee integrity of the profile line. Correcting the septum first, particularly if it is badly bent, is much easier from the standpoint of visibility, hemostasis, and safety.

The hump may be a relative or absolute one. A large Arabic or a Romanesque hump can be characterized as an absolute one. If the profile line sud-

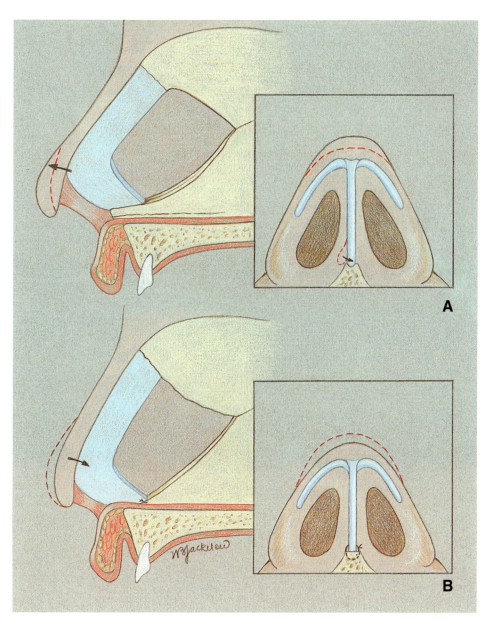

**FIG 24–4.**
**A,** if the dislocated lower edge of the cartilage is freed and replaced within the vomer, this will tend to lift the lower end of the nose. **B,** if it is trimmed, it will tend to drop the lower end of the nose.

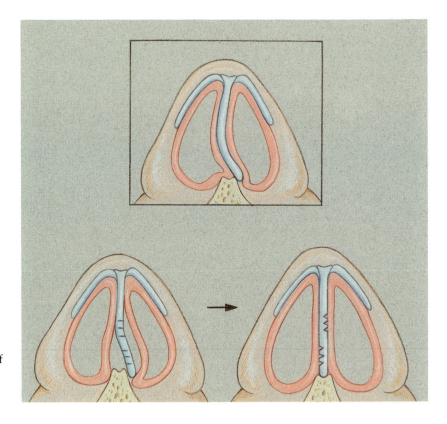

**FIG 24–5.**
Fry has dramatically illustrated the tendency of cartilage to curl to the opposite side from which it is scored. If the deviation is a complex one, both sides should be scored, but only on their concave portion.

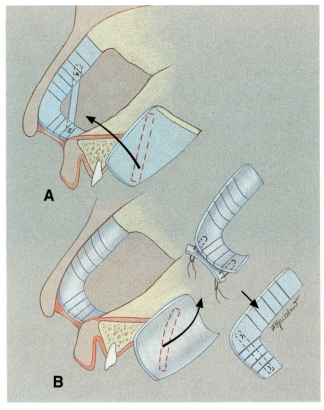

**FIG 24–6.**
In a particularly badly deviated septum it helps to reinforce the scoring by placing a small batten of surplus septal cartilage or vomerine bone **(A)** on the unscored side to act as a reinforcement. Alternatively, one can cut a curved batten out of a segment of curved cartilage that has been resected and suture it on the "convex" side of the remaining septum **(B)**. This strong curve will then act as a "counterspring" and prevent redeviation.

denly dips below the end of the nasal bones, this is a relative hump, which is almost invariably caused by septal abnormality. If the septum has been distorted severely enough to be noticeable externally, almost total removal of the septum will barely affect the profile line. In this nose it is wise to consider using the resected septum or a graft to bridge the sag between the self-supporting tip and the end of the nasal bones.

In severe internal deviations the remaining L-shaped strut may remain deviated or subluxated. If the surgeon fails to straighten it out, he is guaranteed a deviated nose. Until recent years most authors advised various maneuvers to score, cut, crosshatch, or remove strips vertically from the convex side of the deformity, with the idea of allowing the remaining septum to swing back into the midline. There are also a number of maneuvers described to keep it in the original position, but generally speaking, this has been at the best chancy. At least as many noses have redeviated as have maintained the improvement. Gibson and, more recently, Fry have effectively demonstrated the existence of interlocking stresses within cartilage. Most significantly, Fry has dramatically illustrated the tendency of cartilage to curl to the opposite side from which it is scored. Thus the septum should be scored on the concave side (Fig 24–5). If the deviation is a complex one, both sides should be scored, but only on their concave portion. Some surgeons prefer to do this with a morcelizer rather than multiple cuts with an angled blade.

In a particularly badly deviated septum it helps to reinforce the scoring by placing a small batten of surplus septal cartilage or vomerine bone on the unscored side to act as a reinforcement. If possible redeviation is feared, this batten can be placed diagonally across the remaining septum. This maneuver is illustrated in Figure 24–6,A. Alternatively, one can cut a curved batten out of a segment of curved cartilage that has been resected and suture it on the "convex" side of the remaining septum. This strong curve will then act as a "counterspring" and prevent redeviation (Fig 24–6,B).

## TECHNICAL SUGGESTIONS

No one single operative technique can always correct a deformity so infinite in its variables. What must be done is a procedure that will restore function, correct deviation, and prevent saddling, columella retraction, and tip droop.

The principle of the operation is to divide every attachment of the cartilaginous septum except for the mucosal flap on the remaining cartilage on one side. The interlocking stresses in the twisted cartilage must be released. What cannot be straightened must be resected or morcelized. The goal should be maximum mobility with the least removal of tissue possible.

A few caveats may be in order:

1. The secret to avoiding perforation is to elevate the flap at the right level—subperichondrially. In the distal 1 or 2 cm of cartilaginous septum, the mucosa is intimately attached to the cartilage. After an incision is made along the protrusive leading edge, a pair of Converse scissors or a sharp elevator is useful in finding the correct plane. It is easy to start down the wrong one, and this virtually guarantees perforations and tears, particularly along the spurs, crests, and ridges where the mucosa is as thin as wet tissue paper. There is a characteristic gray-blue reflex visible on entering the right plane ("If it ain't blue, it ain't true"). There is also a clean smooth feel on the instrument, which will glide along easily. When the instrument passes from the cartilage to the vertical plate of the ethmoid, there is a characteristic change in the feel of the scraping. It is best to proceed in semicircular upward motions rather than push straight and back. Do not try to go past the angle of deviation or around ridges. This will also produce perforations. (Small perforations are of no consequence unless they are back to back on both mucosal leaves; this will produce a permanent perforation.)

2. Along the inferoanterior aspect of the cartilaginous septum where it fits in the vomerine ridge, it is difficult to pass down from the subperichondrial space of the cartilage to the subperiosteal space of the cartilage to the subperiosteal space of the vomer. Figure 24–7,A and B shows why. The quadrilateral septal cartilage is completely invested by perichondrium, even along its lower edge, which may or may not sit in the vomer groove. The vomer ridge, in turn, has periosteum tightly adherent over it. Therefore after undermining from the roof of the nose to the septovomerine ridge, one should not try to continue inferiorly but back off and begin a new tunnel under the periosteum of the vomer. It is much easier to join these two space without tearing once they have been independently developed.

3. If you use a swivel knife, do not proceed along the vomer first and then up, anteriorly, and

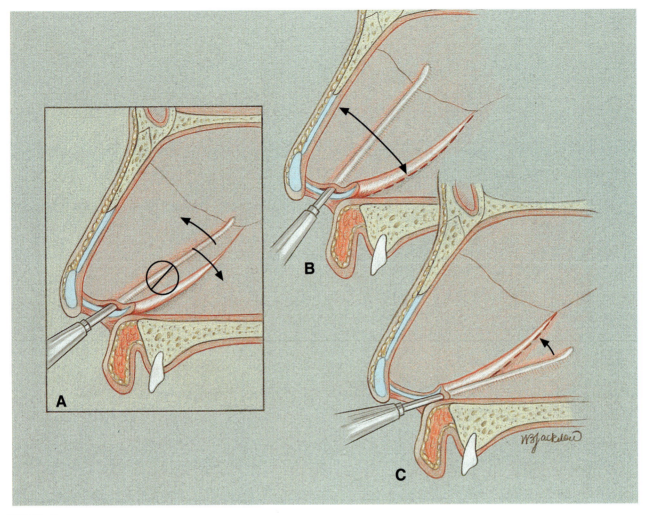

**FIG 24–7.**
**A** and **B,** after undermining from the roof of the nose to the septovomerine ridge, one should not try to continue inferiorly but instead back off and begin a new tunnel under the periosteum of the vomer **(C)**. It is much easier to join these two spaces without tearing once they have been independently developed.

out. You may come up too high and not leave enough dorsal buttress for support. It is much safer to make the vertical cut up to a preselected point in the cartilaginous septum about 1 or 2 cm back from the leading edge. Do not perforate to the opposite perichondrium. Under direct vision, after undermining the subperichondrial space on the opposite side, one can push aside the septal leaves by opening up a speculum with the cartilage between the blades. The dorsal incision line in the cartilage can be started with a pair of angled scissors. Then either with strong shears or a swivel knife proceed posteriorly along a preselected line parallel and about 2 cm below the dorsal profile. When the rostrum of the vertical plate of the ethmoid is reached, use a swivel knife to swing down to the vomer and then back out

along the vomer ridge and out. Strong double-action shears are equally effective (Fig 24–8,A–C).

4. Doing this operation is like making a watch in a drainpipe. The most useful instruments I have found to ease this sometimes difficult procedure are a combination suction-elevator and the angled septal shears. The former eliminates the need to keep changing instruments at critical moments. The latter is much easier to use because it will cut through cartilage and ethmoid plate in one cut.

5. Often a deflected vomer can be greensticked into the midline by placing a 1-mm chisel on the nasal floor and scoring along one side of the base of the deviated vomer ridge. A little pressure by opening a long thin speculum along the floor of the nose may do the trick (Fig 24–9).

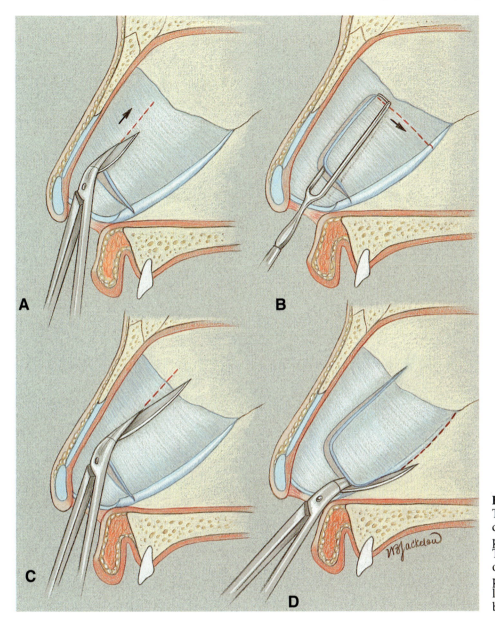

**FIG 24–8.**
The dorsal incision line in the cartilage can be started with a pair of angled scissors (**A**). Then with a swivel knife (**B**) or strong shears (**C**), proceed posteriorly along a preselected line parallel and about 2 cm below the dorsal profile (**D**).

6. If the vertical element of the remaining L-shaped cartilage support is still crooked, do not depend on columellar pockets or transfixation devices to straighten it. Not only will it not work, but it will also carry the tip of the nose with it when it redeviates. Score it on its concave side, and if need be, stiffen it on the intact (convex) side with a thin cartilage batten (see Fig 24–6,A and B).

7. At the end of the procedure if you wish to pack the nose, pack the convex side first. (If the nose deviates to the right, pack the left side first.) Do not use the "cramjam" technique; pack carefully from the floor up with just enough material to put the mucosal leaves back to back. Put in one nasal length at a time, and tamp it down by opening your speculum. Bear in mind that an overall splint will bring things further together and too much packing may tend to separate the nasal bones. Bilateral internal Teflon splints are equally effective but much more comfortable and less messy. The patient can breathe around them, and they can remain in place for as long as 2 weeks.

8. Totally intact, accurately closed mucoperichondrial leaves, if inadequately splinted, may be dangerous. Septal hematomas are not uncommon. If not evacuated properly they can give a thick, ob-

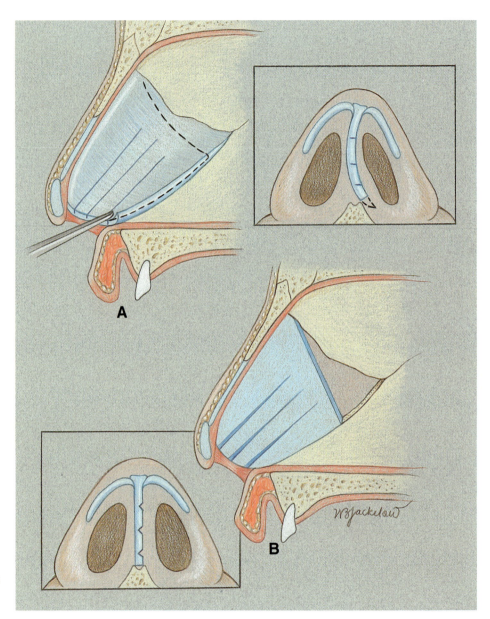

**FIG 24–9.**
**A,** often a deflected vomer can be greensticked into the midline by placing a 1-mm chisel on the nasal floor and scoring along one side of the base of the deviated vomer ridge. **B,** a little pressure by opening a long thin speculum along the floor of the nose may do the trick.

**A**

**B**

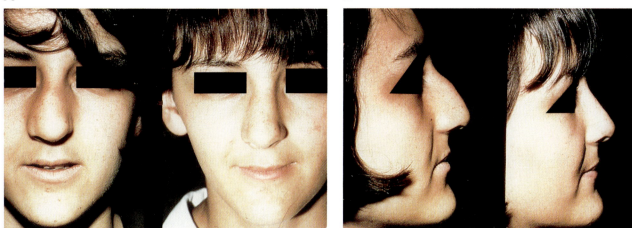

**FIG 24–10.**
**A,** preoperative and postoperative septoplasty (and osteotomies of nasal bone) in a young female (front view). **B,** lateral view.

structive septum. If in doubt, there is no harm in making a couple of stab wounds with a no. 15 blade at separate sites on either side at the base of the mucoperichondrial flaps for drainage.

9. The turbinates are often part of the problem. Time and space do not permit a detailed account of this aspect or airway correction. It may be appropriate to deal with troublesome turbinates at the time of surgery by several simple maneuvers. They can be outfractured by forceful pressure with a long speculum, cauterized along their edge, or trimmed away. Beware of overly enthusiastic treatment for fear of rhinitis sicca as a consequence. Postoperatively the turbinates may respond to intranasal corticoids injected directly into the submucosa in small amounts.

Clinical examples of the type of improvement that can be achieved by the above techniques are as follows. Figure 24–10 is a case of a young girl who complained of right-sided airway obstruction. Examination reveals that the septum and entire nose itself are deviated to the right side. Septoplasty (closing with osteotomies and hump removal) dramatically improved not only the shape of the nose but the airway as well. Figure 24–11 shows a middle-age male who complained of severe airway obstruction. The septum and nasal bones were severely deviated to the left. Postoperative examination shows the improvement that septoplasty (closing with osteotomies) can do to improve the problem. Septoplasty can be and is often combined with aesthetic changes

in the nose. Figure 24–12,A–C shows a young man who complained not only that his nose was too broad and long but also that his airway was obstructed on the left. Physical examination revealed that the caudal septum was sitting on the left vestibule and obstructing the airway. Septoplasty (along with cephalic crux resection, hump removal, and nasal shortening) was performed. Postoperative photographs (Fig 24–12,D–F) show not only improvement in the aesthetic result (greater than 1 year) but also a normal basal view. The caudal edge of the septum is no longer protruding into the left vestibule, and his airway is no longer a problem.

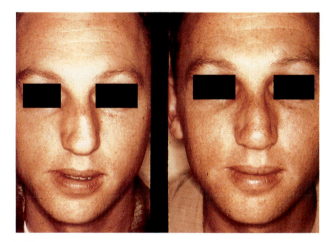

**FIG 24–11.**
Preoperative and postoperative septoplasty in a very severe case of septal deformity causing marked left-sided airway obstruction.

**A**

**B**

**C**

**D**

**E**

**F**

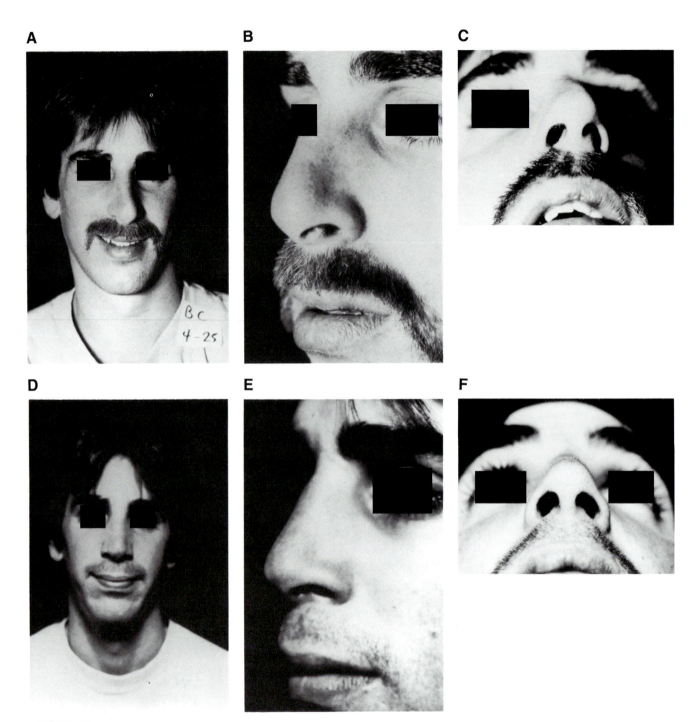

**FIG 24–12.**
**A,** septoplasty is often combined with aesthetic nasal surgery. This is a young male who complained of both left-sided airway obstruction and a nose that was too large in all dimensions. **B,** oblique view. **C,** basal view showing the caudal edge of the septum in the left vestibule. **D,** postoperative (over 1 year) front view. **E,** oblique view. **F,** basal view showing no deviation of the caudal edge of the septum.

# BIBLIOGRAPHY

Becker OJ: Problems of septum in rhinoplastic surgery, *Arch Otolaryngol* 53:622, 1951.

Converse JM: Corrective surgery of nasal deviation, *Arch Otolaryngol* 52:671, 1950.

Dingman R: Correction of nasal deformities due to defects of the septum, *Plast Reconstr Surg* 18:291, 1956.

Fomon S et al: New approach to ventral deflections of nasal septum, *Arch Otolaryngol* 54:356, 1951.

Fomon S et al: Plastic repair of obstructing nasal septum, *Arch Otolaryngol* 47:7, 1948.

Fomon S: Physiological principals in rhinoplasty, *Arch Otolaryngol* 53:256, 1951.

Fry HJH: Interlocked stresses in human nasal septal cartilage, *Br J Plast Surg* 19:276, 1966.

Fry HJH: Nasal skeletal trauma and the interlocked stresses of the nasal septal cartilages, *Br J Plast Surg* 20:146, 1967.

Fry HJH: The importance of the septal cartilage in nasal trauma, *Br J Plast Surg* 20:392, 1967.

Gibson T, David WB: The distortion of autogenous cartilage grafts: Its cause and prevention, *Br J Plast Surg* 10:257, 1958.

Goldman IB: New techniques in surgery of deviated nasal septum, *Arch Otolaryngol* 64:183, 1956.

Goldman IB: Rhinoplastic sequelae causing nasal obstruction, *Arch Otolaryngol* 83:151, 1966.

Gray L: The deviated nasal septum, *J Laryngol Otolaryngol* 79:567, 1965.

Horton CE: Combined septoplasty and rhinoplasty. In Masters FW, Lewis JR Jr, editors: *Symposium on aesthetic surgery of the nose, ears, and chin,* St Louis, 1973, Mosby–Year Book.

Kazanjian VH, Converse JM: *Surgical treatment of facial injuries,* Baltimore, 1974, Williams & Wilkins.

Killian G: Die submucose Fensterresektion der Nasenscheidewand, *Arch Laryngol Rhinol (Berlin)* 16:362, 1904. (The submucous window resection of the nasal septum, *Ann Otol Rhinol Laryngol* 14:363, 1905.)

Metzenbaum M: Replacement of lower end of dislocated septal cartilage versus submucous resection of dislocated end of septal cartilage, *Otolaryngology* 9:282, 1929.

Peer LA: Operation to repair lateral displacement of the lower border of septal cartilage, *Arch Otolaryngol* 25:475, 1937.

Proetz AW: Physiology of nose from the standpoint of plastic surgeon, *Arch Otolaryngol* 39:514, 1944.

Selzer AP: Nasal septum: plastic repair of deviated septum associated with deflected tip, *Arch Otolaryngol* 40:433, 1944.

Steffensen WH: Reconstruction of the nasal septum, *Plast Reconstr Surg* 2:66, 1947.

# PART IV

# *Ancillary Procedures*

# The Forehead: Its Relationship to Nasal Aesthetics and Indications for and Methods of Contour Changing

## Douglas K. Ousterhout, D.D.S., M.D.

Look at any face, what is the first thing you see? It is probably not the nose. I suspect that the majority of times we make eye contact first. Generally the observer's eyes next look at the mouth for what is being said. Then the other structures are observed as we have more time to take in but not analyze the nose, the lips, the chin, the cheeks, the symmetry, skin texture and color, relative degrees of prominence, etc. Depending on our familiarity with the individual, we may even think about that person's beauty, handsomeness, or lack of it. It has been stated by many surgeons that the three most important prominences of the facial area are the nose, the cheeks, and the chin. It is my feeling that these three areas have to a degree been relegated this importance by plastic surgeons because they are the three areas that until recently are the most easily approached and modified. We can augment or reduce the chin, albeit the latter is considerably more difficult. Certainly we can augment or reduce the nose; augmentation of the cheeks is far more common, but the cheeks can also be reduced. But what about the largest surface of the face, the forehead.

Look in any fashion magazine, look at any model, male or female, and do you see an abnormal forehead? Of course not. The foreheads of models are every bit as "perfect" as the rest of their facial structures. If the forehead is too vertical, e.g., Fran-

kenstein the monster, if the frontal sinus is too pneumatized and prominent, if the forehead slants back to much, if it is asymmetrical, or if it shows contour irregularities or signs of trauma or disease, any and all of the above will distract from the beauty or handsomeness of the wearer. Any time there is a deformity of sufficient magnitude to draw our attention to it, it may adversely affect our opinion of that individual.

If the individual has a large forehead, we sometimes consider that individual as being intelligent. If a person has a very short forehead, we may consider it a negative feature. If the frontal sinuses are too pneumatized, it causes the eyes to be deeply set or shadowed, and it may give the person a sinister appearance. If the brows are too far back and do not protect the eyes at all, that is, the brows are behind the globe of the eyes, we may consider that person as not having a sufficient forehead and perhaps even being mentality deficient.

The forehead is the largest area of the face and covers a very large percentage of the total face, even as much as 45%. If from no other point of view than its size, the forehead has considerable importance in total facial appearance.

As much as a small chin may cause a nose to appear larger than it actually is, a retruded forehead can also cause a nose to appear exaggerated in size

(Fig 25–1). A full forehead may work in the reverse and cause the nose to appear somewhat smaller than it truly is. For the benefit of the nose, the forehead should be in balance.

Therefore, the forehead and its harmony with the rest of the face, including the nose and its surrounding structures, is every bit as important as any other single facial feature. The forehead lift, for example, has become a very important part of facial rejuvenation surgery.

It is obviously very important to the wearer, for any deformities present can be just as distracting as other abnormal features. Those who wear bangs frequently do so to hide a long forehead; they have learned that it makes them look better with more harmonious facial proportions.

There are significant ethnic differences that we respect and realize even if we have not taken the time to study them. We know that the prominence of the forehead and brows beyond the cornea is 8 to

**A**

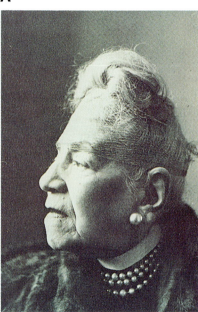

**FIG 25–1.**
**A,** woman with a markedly retruded forehead. **B–D,** three men with different foreheads, from markedly retruded to quite prominent, that create a different effect on nasal size and shape.

**B**

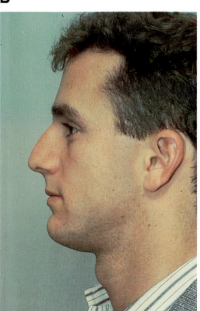

**C**

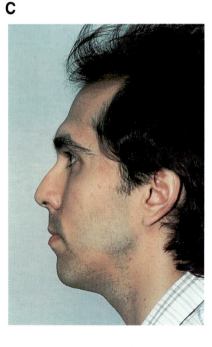

**D**

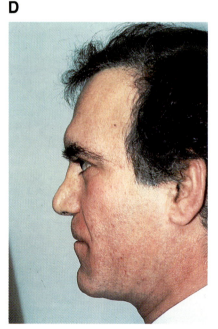

10 mm in the female[16] as opposed to 10 to 14 mm in the male. If the individual is larger in stature, we would then fully anticipate that a greater degree of bossing could be present. Conversely if the individual is small or particularly if the individual is Oriental, we should then fully anticipate that the brows would be back even, to just a few millimeters' projection beyond the cornea, to actually even being slightly behind the cornea. These we accept as being normal. When looking at the forehead of non-Caucasian groups, it is not unusual to see a forehead with more or less posterior slope or with considerably more or less frontal bossing.

Similarly, we now appreciate that there is considerable sexual differences in the shape of the forehead.[13, 14] We appreciate that the male has more brow projection over the eyes secondary to the prominence of the frontal sinuses with increased bony brow bossing as compared with the female and that there is generally an area of flatness above the glabella between the areas of brow bossing. We also appreciate that there may be an area of fullness above this area of flatness along the midline but that this is not necessary for male skull determination. Conversely, the female tends to have little or no frontal bossing and no area of flatness in the midforehead, but in fact the head tends to be continuously convex in both the horizontal and sagittal planes. We know that there is usually no upper forehead midline fullness (Fig 25–2). All of these above factors are important to us in the overall appreciation of normal forehead aesthetics and appreciation of forehead aesthetics in relationship to the remainder of the facial structures.

It is therefore quite obvious that the forehead, due to its size, shape, position, and sexual and ethnic differences, is extremely important in facial aesthetics. Failure to consider it in the overall planing of aesthetic surgery of any other part of the facial skeleton including the nose is to have missed one of the most important areas in obtaining total facial harmony. Marchac, in a chapter on forehead contouring,[3] described a patient who requested nasal surgery but in whom the forehead was actually the problem. The forehead, because of its proximity and actual union at the glabella, must in particular be in harmony with the nose. The manner in which the midforehead and brows flow into the nose is of considerable importance in aesthetics.

It is obvious that for an individual to have the maximum of beauty or handsomeness, it is important that all of the structures of the craniofacial skeleton be in harmony. If it is not in harmony, then anything that prevails, or the opposite, is deficient, will cause a disharmony and with it an associated lessening of that individual's overall appearance.

The questions then are how do we evaluate forehead appearance and if it does not seem to be in harmony with the other structures, how do we modify it? It seems quite impossible to give a cookbook list of forehead-nose harmonious and disharmonious conditions. One must study art and have an appreciation for facial proportions. Tolleth feels that this can be learned by studying art books and learning to sculpt even if only in a primitive way.[15] Anything one does in this regard can only help. Ricketts has described facial proportions based on the golden mean;[12] Kolar[1] has described the face from an anthropologic point of view. It is additionally very important to study the face, especially the beautiful

**A**

**B**

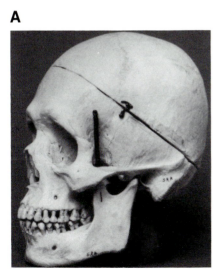
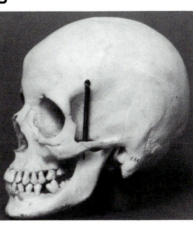

FIG 25–2.
**A,** male skull; **B,** female skull. Note the difference in bossing, the lower midforehead flat area (male characteristic), and the continuous curvature of the forehead both transversely and vertically (female characteristics). (Skulls from the Atkinson Skull Collection, University of the Pacific, San Francisco.) (From Ousterhout DK: *Plast Reconstr Surg* 79:701, 1987. Used by permission.)

and handsome face, from every angle. Where are the curves, where do the temples begin, how do the brows approach the nose? Studying dry skulls, which may or may not have come from "beautiful people," is also of tremendous help. These give one a basis for assisting in decision making. But within all of these analyses, personal feeling will always be a major factor. Beauty will always remain quite personal.

When the decision has been made that a contour modification should be made, either augmentation or reduction, the amount and area of change will dictate the technique. The majority of procedures completed by me have utilized some methylmethacrylate.

If an implant is to be used, then I feel that the rhinoplasty procedure should be completed first so as to avoid contamination of the implant with nasal organisms during the rhinoplasty. Of course, that will not always be possible. An individual may request nasal surgery some time after forehead modification. In either case and whatever one's preference, antibiotics are utilized in every case.

## REDUCTION OF THE FOREHEAD

The majority of procedures that I complete on the forehead involve reduction. These reductions have been divided into three groups based on the evaluation of hundreds of dry skulls, on patient evaluations and the contour deformities generally seen, and on contour changes requested, combined with the methods of contour changing possible.[5, 6]

Group I forehead deformities occur in those individuals in whom there is excessive fullness of the supraorbital rim that needs reduction but in whom there is either no frontal sinus present or in whom the anterior wall of the frontal sinus is thick enough that in reduction of the brow the frontal sinus will not be entered. This group of patients has been the most rare group, only occurring in a few individuals.

Group II forehead deformities are those in which there is excess frontal bossing but the excess is minimal. They will require only a slight reduction, but when that reduction is completed, there will still be a concave area above the bossing that requires filling. This group has been the most common group.

It has occurred in both males and females, but is the one most normally seen in women who have masculine forehead deformities. It requires some re-

duction of the bossing but, more importantly, filling in of the concave or flat area above the bossing with some material. I have used methylmethacrylate as the filling material.

Group III forehead deformities occur in those individuals with excessive bossing of the frontal bone, particularly anterior to the frontal sinus, as seen in hyperpneumatization of the frontal sinus[8]; establishing a normal contour of the forehead will require setting back the anterior wall of the frontal sinuses. This is the most involved operation because it requires osteotomies of the frontal bone, marginal reduction through burring, and then repositioning of the frontal bone in four to six pieces in a more recessed position. I have only seen this condition in males, but I suspect that someday I will see a woman with this condition.

## SURGERY

Surgery is started in all three groups through a bicoronal incision (Fig 25–3,A). The decision as to placement of the incision, within the hair or anterior to the hairline, is a separate issue and will not be discussed here. It generally makes no difference in forehead reduction surgery, but it could be of importance with augmentation, as will be discussed. Shaving off the hair is not necessary, but I generally shave a strip 6 mm wide to avoid pieces of hair falling into the wound. Following the incision the forehead soft tissues are reflected down to the level of the superior orbital rims with some dissection down laterally, (Fig 25–3,B). The pericranium is then incised along the superior margin of the temporalis muscles and across the top just anterior to the bicoronal incision. The pericranium is then reflected forward as a separate layer to expose the orbital rims and protect the supraorbital and trochlear neurovascular bundles (Fig 25–3,C). The temporalis muscles are reflected out of the upper portion of fossa for approximately 2 cm (Fig 25–3,D). This approach is used for all of the forehead procedures, both reduction and augmentation.

In the group I patients the bone is contoured by using methylmethacrylate burred to the desired shape with particular attention to whether this is a male or female or whether one is creating or maintaining the desired sexual characteristics. For the first few times that one does this, it is very handy to have a skull of the appropriate sex in the operating room so that proper contouring can be completed. I

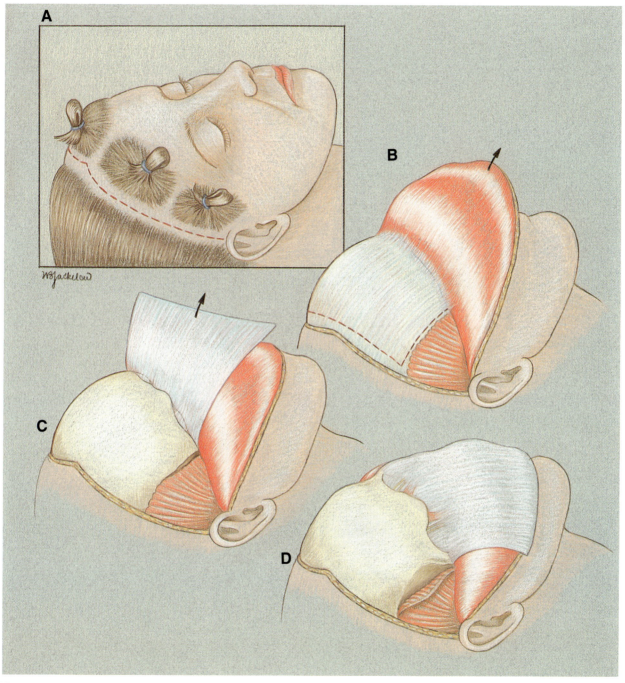

**FIG 25–3.**
**A,** placement of a bicoronal incision, if in the hair. If one plans on using any methylmethacrylate, shave approximately 6 mm of hair at the incision so that no hair will be incorporated in the wound; otherwise, minimal hair is clipped. **B,** dissection of the scalp down to the orbital rim. **C,** the pericranium is dissected forward into the orbits to protect the supraorbital neurovascular bundle. **D,** the temporalis muscles are dissected out of the upper portion of each temporal fossa. (Adapted from Ousterhout DK, editor: *Aesthetic contouring of the craniofacial skeleton,* Boston, 1991, Little Brown.) (Redrawn from M. Dohrmann.)

can assure you that as well as one understands the skull, in the operating room small details are easily forgotten. It is no embarrassment to have a skull available in the operating room that one can view during the operation.

In these conditions, as the circumference of the forehead is being reduced, it is usually necessary to remove a small segment, 5 to 8 mm of scalp, and achieve a slight lift even if a lift is not desired; other-wise the brows will have a tendency to drop down to a lower level.

A representative patient is shown in Figure 25–4. Figure 25–5 shows the area of contour adjustment.

In the group II deformity, after the bone exposure is completed, the bone is reduced as desired, but particular caution is taken not to enter the frontal sinus. As the bone becomes thin but before the

**A**

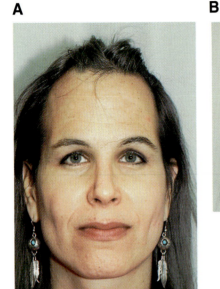

**B**

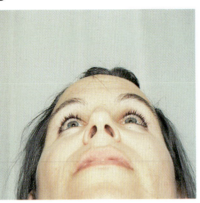

**C**

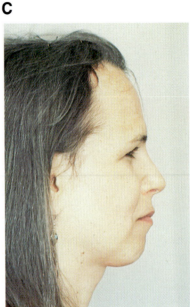

**D**

**E**

**F**

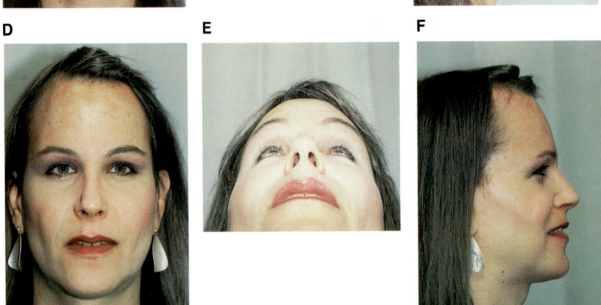

**FIG 25–4.**
Preoperative **(A–C)** and postoperative **(D–F)** views of a female patient who had skull feminization contouring by reduction alone. Because of the long forehead, the bicoronal incision was placed anterior to the hairline. She also had an advancing, sliding genioplasty.

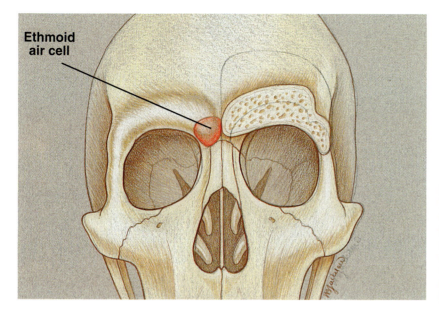

**Ethmoid air cell**

**FIG 25–5.**
Drawing demonstrating the area of the skull reduced *(whiter area)* in the patient seen in Figure 25–4. The area in the *circle* represents an ethmoid air cell seen on a posteroanterior radiograph. (Adapted from Ousterhout DK, editor: *Aesthetic contouring of the craniofacial skeleton*, Boston, 1991, Little Brown.) (Redrawn from M. Dohrmann.)

sinus is entered, the remaining bone over the frontal sinus will appear a bluish red. One must not go beyond that level. If one does accidentally enter the sinus, I think the procedure of choice would be to cut out a square or rectangle around this area and then replace it with a piece of cranial bone taken from posterior of the bicoronal incision in the hair-bearing scalp. This should then be wired carefully into position after cutting it exactly to the proper size. In those type II patients where some methylmethacrylate is utilized to fill in the defect, the methylmethacrylate should not come within a centimeter of the margins of the bone graft. Following surgery in those cases with a bone graft, the anesthesiologist should not use positive-pressure mask breathing, nor should patients be allowed to blow their noses for at least 10 days following surgery to prevent bacterial contamination of the methylmethacrylate.

Once the bony contour is exactly as desired, the concavity above the frontal bossing and below the upper, more normal forehead contour must then be filled. In my experience bone grafts do not work well in this area because they cannot be tapered in nicely to the forehead margins and they will always undergo some degree of resorption, usually considerable. As a result of both of the above, the final aesthetic result over the relatively thin soft tissues of the forehead area do not look perfect with bone grafts. I therefore find that a prosthetic material is the augmentation method of choice. Silicone is not adherent to the skull, and it is difficult to contour on the operating table. Methylmethacrylate has been utilized by me for this purpose for over 16 years on a regular basis without major complication.[2, 7, 10] It is

hard, functions like bone, does not seem to cause any resorption of the underlying bone, and can be contoured perfectly. The only limitation is the sculpturing ability of the surgeon.

In applying the methylmethacrylate to the skull it is necessary to create some method for locking it onto the underlying skull. Figure 25–6 shows the method I have found to be most successful. By creating two to four holes on opposite sides of the skull at an acute angle to each other, the methylmethacrylate will be nicely held in position. If it needs to be removed, e.g., with an infection, the methylmethacrylate could be cut down the middle and easily removed. If one were to utilize screws tapped into the outer table of cranial bone, there may be considerable difficulty removing the material if it were necessary. If one removed too much of the methylmethacrylate by excessive contouring and wanted to add more, it is not a problem. The surface can be roughened and then more methylmethacrylate added directly to the previous material. A few undercuts would be helpful in this circumstance. Again, as with the group I deformities, the final contour is created as indicated in the preoperative evaluation and by physician and patient desires (Fig 25–7).

Figure 25–8 demonstrates preoperative and postoperative results of a Group II patient who had forehead contouring.

Group III deformities are those deformities of a much more severe nature, those in which there is generally hyperpneumatization of the frontal sinus. In these individuals it is not possible to reconstruct the deformity by grinding down the bone since one

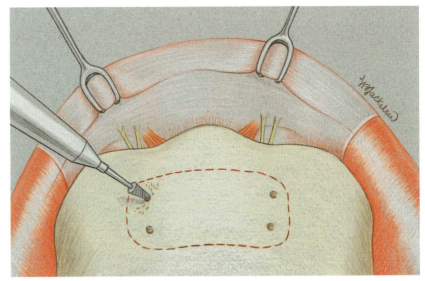

**FIG 25–6.**
Holes are placed in the outer table of the skull such that they are opposing each other and lock the methylmethacrylate onto the skull. (Adapted from Ousterhout DK, editor: *Aesthetic contouring of the craniofacial skeleton*, Boston, 1991, Little Brown.) (Redrawn from M. Dohrmann.)

would enter the frontal sinus prior to the time that the desired contour setback had been achieved. Therefore it is necessary to remove the anterior frontal sinus wall. In this technique the frontal sinus wall is removed either with a Lindemann side-cutting burr (Fig 25–9,A) or with a reciprocating saw; I now prefer the latter. The surrounding areas are then contoured appropriately. The frontal sinus is next completely irrigated free of any bone dust so that the frontal nasal ducts do not become obstructed. The septum between the right and left sides should be removed at least in part so that if a partial duct obstruction were to occur on one side, the sinuses could very easily drain on the contralat-

eral side. The bone that has been removed is then cut into four to six pieces as necessary and repositioned over the sinus. Once the bone has been cut in the appropriate places, it is then stabilized with multiple pieces of 28-gauge wire (Fig 25–9,B). I have not used plates in this area primarily because they can be palpated beneath the relatively thin soft tissues in this area. Microplates might be successful. I have not used any methylmethacrylate as additional contouring in these individuals. I would not want to place methylmethacrylate over the osteotomy sites for fear of contamination. If methylmethacrylate were necessary in this area, I think one would have to come back at least 6 months later to complete the

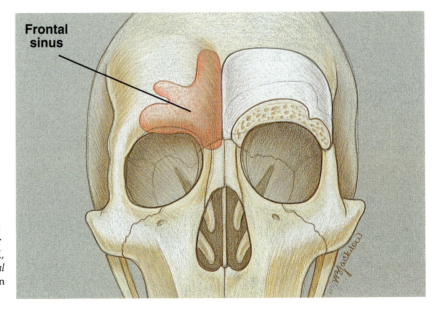

**FIG 25–7.**
The drawing shows the area to be reduced by burring down the excess bone. The *whiter area* is the area augmented with methylmethacrylate filling in the concavity, thus creating a feminine contour. On the right of the forehead *(darker area)*, the area outlined represents the frontal sinus as was seen in this individual on the posteroanterior radiograph. (Adapted from Ousterhout DK, editor: *Aesthetic contouring of the craniofacial skeleton*, Boston, 1991, Little Brown.) (Redrawn from M. Dohrmann.)

contouring. To date no additional contouring has been necessary, and the results of the recession of the frontal sinuses has been very successful. Figure 25–10 shows a group III individual who had recontouring of the forehead. One can readily appreciate the improvement in the forehead contour by this method.

## AUGMENTATION OF THE FOREHEAD

The majority of total forehead augmentations that I have completed have been for major craniofacial congenital abnormalities.[7, 20] There are, however, a group of patients who wish to have a fuller fore-

**A**

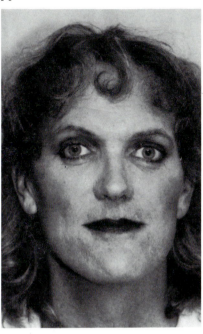

**B**

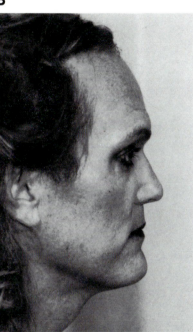

**C**

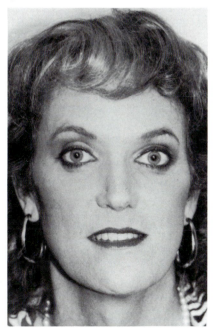

**D**

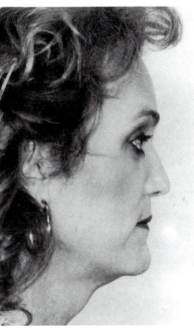

**FIG 25–8.**
Preoperative (**A** and **B**) and postoperative (**C** and **D**) views of a group II female who had feminization of the forehead.

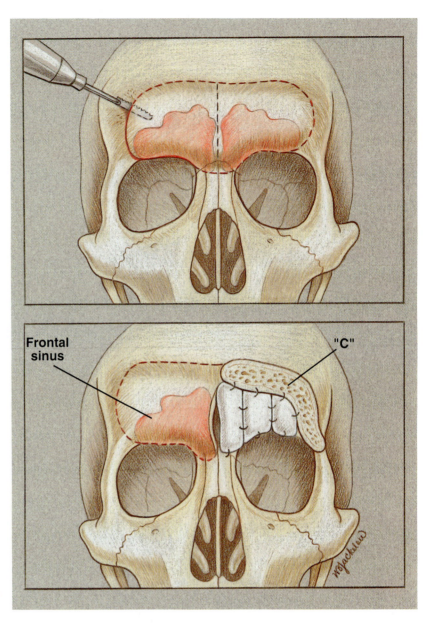

**FIG 25–9.**
**A,** method for taking off the anterior wall of the frontal sinus. **B,** cutting, reconstructing, and stabilizing of the anterior wall after peripheral reduction in order to obtain the desired setback and contour. (Adapted from Ousterhout DK, editor: *Aesthetic contouring of the craniofacial skeleton,* Boston, 1991, Little Brown.) (Redrawn from M. Dohrmann.)

head, both in prominence and in contour, strictly for aesthetic purposes.[9] In this chapter I will only discuss those cases that are aesthetic problems and not reconstructive in the usual sense.

The patients have primarily been of two types. Orientals who do not necessarily want to look occidental but who find that their forehead retrusion is greater than they would like represent the first type. In the average occidental female the normal forehead protrusion beyond the cornea of the eye is approximately 8 to 10 mm, obviously somewhat more in the average male. In the Oriental this distance is considerably less. It is not at all unusual to see an Oriental in whom the brows are even with or actually behind the prominence of the eyes. On occasion

they present for augmentation of this area, not to have the occidental degree of protrusion but to get the brows into a slightly more prominent position. In the occidental the concern has been one of contour where there are congenital irregularities, narrowness of the bitemporal area, particularly at the superior temporal line, and grooving of the forehead, all of which subtract from the individual's appearance.

Again, because of the problems of using autogenous materials, i.e., bone, and the resorption that will occur following augmentation with bone as well as the morbidity associated with harvesting a large amount of bone graft, this procedure has been completed primarily with methylmethacrylate. It is rela-

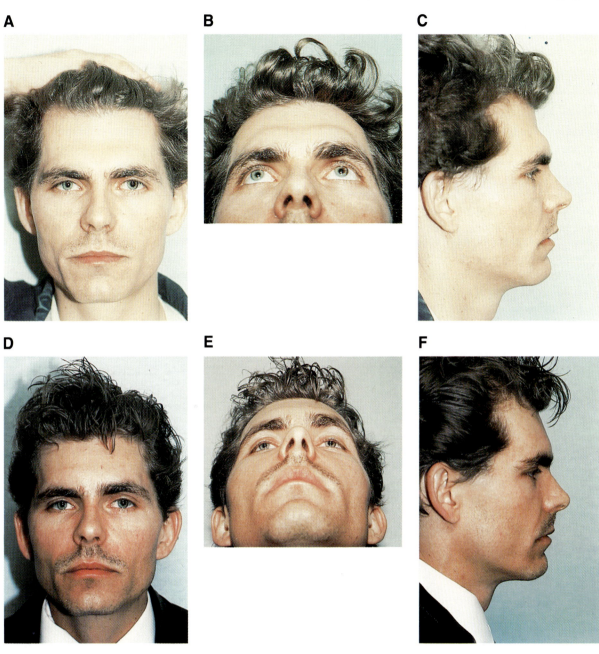

**FIG 25–10.**
Preoperative **(A–C)** and postoperative **(D–F)** views of a forehead reduction in a patient with a group III contour deformity.

tively easy to apply, can be contoured to any desired shape, can be further augmented easily if the contour is at first not acceptable, does not undergo resorption, and can be completed under local anesthesia. The only major, potential problem present is that of infection, but to date, after utilizing this material for over 16 years and being very careful, no infections have occurred, and no implants have had to be removed for complications of surgery. There is no

other material presently available that works as well as methylmethacrylate.[2] I do strongly suspect that over the following years new materials will become available. Not only will these new materials be osteoconductive, but they probably will also be osteoinductive. When such a material becomes available and if it is easily utilized, it certainly will be the material of choice. I strongly suspect that sometime in the next century a material in paste form will become available that can be applied to bone and very quickly become hard and eventually turn into bone. It may even be a tissue culture of bone.

## SURGERY

The exposure to the forehead is exactly as previously described, with the following exception. If the forehead augmentation is going to be fairly long and extend posterosuperiorly, it is important that it not overlap the forehead incision. Therefore in certain individuals it would not be possible to complete the augmentation by utilizing a prehairline incision. My concern is that if the incision were too close to the margin of the methylmethacrylate or actually even overlapped it, a relatively mild wound infection, perhaps even spitting of a suture, could cause an infection to occur and involve the implant. It is very important that the implant not be utilized within 6 months of an infection, beneath a skin graft, or under a stellate scar that is thin and retracted.[17, 19]

Figure 25–3 shows the exposure. The methylmethacrylate is then applied directly to the skull after any necessary retention holes are created (see Fig 25–6). With a wide forehead implant, particularly if it overlaps into the temporal fossa bilaterally, retention holes are generally not necessary.

If one has not utilized methylmethacrylate before, I would recommend a trial in the laboratory in which the methylmethacrylate is applied to the underside, convex surface of a porcelain mixing bowl. One can then rapidly learn the consistency necessary for applying this material but maintaining posi-

tion without having material run freely into the temporal fossa or orbital spaces. This consistency is correct if the material, when pulled, develops fine strands, "angel's hair." The future position of the methylmethacrylate must be well established before applying it to the surface. A gas-sterilized pencil works very nicely to mark the skull. A periodontal probe, an instrument that is readily available through instrument companies, is very handy for establishing the thickness of the material. One can also use a hypodermic needle with a curved hemostat clamped across the needle at the appropriate level so that one knows exactly the thickness of the methylmethacrylate that is being established over the forehead.

The methylmethacrylate is applied at exactly the right time and contoured as much as possible with one's fingers and some flat instruments, the excess cut off as best possible (Fig 25–11). Then, just as the material becomes very hard, the temperature will rise secondary to the heat of polymerization. At this time the area must be copiously irrigated with cool saline so that there is no burning of the surrounding tissues.

Once the material is cool, then the final contouring can be completed. This contouring is best completed with a methylmethacrylate-type burr, a rather coarse burr (Fig 25–12). During the contouring, do not irrigate the surface because there is no burning of the methylmethacrylate from the heat of the burr and, more importantly, all the little filings from the material being burred away may get in the crevices. When the contouring is completed, first wipe off the filings, and then copiously irrigate the tissues to

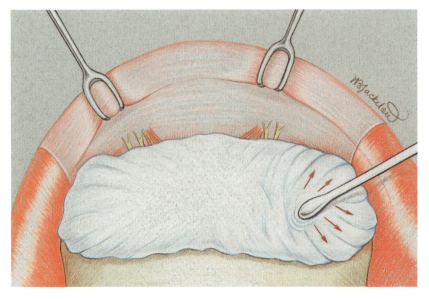

**FIG 25–11.**
Drawing depicting the application of the methylmethacrylate directly to the skull. (Adapted from Ousterhout DK, editor: *Aesthetic contouring of the craniofacial skeleton*, Boston, 1991, Little Brown.) (Redrawn from M. Dohrmann.)

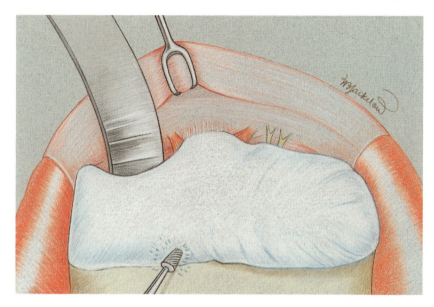

**FIG 25-12.**
Drawing depicting the contouring of the methylmethacrylate with a course rotating burr until the final desired contour is obtained. (Adapted from Ousterhout DK, editor: *Aesthetic contouring of the craniofacial skeleton,* Boston, 1991, Little Brown.) (Redrawn from M. Dohrmann.)

eliminate every last residual piece of material. It is very handy during the grinding process to place moist sponges and towels around the edges of the area being contoured, not close enough to allow them to be caught in the burr but close enough that it will prevent the filings from being too widely dispersed. It will save time in the final cleanup phase.

When the contouring is complete and the tissue eliminated of all free methylmethacrylate, closure is completed. The temporalis muscles are first stabilized to the methylmethacrylate. Numerous holes can be placed along the margin and the temporalis muscle stabilized with 3-0 or 4-0 sutures as necessary (Fig 25-13,A). It may be necessary to elevate the temporalis muscles out of the fossa and rotate it forward to the anterior edge of the plastic to avoid creating a hollowness in the anterior temporal area. Then the pericranium is returned to position; it will not fit adequately because the convexity has now increased, but it can be stabilized as best as possible to the temporalis muscles bilaterally with 4-0 sutures (Fig 25-13,B). When the convexity over the skull is significantly increased, scalp closure may be more difficult. In these cases relaxation of the galea anteriorly by transecting it at multiple levels while protecting the neurovascular bundle is indicated (Fig 25-13,C). On rare occasion with very large augmentations it has been necessary to also dissect posterior to the bicoronal incision and release the scalp posteriorly. I have never had a case, even if the implant has been as thick as 27 mm, obviously a tremendous increase in the circumference of the forehead, that I could not close. The scalp is then returned to position and closed in the usual way. I generally use

deep sutures of 3-0 degradable material followed by staples.

Figures 25-14 and 25-15 show the results of two patients in whom the forehead was contoured by applying methylmethacrylate directly to the skull.

This basic technique can also be utilized for masculinization and has been completed by Dr. Gerald Verdi of Louisville, Kentucky. In this case the male felt that his forehead was too feminine and wanted his supraorbital rims to be built up, and in exactly the same manner methylmethacrylate was utilized to create more frontal bossing.

## RESULTS

The results of all the surgeries described above have been universally pleasing. On two patients with total forehead augmentation I had to go back and do additional contouring, but there has not been a problem from this. In general, however, the first operation has been the only operation necessary. I have also had one Oriental patient who 3 years after placement of the implant, during which time he seemed to be very pleased, decided that he no longer wanted it. I think this feeling was partly precipitated by media statements regarding the problems of implants and possible carcinogenesis, a totally fallacious statement. There has never been any relationship between carcinogenesis and methylmethacrylate. Nonetheless, he became very concerned about his implant and asked that it be removed. When it was removed, interestingly there

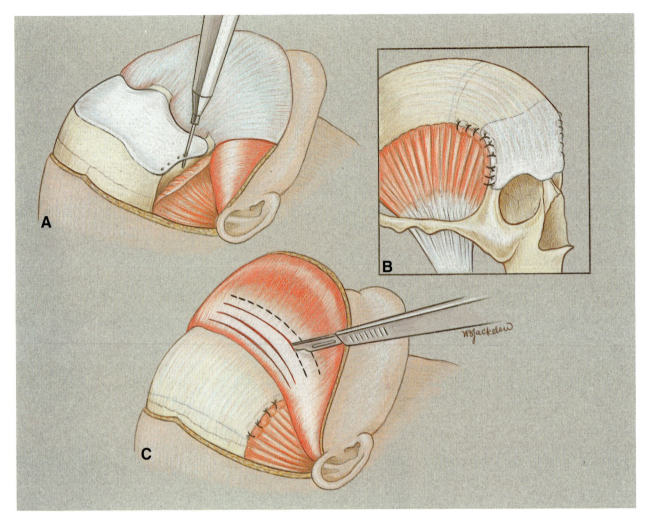

**FIG 25–13.**
**A,** drawing depicting the placement of holes at the edge of the cranioplasty for stabilization of the temporalis muscle to it. **B,** repositioning of the pericranium and stabilization of it to the temporalis muscle as much as possible. **C,** scoring the galea to allow closure of the bicoronal incision without undue tension. Attention must be given to protecting the supraorbital neurovascular bundle. (Adapted from Ousterhout DK, editor: *Aesthetic contouring of the craniofacial skeleton*, Boston, 1991, Little Brown.) (Redrawn from M. Dohrmann.)

was no resorption of bone underlying a total forehead prosthesis. Unfortunately, there are no photographs adequate for publishing.

Patient acceptance has been extremely high and qualifies as one of the more successful cosmetic procedures that we can complete.

## COMPLICATIONS

Complications have been minimal from the surgery. As stated throughout this chapter, there have been no cases of infection.

I have been extremely careful in my patient se-

lection and in completing the surgery and ensuring that the patients take an adequate dose of antibiotics after surgery. There has been no evidence of any migrations of the implants, late seromas, or other problems. There is no difference in the sensory deficit occurring with this surgery than what occurs in any standard forehead lift procedure.

There has been an occasional patient, five, in which a seroma developed in the soft-tissue space between the prosthesis and the scalp. This usually occurs immediately following the surgery. Originally I carefully aspirated this fluid, but in general it kept recurring, albeit in smaller amounts, until around the eighth or ninth day it disappeared completely.

**A**

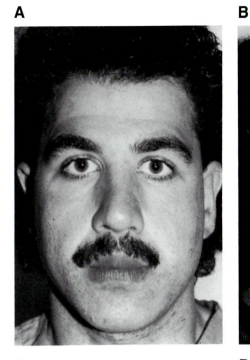

**B**

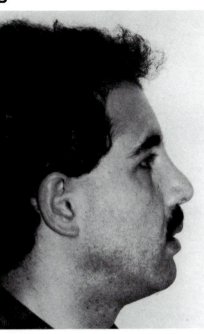

**C**

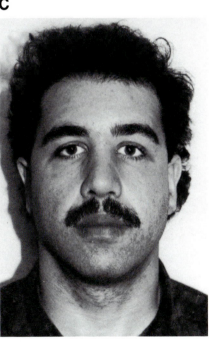

**D**

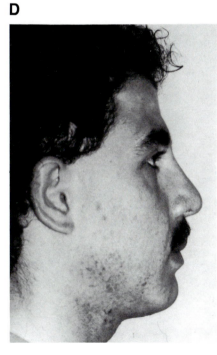

**FIG 25–14.**
Preoperative **(A and B)** and postoperative **(C and D)** views of an individual who had forehead augmentation with methylmethacrylate applied directly to the skull. (From Ousterhout DK, editor: *Aesthetic contouring of the craniofacial skeleton,* Boston, 1991, Little Brown. Used by permission.)

Now I do nothing, and it goes away at 8 or 9 days postsurgery on its own. By leaving it we have reduced the possibility of bringing in an infecting organism with the needle sticks. I formerly thought that the seromas were associated with decreased diligence at removing all of the debris from contouring the methylmethacrylate, but I now think that it is just something that occurs in an occasional individual. Occasionally there may also be some burning around the eyes for a few days following the surgery. This may indeed be associated with adequacy of debridement. Since the very first few cases completed back in the mid-70s this problem has not occurred.

A       B

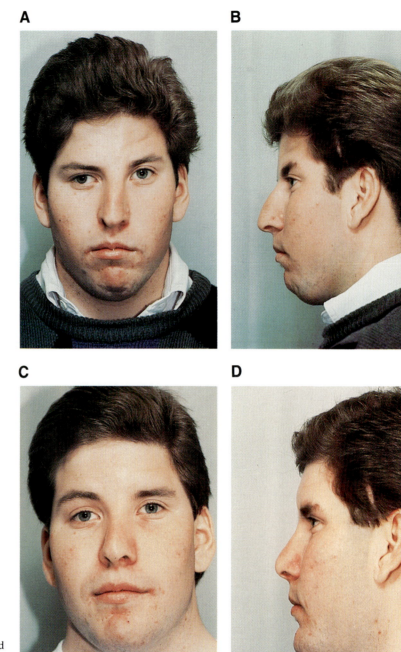

C       D

**FIG 25–15.**
Preoperative (**A** and **B**) and postoperative (**C** and **D**) views of an individual who had forehead augmentation with methylmethacrylate applied directly to the skull. The patient has also had a rhinoplasty and augmenting sliding genioplasty. (Adapted from Ousterhout DK, editor: *Aesthetic contouring of the craniofacial skeleton,* Boston, 1991, Little Brown. Used by permission.)

## CONCLUSIONS

The forehead is a very significant part of the facial surface area, and as such it represents an important part of facial aesthetics.[4, 6, 9, 18] Its proximity to the nose and its union at the nose through the area of the glabella are both very important in enhancing to-tal facial appearance. The nose has an importance in part inversely proportional to the fullness of the forehead. Forehead shape becomes very important in the obviousness of nasal contour. As the chin is often retruded in those with prominent noses, the forehead oftentimes is retruded as well. Obviously improving the chin is extremely important in facial contour in those individuals with such prominent noses; I also believe that contouring the forehead is of importance in such individuals.

The methods of reduction and augmentation of the forehead have been described. These techniques described are available to any plastic surgeon capable of completing a forehead lift. One does not need to be a craniofacial surgeon, except perhaps for the group III forehead reduction patients, a relatively rare problem.

The contouring techniques described offer a great enhancement in facial aesthetics and are extremely well accepted by patients who have such procedures completed. The problem must be corrected, but the surgeon should stay on the side of conservatism. It is extremely important to realize that the self-image is being changed and therefore the surgeon must be working with a mentally stable patient. This is of course true with nose and chin surgery. It is very true with forehead modification as well.[11]

## REFERENCES

1. Kolar JC: Anthropology of the facial skeleton. In Ousterhout DK, editor: *Aesthetic contouring of the craniofacial skeleton*, Boston, 1991, Little Brown.
2. Manson PN, Crawley WA, Hoopes JA: Frontal cranioplasty: risk factors and choice of cranial vault reconstructive material, *Plast Reconstr Surg* 77:888, 1986.
3. Marchac D: Aesthetic contouring of the forehead utilizing bone grafts and osteotomies. In Ousterhout DK, editor: *Aesthetic contouring of the craniofacial skeleton*, Boston, 1991, Little Brown.
4. Ortiz-Monasterio F: Aesthetic surgery of facial skeleton. In Whitaker LA, editor: *Clinics in plastic surgery: aesthetic surgery of the facial skeleton*, Philadelphia, 1991, Saunders, pp 18–19.
5. Ousterhout DK: Brow and forehead reduction, including feminization of the forehead. In Ousterhout DK, editor: *Aesthetic contouring of the craniofacial skeleton*, Boston, 1991, Little Brown.
6. Ousterhout DK: Feminization of the forehead contour changing to improve female aesthetics, *Plast Reconstr Surg* 79:701, 1987.
7. Ousterhout DK, Baker S, Zlotolow I: Methylmethacrylate onlay implants in the treatment of forehead deformities secondary to craniosynostosis, *J Maxillofac Surg* 8:228, 1980.
8. Ousterhout DK, Penoff JH: Surgical treatment of facial deformity secondary to acromegaly, *Ann Plast Surg* 7:68, 1981.
9. Ousterhout DK, Zlotolow IM: Aesthetic improvement of the forehead utilizing methylmethacrylate onlay implants. *Aesthetic Plast Surg* 14:281, 1990.
10. Ousterhout DK, Zlotolow IM: Prosthetic forehead augmentation. In Ousterhout DK, editor: *Aesthetic contouring of craniofacial skeleton*, Boston, 1991, Little Brown.
11. Pruzinsky T, Persing J: Psychological perspectives on aesthetic applications of reconstructive surgery techniques. In Ousterhout DK, editor: *Aesthetic contouring of the craniofacial skeleton*, Boston, 1991, Little Brown.
12. Ricketts R: The science and art of esthetic recontouring of the face. In Ousterhout DK, editor: *Aesthetic contouring of the craniofacial skeleton*, Boston, 1991, Little Brown.
13. Stewart TD: Sex determination of the skeleton by guess and measurement, *Am J Phys Anthropol* 12:385, 1954.
14. Thieme FP, Schull WJ: Sex determination from the skeleton, *Hum Biol* 29:242, 1957.
15. Tolleth H: Facial contours and proportions from an artist's point of view. In Ousterhout DK, editor: *Aesthetic contouring of the craniofacial skeleton*, Boston, 1991, Little Brown.
16. Whitaker LA, Morales L, Farkas LG: Aesthetic surgery of the supraobrital ridge and forehead structures, *Plast Reconstr Surg* 78:23–32, 1986.
17. White JC: Late complications following cranioplasty with alloplastic plates, *Ann Surg* 128:743, 1948.
18. Wolfe SA: Correction of the "simian" forehead deformity. *Aesthetic Plast Surg* 2:343, 1978.
19. Woolf JI, Walker AE: Cranioplasty: collective review, *Int Abstr Surg* 81:1, 1945.
20. Zlotolow IM, Ousterhout DK: Methylmethacrylate forehead onlay implants in the treatment of upper facial deformities utilizing a 3D graphic computer aided designed/computer aided machined (CAD/CAM) system, *Maxillofac Prosthet* 10:18, 1987.

# Genioplasty

James M. Stuzin, M.D.

Henry K. Kawamoto, M.D.

Part of the evaluation of the patient seeking rhinoplasty should involve an analysis of chin position in relation to both profile and frontal aesthetics. Similar to the large variations in contour seen among patients seeking rhinoplasty, a great deal of individual variation is evident from patient to patient regarding chin contour. Some patients present with a retrusive chin. Other patients will exhibit chins that appear long in the vertical diminsion, while still other patients will have a prognathic appearance to their chin. As surgeons must individualize their approach to rhinoplasty, in a similar fashion, an individualization of analysis and planning in aesthetic contouring of the chin warrants similar consideration.

*All chins are not alike.* We emphasize that when looking at a patient with a retrusive chin, simply do not think "chin implant". While a chin implant may provide a good solution for a particular patient's problem, prior to undertaking the procedure, it is important to first analyze the deformity. Following a proper analysis, treatment objectives can be planned in a precise fashion. Remember, if you make the wrong diagnosis, you will perform the wrong operation every time.

## ANALYSIS OF DEFORMITY

There are many methods of analyzing the relationship of the chin to facial aesthetics. The relationships we have found most useful in accurately analyzing chin aesthetics in relation to the rest of the face include (1) the soft-tissue relationships, (2) the bony (or hard-tissue) relationships, and (3) dental relationships.

## SOFT-TISSUE ANALYSIS—HORIZONTAL RELATIONSHIPS (PROFILE)

The horizontal relationships of the face are best analyzed on a profile view. It is important when analyzing the patient's profile to begin with the chin in the neutral position. Obviously, the degree of chin projection will vary tremendously depending on whether the head is either flexed or extended, and for this reason, orienting the chin to a standard reference line is useful. The reference line that we find most helpful is known as the Frankfurt horizontal. This can be quickly established by placing the superior aspect of the external auditory meatus at the same horizontal level with the infraorbital rim. Once the head is oriented to this standard reference line, accurate evaluations of where the chin lies in relation to the rest of the face can be quickly established.

With the head oriented to the Frankfurt horizontal, three reference lines that we have found helpful in evaluating horizontal relationships include (1) the facial plane, (2) the subnasale perpendicular, and (3) the aesthetic line.

### Facial Plane

The facial plane determines the position of the soft-tissue chin point in relation to the root of the nose. Once the face is oriented to the Frankfurt horizontal, an imaginary line can be drawn from the nasion (nasal radix) to the most prominent portion of the chin pad (soft-tissue pogonion).[5] The angle that is established between the Frankfurt horizontal and the facial plane is known as the facial angle and can be accurately measured on standard photographs of the patient in a profile view. The ideal facial angle is 90 degrees in a male and between 88 and 89 degrees in the female (Fig 26–1).

## Subnasale Perpendicular

The subnasale perpendicular is a useful reference line in that it will not only tell you whether the chin is either protrusive or retrusive in relation to the midface but will also provide a fairly accurate quantitative measurement of the amount of retrusion or protrusion that exists. The subnasale perpendicular is again measured with the profile oriented to the Frankfurt horizontal. A perpendicular drawn from the base of the columella–upper lip complex inferiorly establishes the subnasale perpendicular. In the ideally balanced profile, the soft-tissue chin pad should sit either on the subnasale perpendicular or, at the most, 4 mm posterior to this reference line. A chin lying more than 4 mm behind this reference line suggests either a retrusive chin or an overly prominent midface. Conversely, a chin lying anterior to this reference line suggests either a protrusive chin or a retrusive midface[2] (Fig 26–2).

The advantage of using the subnasale perpen-

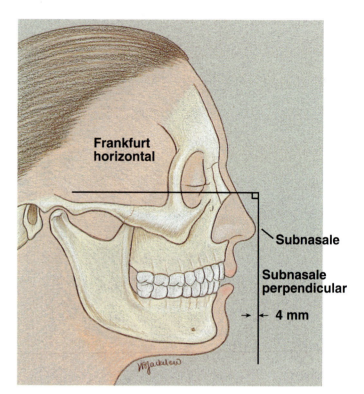

**FIG 26–2.**
The subnasale perpendicular is again determined with the patient oriented to the Frankfurt horizontal. A perpendicular drawn from the base of the columella–upper lip complex inferiorly establishes the subnasale perpendicular. In the aesthetically balanced profile, the soft-tissue chin pad should lie within 4 mm of the subnasale perpendicular.

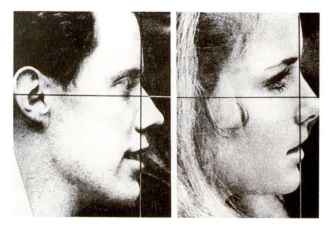

**FIG 26–1.**
The soft-tissue facial plane is determined after orienting the face to the Frankfurt horizontal. Connecting a line from the soft-tissue nasion to the soft-tissue pogonion determines the facial plane. The angle between the facial plane and the Frankfurt horizontal should measure between 88 and 90 degrees. (From Gonzalez-Villoa M, Stevens E: *Plast Reconstr Surg* 1968; 41:477. Used with permission.)

dicular in evaluating the patient's profile is that it gives you a very simple quantitative measurement of how much augmentation will be required in the patient with a retrusive chin. This measurement commonly correlates with those values derived from cephalometric analysis.

## The Aesthetic Line (E Line)

The aesthetic line, or the E line of Ricketts, helps to establish the relationship of the chin to the tip of the nose as well as to the upper and lower lips. This line is again derived with the patient oriented to the Frankfurt horizontal. It is determined by connecting a line from the tip of the nose to the tip of the soft-tissue chin pad.[10, 11] In the aesthetically ideal patient, both the upper and lower lips should lie slightly behind the aesthetic line, with the lower lip slightly closer to the E line than the upper lip (Fig 26–3). When the upper and lower lips sit anterior to the E line, this is known as bilabial protrusion and is usually associated with a convex midface and a

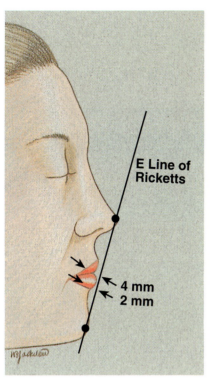

**FIG 26–3.**
The esthetic line (E line of Ricketts) is determined by drawing a tangent from the tip of the nose to the most prominent portion of the soft-tissue chin pad. In the aesthetically ideal patient, both the upper and lower lips should lie slightly behind the aesthetic line, with the lower lip slightly closer to the E line than the upper lip.

retrusive chin (Fig 26–4). Conversely, when both lips lie posterior to the E line, this is known as bilabial retrusion and is associated with a concave midface and a prognathic appearance of the chin (Fig 26–5).

## SOFT TISSUE ANALYSIS

### Vertical Relationships—Frontal

The vertical relationships of the face are best analyzed on frontal views. Within the literature, there are numerous ratios and measurements that can be measured when deciding on whether the face is vertically balanced. While these ratios and measurements tend to be accurate, we have found them to be a bit cumbersome to measure when evaluating the patient. As an alternative to direct measurement, we have found the use of the golden divider, as devised by Dr. Ricketts, to be both simple and accurate when analyzing vertical relationships within the face.

It has been recognized since ancient times that absolute symmetry is boring. Rather, what the eye finds aesthetically beautiful is not symmetrical relationships, but rather proportions that are balanced. When analyzing these proportions mathematically, it appears that a relationship of 1 to 1.618, known as the golden proportion, is what the human eye finds aesthetically beautiful (Fig 26–6). Dr. Ricketts, in his extensive analysis of cephalometrics in the beautiful face, determined that these golden proportions exist throughout the face.[10] With the understanding that these proportions are present, Dr. Ricketts designed a divider that produces two segments always in a relationship with the proportion of 1 to 1.618 (Fig 26–7). This divider makes the determination of vertical relationships quite simple and can be used when examining patients directly, when evaluating their photographs, or during cephalometric analysis. The golden proportions most useful when evaluat-

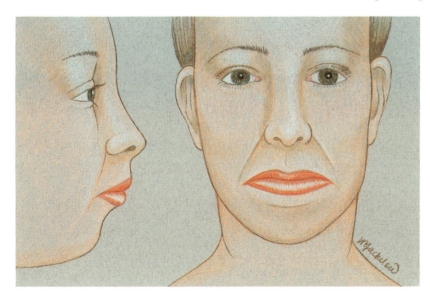

**FIG 26–4.**
Bilabial protrusion is seen when the upper and lower lips both sit anterior to the E line. This is usually associated with a convex midface and a retrusive chin.

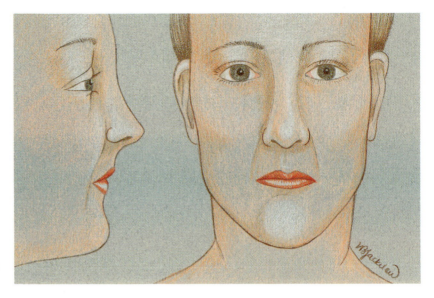

**FIG 26–5.**
Bilabial retrusion is seen when both the upper and lower lips are substantially behind the E line. This situation is associated with a concave midface and a prognathic appearance of the chin.

ing vertical relationships include (1) total facial height (the distance from the forehead to the medial canthus should be golden to the rest of the face (ratio of 1:1.618), (2) the height of the lower two thirds of the face (the distance from the medial canthus to the alar base should be golden to the rest of the

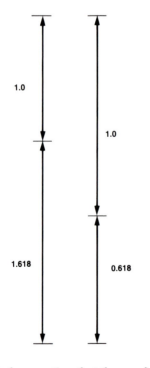

**FIG 26–6.**
The mathematical proportion that the eye finds aesthetically beautiful is known as the golden proportion. The Greeks were the first to realize that aesthetic relationships could be quantitatively defined and noted that the eye found the ratio 1:1.618 to be aesthetically pleasing. Of note, the reciprocal of this ratio produces a mathematical relationship of 1:0.618.

face), and (3) the height of the lower third of the face (the distance from the alar base to the base of the upper lip should be golden to the rest of the face) (Fig 26–8).

The use of the golden divider simplifies evaluation of facial height relationships. This caliper can be placed on the landmarks described and provide an accurate analysis of whether vertical relationships are aesthetically proportioned. Not only will the golden divider allow the surgeon to determine whether these relationships are out of proportion, but it will also provide an accurate quantitative measure of the amount of vertical discrepancy that exists (Figs 26–9 and 26–10).

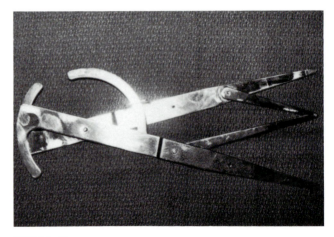

**FIG 26–7.**
The golden divider is a useful device to determine whether the aesthetically balanced vertical relationships exist within the face. This divider is essentially a three-pronged compass, the two segments that the compass defines always being in a relationship of 1:1.618.

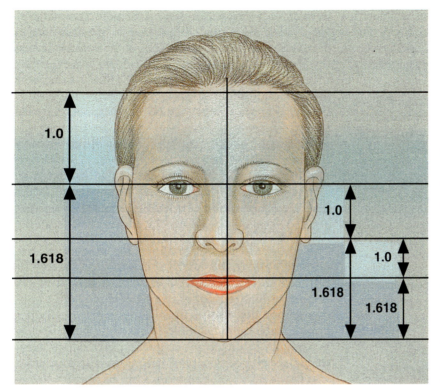

**FIG 26–8.**
The measurement of the golden proportions is quite useful when evaluating vertical relationships within the face. It is noteworthy to realize that in terms of vertical height, the distance from the top of the forehead to the medial canthus is golden to the rest of the face (ratio of 1:1.618). In terms of the height of the lower two thirds of the face, the distance from the medial canthus to the alar base should be golden to the rest of the face (ratio of 1:1.618). Finally, in analyzing the height of the lower third of the face, the distance of the alar base to the base of the upper lip should be golden to the rest of the face (ratio of 1:1.618).

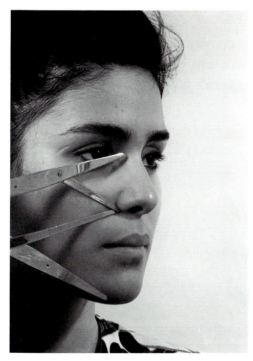

**FIG 26–9.**
The golden divider makes it quite simple to determine whether the golden relationships exist. In the aesthetically balanced face, it is simple to determine that the distance from the medial canthus to the alar base is in golden proportion to the lower portion of the face (ratio of 1:1.618).

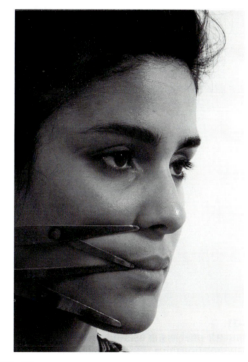

**FIG 26–10.**
In the aesthetically pleasing face, lower facial height is balanced. In this photograph, by using the golden divider it is simple to determine that the distance from the alar base to the base of the upper lip is golden to the rest of the face (ratio of 1:1.618).

With advancing age and weight gain there is a predisposition of fat to accumulate in the neck and lower third of the face over the mandible and preauricular area. This fullness can be viewed as changing the facial triangle from a base-up to a base-down appearance (Fig 27–3,A and B). A base-down triangle is less desirable and creates a tired, less attractive appearance. With the use of judicious liposculpting in the lower part of the face and neck over the mandible and the preauricular sites in conjunction with rhytidoplasty a more pleasing base-up triangle can again be achieved (Fig 27–4,A–D).

The face is not suctioned all over, but certain sites are selectively treated by lipoplasty. The sites most commonly treated are the ones in which the fat tends to accumulate, namely, lateral to the nasolabial creases, in the preauricular area and nasolabial creases, and in the buccinator fat pad. In a select number of patients the fullness in the nasolabial creases exists and cannot be eliminated by the lateral pull of the face-lift. This fullness is more prominent near the nose. A modest flattening achieves a more harmonious facial appearance (Fig 27–5,A–D). This procedure is not done in all patients. If overdone, this flattening of appearance will create an unnatural and undesirable look.

This site can be approached from multiple incisions in close proximity to the site. The one I most commonly use is a small incision beneath the chin that I use to aspirate the central portion of the neck. Through one of these incisions a small cannula, 2

mm, can be passed over the mandible and along the nasolabial crease. If a complementary incision is needed, it is placed high in the nasolabial crease and the cannula passed downward to remove any residual fat present along the nasolabial crease or below the commissure of the mouth.

Another incision advocated is within the nasal mucosa. I have not commonly used this incision and prefer the intact skin. A small, judiciously placed incision is inconspicuous.

On occasion, there is a slight fullness lateral to the marionette deformity after the face-lift. This can be easily treated under local anesthesia with a very small cannula, 2 mm, and aspiration of a very small amount of fat. Precision is of the utmost importance in removing facial subcutaneous fat. Any contouring defect is readily apparent and very difficult to conceal. Important aspects of the procedure are a small-diameter cannula and careful removing of the fat. Hetter, in LSNA (Lipolysis Society of North America) courses, has advocated counting the number of strokes on each site. Although I do not share this pedantic approach in other sites, I am in agreement with this concept in dealing with the small areas about the face and use the method of counting strokes.

Recently I have switched to the syringe aspirator in the face. The syringe offers advantages of careful measurement of even a small amount of fat. It offers ease of use and measurement of the amount of fat aspirate and provides more precision than with the pump aspirator.

**A**

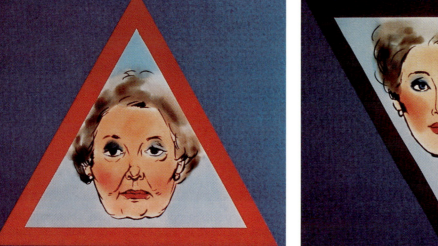

**B**

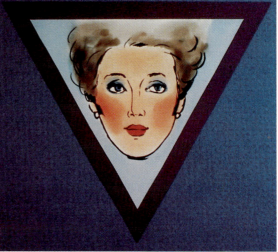

**FIG 27–3.**
A graphic demonstration of the "base-down" **(A)** and the "base-up" **(B)** face with removal of subcutaneous fat.

**A**

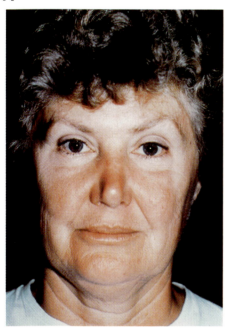

**C**

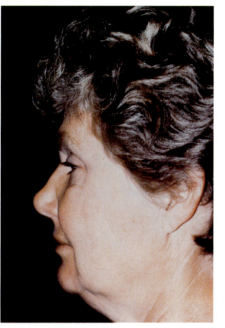

**B**

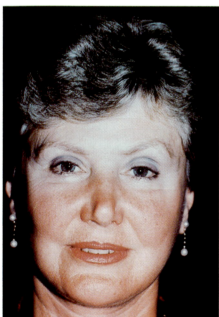

**D**

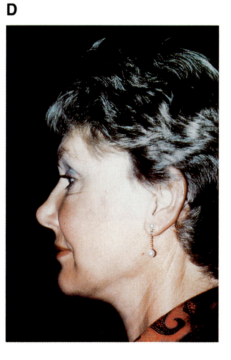

**FIG 27–4.**
A 54-year-old woman who underwent lipoplasty of the face and neck in combination with rhytidectomy. Preoperative views (**A** and **C**) demonstrate fullness in the lower portion of the face and neck. Postoperative results (**B** and **C**) after removal of 40 cc of fat aspirate and a skin tightening procedure show reduced volume in the lower part of the face and neck, better definition of the jawline, and a thinner "base-up" facial configuration.

## QUALITIES OF IDEAL FACIAL IMPLANTS

The size and shape of implants are the crucial factors in creating normal facial anatomy. The inadequacy of earlier implants in the malar and mandible region was due to a deficiency in these two elements (Figs 28–4 and 28–5). Through appropriate selection of implants, the potential for mobility and malposition is diminished to an almost negligible degree.

Ideal implants should be easily implantable, nonpalpable, readily exchangeable, malleable and conformable, acceptable to the body, forgivable to infection, and modifiable by the surgeon (Table 28–1). The silicone or Silastic implant appears to meet these characteristics better than other materials.[8, 9] Smooth silicone implants placed directly on bone become rapidly fixed and securely surrounded by fibrosis and capsule formation. They can readily be removed and exchanged when desirable or necessary. Porous implants that permit ingrowth, fenestrated implants, and implants that embody a cloth backing or fixation have a higher predilection for infection.[10] They are also less advantageous in regard to exchangeability and modifiability. This is also true of more permanent materials such as hydroxyapatite, which is very difficult to modify or remove.

Technical limitations in the use of facial implants still prevail. Differential augmentation and alteration of the facial skeletal form are in an early phase of de-

**TABLE 28–1.**

Comparison of Ideal Qualities of the Most Commonly Used Facial Implant Materials

| Ideal Qualities | Materials | | |
|---|---|---|---|
| | Silastic | Proplast | Other |
| Exchangeable | + + + + | + | – |
| Conformable | + + + + | + + | + + |
| Modifiable | + + + | + + + + | – |
| Host acceptable | + + + + | + + | + + |
| Nonpalpable | + + + | + | + |
| Insertable | + + + + | + + + | + + |

velopment. For the choice of correct size, shape, and placement of implants, the surgeon must still rely solely on his own judgment and artistic perspective. The advent of computerized technology for manufacturing implants and for designing and creating implants customized to the needs of individual patients is just around the corner. Meanwhile, the highest item on the list of problems associated with facial implant augmentation is patient and physician dissatisfaction with the results.[9]

The success of recent anatomic facial implants is, in large part, due to their conformability to the facial skeleton. Current technology is producing implants whose posterior aspect can be accurately molded to the specific shape and universal form of the human skull, both in the malar and premandible regions. The expansion of implant size and shape to volumetrically fit the dimensions of the face minimizes movability and malposition in the most efficient manner. Adherence to these principles increases successful results.

The most satisfying features of a facial implant composed of smooth silicone are its acceptance by the human body and its resistance to infection. It is common knowledge that silicone breast implants surrounded by infection can sometimes be "saved" by various extravagant means. Resolution of inflammation, cellulitis, and abscesses occurring after facial implants have been inserted is very possible by promptly and adequately using antibiotics and perhaps even drainage techniques.[9] This is not to say that plastic surgeons should be cavalier in expecting this eventuality for cure. Indeed, disastrous consequences have been reported relative to facial implant infections. It should be pointed out, however, that the favorable quality of silicone facial implants provides a margin of safety regarding tissue contamination. This feature offers the surgeon a significant advantage.

In order to be inserted through small apertures

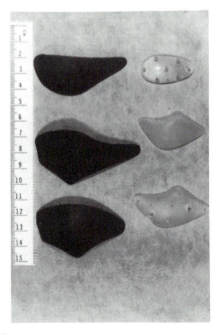

**FIG 28–5.**
*Left,* newer models of malar implants, 1980. *Right,* old-style malar implants.

in the soft-tissue envelope of the face, facial implants must have malleability and compressibility. As the size and surface area of contemporary implants has increased, these qualities have become even more important. It is often necessary to place implants as large as 10 to 20 $cm^2$ onto the malar bone or the mandible of the facial skeleton. Silicone rubber implants fabricated into a suitable medium-grade consistency make it possible to perform this procedure with great facility.

Finally, the easy modifiability of silicone implants works in the surgeon's favor, especially when a formidable barrier is encountered during the operation. Instead of enforcing a traumatic dissection upon an area of anatomy where nerve damage is imminent, the surgeon can easily diminish the implants or alter their configuration without affecting the resulting contour.

## PREOPERATIVE PLANNING

Preoperative planning for all plastic and reconstructive surgery is the determining factor for achieving successful results. Preoperative planning for aesthetic surgery must include accurate and definitive communication with the patient. The perception and the expectations of the patient must be strictly duplicated by the surgeon. For traditional surgery on aging patients, communication with their needs and wishes is relatively simple: they wish to have their own youthful contours and facial features restored as completely as possible. With the passing years, people become accommodated to the slow and gradual changes that age brings about in the soft-tissue contours of their faces. Consequently, the technical limitations of routine facial aesthetic surgery are acceptable to them because they usually can perceive significant postoperative improvements. Human beings who have lived for four or more decades would be shocked to find themselves once again given the facial image of 20-year-olds. Current techniques for altering skeletal contour and facial promontories create a potential radical departure from the patient's own inherited anatomic configuration. Following facial implant surgery, patients must live with entirely different visual and perceptual images of themselves. Today's patients have specific ideas about how they would like their facial configuration to look. They frequently wish to imitate the currently established standards of beauty as exemplified in strong, bold, well-defined features and classic contours. The plastic surgeon's challenge is to meet

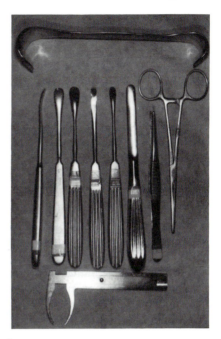

**FIG 28–6.**
Instrument set for facial augmentation.

these expectations as closely as possible in order to satisfy the patient. Although aesthetic surgery has at its command an assorted menu of tools such as cephalometrics, the "zero meridian" concept,[2] CE-MAX (Fremont, Calif), magnetic resonance imaging (MRI), and computer-imaging techniques, precise implementation of facial form presently remains difficult, at best. The surgeon should use every available method to comprehend the precise image of facial form that the patient desires before he attempts to duplicate it. For consultation purposes, patients are encouraged either to modify photographic images of themselves or to provide from fashion magazines or other sources examples of facial contours that they consider appropriate and fitting for themselves. They are encouraged to find faces that they feel look very similar to their own but that have more attractive qualities in those anatomic areas they are seeking to improve. Most patients present fairly realistic images. When they do not, it is easy to discover the expectations that cannot be met. Obviously, the surgeon should not undertake what he is not certain he can accomplish.

Additionally, it is important to focus on specific details of zonal anatomy during the patient consultations (see Fig 28–1). For purposes of technical implementation, the surgeon must know whether enhancement should occur mostly in malar zones 1 or 2 or whether it is submalar zone roundness and fullness that the patient is seeking. Similarly, he must

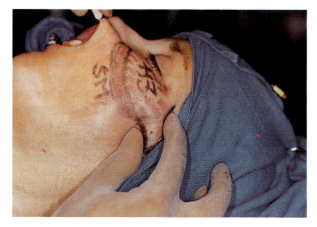

**FIG 28–8.**
Malar augmentation, intraoral route. The malar space dissection is controlled by manual palpation of its bony limits.

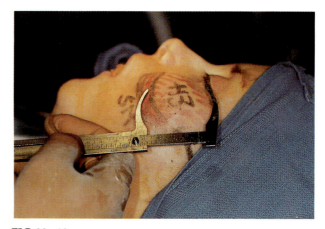

**FIG 28–10.**
Malar augmentation, intraoral route. Accurate measurements of the malar space and the alloplastic implant may be made and modified during surgery.

mammoplasty, the necessary anatomic space remains the same, no matter which incisional approach and entrance wound is utilized. Only a small number of particular maneuvers to secure accurate placement and positioning may vary during each alternative approach. The most important decision should occur prior to the operation, and that decision is the choice of the implant size and shape.

The various routes for entering the malar space, including the submalar region, are as follows: (1) intraoral (Figs 28–7 to 28–13), (2) lower blepharoplasty (subcilial) (Figs 28–14 to 28–16), (3) rhytidectomy (Figs 28–17 to 28–22), (4) zygomaticotemporal, and (5) transcoronal. I am certain that a transconjunctival route is possible and may become a method of choice for the future. At the present time, I have not utilized it.

The intraoral route has been the most frequent and traditional approach to maxillary malar and midface augmentation. The incision is 1 cm long and is made through the mucosa in a vertically oblique direction (see Fig 28–7). It is located over the anterior buttress of the maxilla, just above the first molar and approximately 2 cm medial to the orifice of Stensen's duct. A subperiosteal spatula-shaped elevator with a 1-cm-wide blade is thrust directly through the zygomaticus muscle onto bone in an oblique orientation at the inferior base of the maxillary buttress and at the apex of the gingival-buccal sulcus. The overlying soft tissues are swept obliquely upward over the maxillary eminence by maintaining the elevator directly on bone. The elevator should always be maintained on the bony margin along the

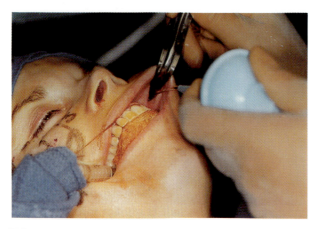

**FIG 28–9.**
Malar augmentation, intraoral route. Continuous antibiotic irrigation of the wound minimizes infection.

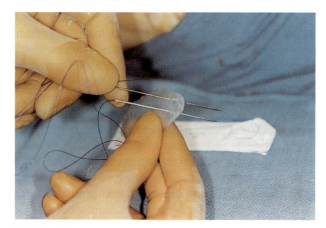

**FIG 28–11.**
Malar augmentation, intraoral route. A 2–0 Prolene suture on two, 4-in. Keith needles is passed through the posterior tail of the implant.

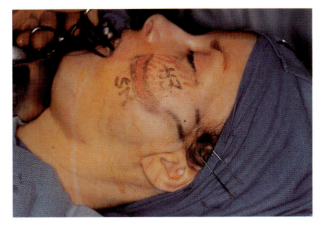

**FIG 28–12.**
Malar augmentation, intraoral route. A 2–0 Prolene traction suture on a Keith needle is passed through the temporoscalp with a long needle holder.

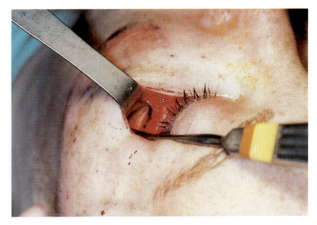

**FIG 28–14.**
Malar augmentation, blepharoplasty approach. Tissues are elevated from bone within the malar space.

inferior border of the malar eminence and zygomatic arch. Manual palpation is performed on the previously marked design of the malar space on the skin while the underlying elevator mobilizes the tissues directly from the bone. This maneuver includes palpating the orbital rim and the upper and lower borders of the zygoma as the elevator creates the subperiosteal space in these areas. Once bony margins are reached, further space expansion is performed only by means of a rounded, blunter spatula-shaped elevator (see Fig 28–6). No dissection should occur into the soft tissues with a penetrating and forceful motion. No dissection should occur directly into the area of the infraorbital nerve. When desired, the periosteum may be mobilized, both lateral and inferior to the infraorbital foramen, with a careful scraping

motion until the nerve and foramen are visualized. This is rarely indicated. Frequent irrigation is performed with antibiotic solution (bacitracin, (see Fig 28–9). 1:20,000) once the space is mobilized, the chosen implant is introduced with a long, straight, nonserrated clamp placed transversely across the upper end of the implant and inserted into the posterior zygomatic tunnel. Should buckling of the implant occur, correct positioning can be ensured by using a Russian forceps in combination with a spatula-shaped periosteal elevator passed both anterior and posterior to the implant. Fiber-optic Aufricht retractors to illuminate the interior of the space reveal the internal anatomy and confirm the correct position of the implant. In the submalar zone, the soft tissues are swept off the shiny, white, glistening, fibrous tendon of the masseter muscle in an inferior

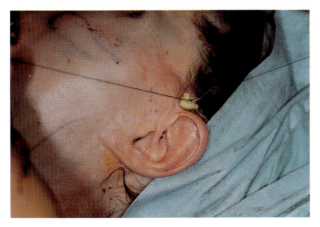

**FIG 28–13.**
Malar augmentation, intraoral route. A 2–0 Prolene traction suture is secured over a bolus stent for 2 to 3 days.

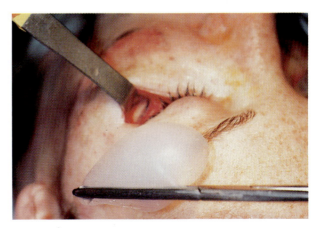

**FIG 28–15.**
Malar augmentation, blepharoplasty approach. An implant is about to be inserted by using a straight, nonserrated clamp across this entire transverse diameter.

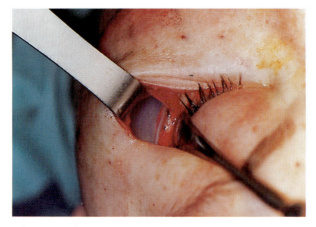

**FIG 28–16.**
Malar augmentation, blepharoplasty approach. The implant is in its proper position, 4 mm below the orbital rim.

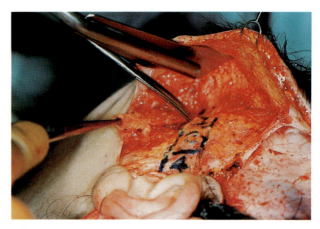

**FIG 28–18.**
Malar augmentation, rhytidectomy approach. Entrance to the malar space, zone 1, is through the "safe area" by direct transverse penetration onto bone.

and outward direction. This opens up the submalar space for approximately 1 to 2 cm, depending on the desired choice of cheek shape and the corresponding implant necessary to achieve it. When any portion of the submalar or inframalar region is augmented by a single implant or a total malar shell, a lower, rounder, and fuller facial contour is created. This occurs by volumetric filling of the midface in the submalar triangle.

When adequate anesthesia techniques are used, as noted above, visualization of the skeletal anatomy and musculature is excellent through the intraoral approach. This exposure facilitates accurate implant placement into zones 1, 2, and 5 (submalar). It permits the operator to place a spatula-shaped elevator above and below the implant to make certain that its edges are not buckled or that the zygomatic exten-

sion of the implant is not curled. It is not necessary to visualize the infraorbital nerve, but it is easy to do so when indicated or when an implant is designed for the paranasal zone 3.

Complications from the intraoral approach include dysesthesias from damage to the infraorbital nerve or motor dysfunction of the orbicularis oris musculature. Nerve symptoms may be attributed to (1) transection of small branches in the lip during the incision, (2) direct damage to the major nerve bundle during dissection, or (3) pressure impingement on the nerve from the implant. These complications, however, are rare and should almost be non-existent when the above basic guidelines to dissection are applied. Closure of this vertical intraoral incision is secure because the muscle pillars of the zygomaticus that overlie the maxillary buttress can

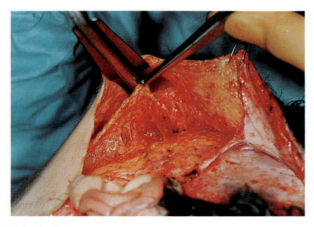

**FIG 28–17.**
Malar augmentation, rhytidectomy approach: deep-plane SMAS dissection over the malar region.

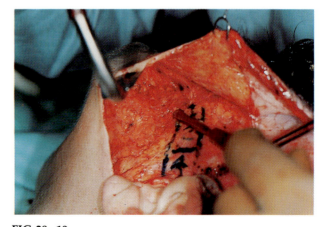

**FIG 28–19.**
Malar augmentation, rhytidectomy approach: dissection of zone 1 and into the submalar zone (zone 5).

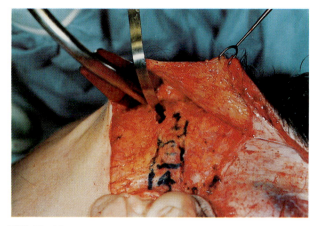

**FIG 28–20.**
Malar augmentation, rhytidectomy approach. A narrow malleable ribbon retraction may be used to visualize the malar space dissection.

be firmly reapproximated with sutures to provide a sturdy two-layer closure. Traditional transverse incisions through these muscles produce traumatic transection that results in transient and perhaps even permanent damage to function. This can inhibit normal lip elevation. Another significant disadvantage of the customary intraoral approach is that it produces a weakness in this inferior aspect of the dissection space, thereby increasing possibilities of rotational asymmetries and descent of the implant into an undesirable medial, inferior position.

## SUBCILIAL BLEPHAROPLASTY APPROACH

In the subcilial blepharoplasty approach, an ordinary blepharoplasty incision may be utilized 3 mm

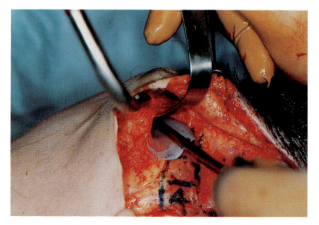

**FIG 28–21.**
Malar augmentation, rhytidectomy approach. Insertion of the malar shell is facilitated by a ribbon retractor.

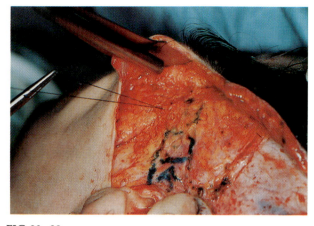

**FIG 28–22.**
Malar augmentation, rhytidectomy approach: final closure over the malar space.

below the lash line and limited in its lateral extension to avoid scars in the lateral canthal region. This approach may be used either in conjunction with routine blepharoplasty or as an independent route of entry for a malar implant. When used for implant placement alone, the incision is limited to a length of 10 to 15 mm. It is designed only in the middle to lateral third of the lower eyelid in the subcilial region. There is no contamination by intraoral organisms with this incision. Moreover, the dissection inferiorly develops no floor weakness (see Fig 28–14). Instead, it provides a sturdy shelf upon which the implant rests. During this dissection, the infraorbital nerve is also intentionally avoided. An incision is made in the periosteum 3 to 4 mm anterior to the orbital rim along its lateral aspect in order to obviate potential adhesions that may result in ectropion and lower lid contracture. A skin flap should *never* be used because it always shrinks and predisposes to excessive eyelid retraction. By utilizing a skin *muscle* flap approach, however, there should be no trauma to the orbicularis muscle.

Excessive muscle damage with bleeding into lid tissues stimulates fibrosis and contracture within the middle lamella of the lower eyelid and produces ectropion. Standard lateral canthopexy techniques are used to minimize this possibility. Resection of the skin and muscle flap should be conservative, i.e., minimal to zero excision, because of additional traction forces exerted on the lower eyelid from the volume expansion under the malar zygomatic tissues by the implant.

The greatest advantage of the subcilial blepharoplasty approach is the opportunity for correct positioning (see Figs 28–15 and 28–16). The surgeon is able to directly observe the relationship of the implant to the inferior orbital rim. The greatest disadvantage of this approach is the potential for creating morbid distortions of the eyelid anatomy, as described above.

## THE RHYTIDECTOMY APPROACH

Zone 1 of the malar region is a safe zone for penetration through the SMAS into the malar space. There are no significant branches of the facial nerve in that region. Once the rhytidectomy flap is elevated over zones 1 and 2, the roof of the malar space can be directly penetrated through the SMAS with a small, sharp elevator onto the malar bone (see Figs 28–17 and 28–18). This may be done either medial or lateral to the zygomaticus origins. The seventh nerve branches to the frontalis muscle run more proximal over the middle third of the zygomatic arch, and the motor nerve to the orbicularis oculi is more superior. By creating a transverse aperture that parallels facial nerve fibers, there is minimal risk of impairing the motor function. Once the bone level is reached, a standard subperiosteal dissection and expansion of the malar space are accomplished as described previously. It is important to remember that dissection backward along the zygomatic arch is necessary in order to position a malar shell implant comfortably and correctly without a buckling of the lateral tail (see Fig 28–20).

Rhytidectomy insertion offers a twofold advantage: first, a readily accessible sterile entry wound and, second, a reasonable opportunity for accurate placement accompanied by direct palpation and observation (see Figs 28–21 and 28–22). This approach has not been utilized frequently by me. Nevertheless, because it provides great accuracy in placement and minimal occurrence of asymmetries, it should be seriously and personally evaluated by all surgeons who undertake malar-plasty.

## TEMPORAL ZYGOMATIC AND CORONAL APPROACH

Craniofacial surgery has contributed to the success and accuracy of approaching the malar zygomatic region by means of coronoplasty. I have not mastered this method at the present time. Craniofacial-subperiosteal face-lifting, as reported in recent years, has a frequent incidence of frontalis nerve damage that is often permanent. This complication represents a significant deterrent for the casual surgeon. Additional future experience with a craniofacial approach to the malar zygomatic region will most likely increase the utilization of this method of malar-zygomatic augmentation.

## CHOOSING MALAR/SUBMALAR IMPLANTS

Patients have very precise visual images of the cheek contour they wish to emulate. As has been mentioned earlier, detailed preoperative discussions are necessary in order for the surgeon to fully compre-

**A** 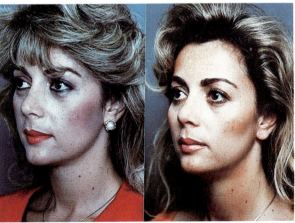 **B**

**FIG 28–23.**
**A** and **B,** 27-year-old female 1 year following malar shell augmentation of zone 1 and submalar zone 5.

hend the subtleties and nuances of the patient's desires and expectations with regard to shape. I request my patients to bring photographic images from fashion magazines. Contrary to standard residency teaching, this clarifies my understanding of the patient's expectations by giving me an invaluable visual image to discuss with the patient. Computer-imaging techniques are, of course, limited because of the very possible inability of the surgeon to technically match the patient's desired visual image. Nevertheless, computer imaging can be useful. In the final analysis, however, it is the discretion of the surgeon that must dictate his choice of size, shape, and location of implants. It is his clinical judgment that accomplishes a successful approximation of the patient's desired goal.

Basic decisions must be made concerning the anatomic zones to be augmented. Implants that fill the upper and lateral malar zygomatic areas of zones 1 and 2 create a sharp, high, and angular appearance.

Implants that augment the lower aspect of these zones down into submalar zone 5 create a lower, full, round cheek form (Figs 28–23 to 28–26; see also Fig 28–34). Implants that can produce either type of facial contour are presently available in varying sizes and shapes. To augment only the submalar zone requires isolated alloplastic implant shell. Routinely this implant is placed through an intraoral approach and with full visualization of the masseter muscle floor upon which it must be placed. A submalar implant is basically an anatomic extension of the patient's malar-zygomatic bone. Depending upon the thickness that has been chosen (4 to 6 mm), this implant adds volume to the canine fossa, as well as along the medial and inferior aspect of the patient's virgin bony malar-zygomatic eminence. It specifically increases midfacial cheek contour medially and inferiorly, provided that the patient already has adequate upper malar-zygomatic volume in zones 1 and 2. The anatomic "submalar triangle" (zone 5) can be

**A**

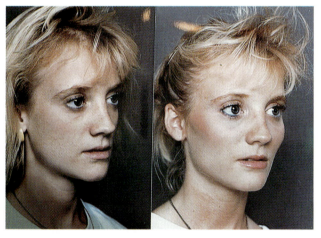

**B**

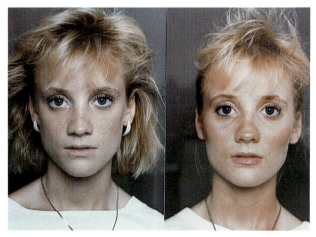

**C**

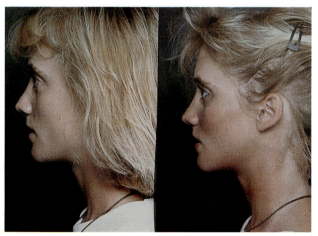

FIG 28–24.
A–C, 21-year-old female with malar shell augmentation into zones 1 and 2 and submalar zone 5.

**A**                                    **B**

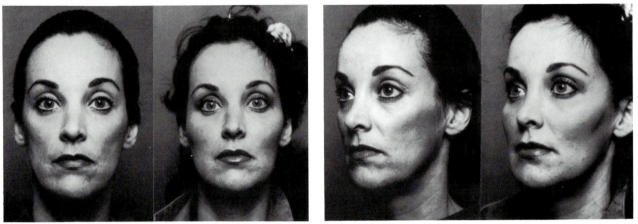

**FIG 28–25.**
**A** and **B,** 35-year-old female with Silastic implants in malar zone 1, submalar zone 5, and the premandible zone (posterolateral).

variably filled by altering the thickness of the implant.

## TECHNIQUES TO ENSURE ACCURACY OF PLACEMENT

The basic shape of anatomically contoured malar shells and premandible implants has been designed to fit the facial skeleton (see Figs 28–3 and 28–4). By virtue of their size and the configuration of their posterior surface, these implants have limited capacity for rotational malposition. Accuracy of position is more important in the malar region than in the premandible region. The soft tissues of the central mentum and midlateral zones are usually thick enough to obscure a mild malpositional or rotational deformity. In the midlateral zone, where the subcutaneous tissues overlie the mandible, just anterior to the thick volume of the masseter muscle, the posterior tail of the implant may be significantly prominent, either visually or by palpation. This can be troublesome to the patient, even though a slightly abnormal position may be nearly imperceptible. It is for these reasons that Silastic implants have been manufactured that have thinly tapered, nearly nonpalpable margins (see Fig 28–3). Malposition of an implant is not difficult to correct, but it requires a redissection of the standard premandible space so that the implant can be manually replaced in the correct position. Although it is possible to use suture fixation of the implant either percutaneously or intraorally, I have not found these methods necessary. Fenestration of the implants either peripherally or centrally, as well as texturing of them, may minimize rotational displacement but complicates removal, replacement, or repositioning. The main cause of this problem, in my opinion, is the technical dissection of an asymmetrical space, along with abnormal placement at the very outset.

Accurate placement of malar implants can be ensured by visually relating the position of the implant to the internal anatomy. Such visualization can be facilitated through an intraoral approach with fiberoptic instrumentation and adequate anesthesia techniques, as described previously. Further security can be obtained by suturing the malar or submalar implant to the fibers of the masseter tendon anteriorly. Accuracy of posterolateral placement by traction sutures through the implant tail greatly assists in precise positioning of a malar and submalar implant. This can be accomplished by means of 2–0 Surgibond sutures swaged on 8-in. arthroscopy needles, which are used to penetrate transcutaneously and posteriorly from within the malar space to behind the temporal hairline (see Figs 28–11 and 28–12). These sutures are tied over a tonsil sponge for 2 or 3 days (see Fig 28–13). Although not absolutely necessary, this technique, developed over the past year, appears to provide the extra small percentage of accuracy necessary to "guarantee" symmetrical contour. The subcilial blepharoplasty approach offers the surgeon an opportunity to visually supervise placement and confirm the accuracy of positioning.

**A**

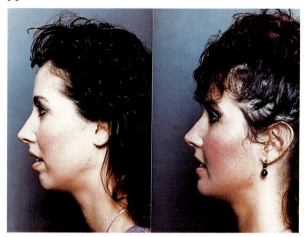

**B**

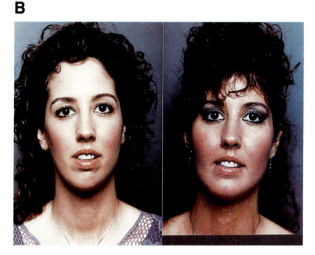

**C**

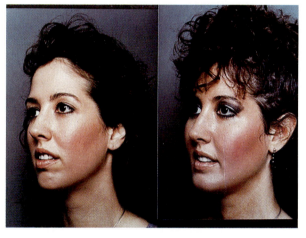

**FIG 28–26.**
A–C, 34-year-old female with marked facial asymmetry corrected by different-sized malar and submalar implants as well as different-sized central and lateral mandibular implants.

## PREMANDIBLE AUGMENTATION

Augmentation of the premandible region follows the same basic principles. Extending a centrally placed implant into the midlateral and posterolateral zones only requires dissection along the inferior mandibular border into the "safe zone" posterior to the mental nerve. There is significant constriction and adherence of the tissues to the bone surrounding the mental foramen. Once these are released, dissection of the tissues from the posterolateral zone occurs with ease.

Operations to augment the central mandible for aesthetic purposes have existed for 30 years. Plastic surgeons have well understood and have accepted the advantages of improved nasomentum profile relationships. Within the last 5 to 10 years, premandible augmentation concepts have developed that can extend central chin implants over a larger surface area of the premandible, as well as into a more anatomic contour (see Fig 28–4). These new implants and techniques make it possible to alter the shape and size of the midlateral and posterior aspects of the mandible, as well as to lengthen the submandibular segment vertically.

Access to the premandible space can be achieved by either the standard intraoral route or the submental route. I reserve the submental approach exclusively for operations that require additional surgery in the submental and submandibular region, such as liposculpturing and plastymal contouring. Otherwise, my routine approach is intraoral.

In both approaches, the incisions are transverse and are 2 cm in length (Fig 28–27). The intraoral transverse incision is through mucosa only. The mentalis muscles are then divided vertically through their midline raphe to avoid transection of the muscle bellies and total detachment from their bony ori-

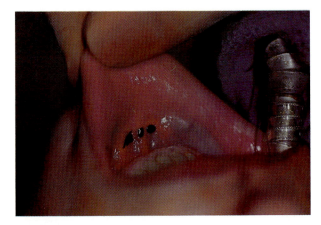

**FIG 28–27.**
Premandible augmentation, intraoral approach. The 2-cm mucosal incision is designed transversely 1 cm from the gingival labial sulcus.

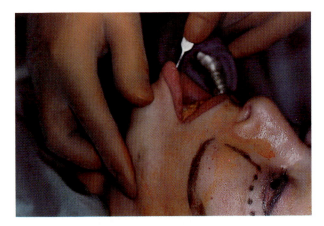

**FIG 28–28.**
Premandible augmentation, intraoral approach. A subperiosteal tunnel is created along the lower border of the mandible beneath the mental nerve by using the opposite hand to guide the elevator.

gins. This aperture provides direct access downward onto the bony plane and eliminates the muscle weakening that occurs with customary transection methods. Incisions that transect muscle fibers not only lead to inadequate closure but may also create weakness and laxity of the mentalis muscle, thereby contributing to a potential for chin ptosis. Ptosis of the mentalis musculature and soft-tissue mound of the central mentum is described in the literature as one of the controversial aspects of alloplastic implants. Indeed, the possibility for deformities such as central drooping and witch's chin does exist. They can be prevented, however, by using the previously described vertical entrance wound and securely approximating the mentalis muscle pillars during closure. The mentalis muscle can easily stretch to accommodate the introduction of large, extended anatomic implants.

By adhering to the principle of subperiosteal elevation on bone, the muscle attachments are elevated from their origins along the inferior margin of the mandible. This is a safe area that does not endanger the mental nerve (Fig 28–28; see also Fig 28–31). The mandibular branch of facial nerve VII does, however, cross just anterior to the midportion of the mandible in the midlateral zone. Consequently, it is important not to traumatize the tissues that overlie and constitute the roof of the premandible space in that region. The mental nerve and foramen can vary in number and location. Reported anatomic variations consist of multiple foramina existing between 1.5 to 4.5 cm from the midline in a certain percentage of individuals.[7] The bony configuration of the foramen, however, directs the mental nerve in a superior path upward into the lower lip. Dissections

that remain inferior to the foramen and along the lower border of the mandible will avoid significant danger of nerve damage.

In my personal series, I inadvertently placed a premandible implant superior to the mental nerves bilaterally. The immediate result was compression symptoms in the form of anesthesia of the lower lip. Fortunately, other facial procedures that were performed at the same time (rhytidectomy and blepharoplasty) obscured the diagnosis until the swelling had diminished. The implant was repositioned beneath the nerves on the ninth postoperative day. Replacement of an implant or repositioning can easily be done within the first 10 to 14 days. By applying the basic principles of wound healing that have been taught during residency, the surgeon is able to reenter the premandible or malar space to replace or reposition implants prior to the rapid increase in wound tensile strength, which occurs from 14 to 21 days after the operation.[6] Although dysesthesias and paresthesias in small or sometimes larger areas of distribution of the mental nerve are quite common following alloplastic chin and premandible augmentation, the symptoms are mostly temporary and generally subside within 4 to 6 weeks.

Clinically there appears to be a definite correlation between the occurrence of nerve symptoms and the degree of difficulty that the surgeon experiences in placing the implant. There is no correlation, however, with the size and shape of the implant. Extended alloplastic anatomic-contoured implants contain specific notches designed to avoid pressure around the mental foramen. This notch extends 1½

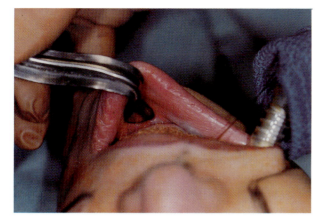

**FIG 28–29.**
Premandible augmentation, intraoral approach. A fiber-optic lighted retractor is used to visualize the mental nerve.

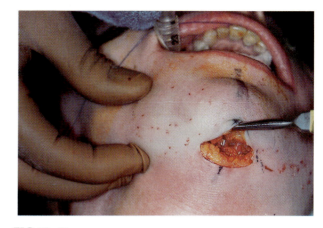

**FIG 28–31.**
Premandible augmentation, submental approach. Subperiosteal elevation into the midlateral zone beneath the mental nerve by using manual palpation is shown.

to 3½ cm from the midline to provide for normal anatomic variations in the location of the mental foramen, which is located 8 to 10 mm up from the lower mandibular margin. It therefore allows the surgeon an excellent margin of safety.

Additional incisions may be made posterior to the mental nerve to accurately place lateral mandibular bars and implants that extend into the midlateral and posterolateral zones. A small 1-cm vertical mucosal incision made in front of the first molar followed by direct penetration through the muscle onto the mandibular bone allows access to and easy dissection of the premandible space beneath. This aperture, while assisting in accurate placement of the lateral mandibular bars, also facilitates positioning the posterior extensions of other implants to simulta-

neously augment both the central mentum and the midlateral zones anteriorly.

As has already been mentioned, integrity of the mental nerve and easy positioning of the implant beneath it can be ensured through fiber-optic techniques (Fig 28–29). A narrow malleable ribbon retractor is utilized to distract the soft tissues for the placement of premandible implants into their tunnels. To position a long, extended premandible implant, it is essential to create a tunnel or space that is longer posteriorly than the length of the implant. This permits the implant to be inserted from the central incision far into one side and then be folded upon itself to be introduced into the opposite mandibular tunnel (Figs 28–30 to 28–33). Careful palpation, lateral positioning, and observing the central marking of the implant directly over the cen-

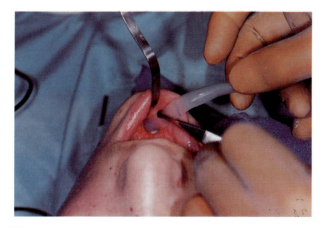

**FIG 28–30.**
Premandible augmentation, intraoral approach. The Silastic extended anatomic implant is placed in the lateral tunnel with assistance from a narrow malleable ribbon retractor.

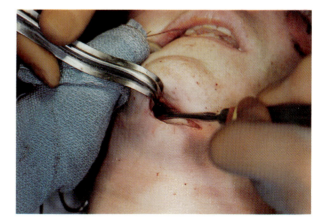

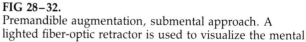

**FIG 28–32.**
Premandible augmentation, submental approach. A lighted fiber-optic retractor is used to visualize the mental nerve and foramen.

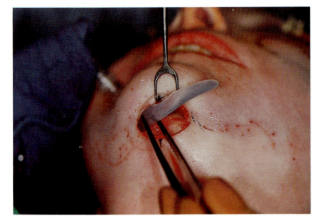

**FIG 28–33.**
Premandible augmentation, submental approach. An extended anatomic implant is inserted into the lateral subperiosteal tunnel beneath the mental nerve.

tral mental protuberance are keys to accurate placement.

Posterolateral implants are placed through either a midlateral or a posterolateral incision. The posterolateral incision is transverse and is located approximately 1½ to 2 cm anterior and adjacent to the angle of the mandible. Appropriate space for placement is created by making a direct dissection onto the bone and subperiosteally beneath the masseter muscle. A curved elevator is used to dissect around the internal and posterior aspects of the ascending ramus in the angle region. In this way, implants that are designed to fit securely around the angle of the mandible can be accurately positioned. As with all facial implant incisions, a two-layer closure of muscle and mucosa is optimum.

## CHOOSING PREMANDIBLE IMPLANTS

Implants can be designed to augment every zone of the premandible space. There is very little indication for a central mentum implant. This almost always creates a central mound deformity with an adjacent "anteromandibular sulcus" and potential "witch's chin" or "drooping" appearance. By extending the implant into the midlateral zone, anterior widening and broadness can be achieved (Figs 28–34 and 28–35). Volumetric expansion of the midlateral and posterolateral zones creates just that, widening of the lower-third facial contour in those anatomic premandible zones. The angle of the jaw can be markedly accentuated with a posterior mandibular implant. Traditionally, a premandible or chin implant has never been used to lengthen the vertical dimension of facial contour. Osteotomies have been the procedure of choice. Now implants have been designed that wrap around the inferior margin of the mandible in the central mentum and midlateral zones to augment and enhance the vertical dimension of the face by 3 to 5 mm. When indicated, these implants produce profound improvement (Fig 28–36). They also contribute to correction of the anteromandibular prejowl sulcus, or "marionette groove," of the aging face.

## CONCLUSIONS

Infinite variations in facial contour can now be achieved with creative alloplastic facial implantation

**A**

**B**

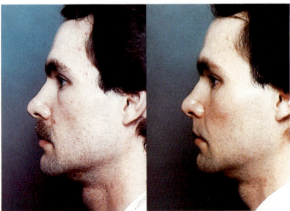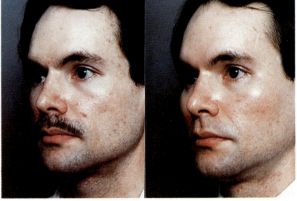

**FIG 28–34.**
**A** and **B,** 36-year-old male with malar shell implants in malar zones 1 and 2 and submalar zone 5.

A

B

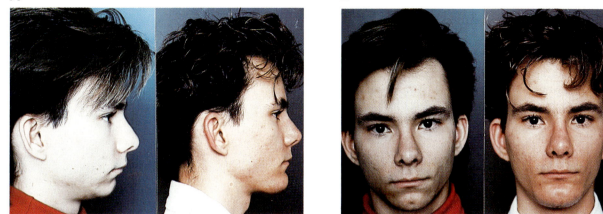

**FIG 28–35.**
**A** and **B,** 22-year-old male 1 year following a large extended anatomic premandibular implant in the central mentum and midlateral zones.

in both the malar and premandible regions. By utilizing basic principles and techniques as well as the concepts of zonal anatomy described herein, augmentation of the facial skeleton can be accomplished with a minimum of complications. Paramount in determining facial contour and in minimizing the patient's dissatisfaction is the choice of the size and shape of the implant and its correct positioning with the proper facial skeletal zone. Implants are available or can be customized by the surgeon to create a variety of contours and to fulfill almost any need. CEMAX and MRI computer technology are rapidly leading to the manufacture of elegant, customized implants with which the surgeon can optimally im-

prove each patient's aesthetic or reconstructive facial balance.

Augmentation of the facial skeleton is the fourth plane of surgical conquest in the 1990s. Historically and initially, skin elevation and tightening provided the only option for the aging face, and a two-dimensional one at that. The evolution of aesthetic surgery of the face that took place in the 1970s and 1980s created techniques for fat sculpturing and liposuction. Further and significant improvements in rhytidectomy have been provided by the SMAS techniques.

Skeletal augmentation now represents the final phase for improvement of the facial contour. It cre-

A

B

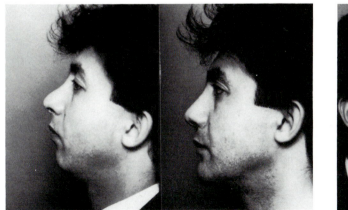
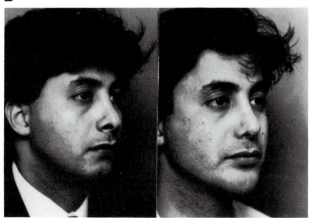

**FIG 28–36.**
**A** and **B,** 35-year-old male who required more vertical length and anterior jawline projection. A large extended anatomic implant fills the central mentum and midlateral zones and submandibular zone 5.

ates the most basic and most stable architectural foundation. By modifying the skeletal framework in a three-dimensional manner with volume-mass alloplastic implants, it is possible to alter inherited facial images as well as complement the deterioration, sagging, and diminution of facial tissues that come with age. Progress in developing implants is continuing. Implants are being designed and implemented for the temporal region; the supraorbital, lateral orbital, and frontal ridges; the medial infraorbital groove; and the nasojugal sulcus.

There is virtually no aspect of the facial skeleton that cannot be augmented satisfactorily by means of the technical principles described in this chapter. It can truthfully be said that alloplastic implants may become the "open sesame" of aesthetic surgery—the door by which almost magical improvements can be made, depending upon the imagination and skill of the surgeon.

## Acknowledgment

I gratefully acknowledge the superb assistance of my father Anthony and Dr. Sekhar with regard to the editing and technical production of this manuscript.

## BIBLIOGRAPHY

Binder WJ: Submalar augmentation, an alternative to facelift surgery, *Arch Otolaryngol Head Neck Surg* 115:797, 1989.

Gonzalez-Ulloa M: Basic studies in preparation for profileplasty. In Wallace AB, editor: *Transactions of the Second International Congress of Plastic Surgery*, Baltimore, 1961, Williams & Wilkins.

Gonzales-Ulloa M: Building out of the malar prominences as an addition to rhytidectomy, *Plast Reconstr Surg* 53:293, 1974.

Hinderer U: Profileplasty, *Int Micr J Aesthetic Plast Surg* Card 1 No 1, 1971.

Millard RD: Adjunct in augmentation mentoplasty and corrective rhinoplasty, *Plast Reconstr Surg* 36:9, 1965.

Peacock EE Jr, Van Winkle W Jr: *Wound repair*, ed 2, Philadelphia, 1976, Saunders.

Serman NJ: Differentiation of double mental foramina from extra bony coursing of the incisive branch of the mandibular nerve—an anatomic study, *Dent Med* 1987; 5:20–22.

Terino EO: Malar mandible and chin augmentation by alloplastic techniques. In Ousterhout D, editor: *Aesthetic contouring of the cranial facial skeleton*, Boston, 1991, Little Brown.

Terino EO: Complications of chin and malar augmentation. In Peck G, editor: *Complications and problems in aesthetic plastic surgery*, New York, 1991, Gower Medical.

Whitaker LA: Aesthetic augmentation of the malar midface structures, *Plast Reconstr Surg.* 80:387, 1987.

# Index